Telehealth in the Developing World

Telehealth in the Developing World

Edited by

Richard Wootton

Scottish Centre for Telehealth, Aberdeen, UK;
University of Queensland, Brisbane, Australia

Nivritti G Patil

University of Hong Kong, Hong Kong, China

Richard E Scott

University of Calgary, Calgary, Canada

Kendall Ho

University of British Columbia, Vancouver, Canada

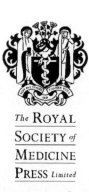

The ROYAL
SOCIETY *of*
MEDICINE
PRESS *Limited*

International Development Research Centre
Ottawa • Cairo • Dakar • Montevideo • Nairobi • New Delhi • Singapore

© 2009 Royal Society of Medicine Press Ltd
Reprinted 2009
Co-published by

1 Wimpole Street, London W1G 0AE, UK
Tel: +44 (0)20 7290 2921
Fax: +44 (0)20 7290 2929
Email: publishing@rsm.ac.uk
Website: www.rsmpress.co.uk

International Development Research Centre
PO Box 8500, Ottawa, ON K1G 3H9, Canada
Email: info@idrc.ca
Website: www.idrc.ca

This publication has been generously supported by a grant from the International Development Research Centre, Canada; with additional contributions from HiiTeC and the Faculty of Medicine, University of Hong Kong.

British Library Cataloguing in Publication Data
A catalogue record for this book is available from the British Library

ISBN 978-1-85315-784-4
E-ISBN 978-1-55250-396-6

Distribution in Europe and Rest of World:
Marston Book Services Ltd
PO Box 269
Abingdon
Oxon OX14 4YN, UK
Tel: +44 (0)1235 465500
Fax: +44 (0)1235 465555
Email: direct.order@marston.co.uk

Distribution in the USA and Canada:
Royal Society of Medicine Press Ltd
c/o BookMasters Inc
30 Amberwood Parkway
Ashland, OH 44805, USA
Tel: +1 800 247 6553/+1 800 266 5564
Fax: +1 419 281 6883
Email: orders@bookmasters.com

Distribution in Australia and New Zealand:
Elsevier Australia
30–52 Smidmore Street
Marrickville NSW 2204, Australia
Tel: +61 2 9517 8999
Fax: +61 2 9517 2249
Email: service@elsevier.com.au

Typeset by Saxon Graphics Ltd, Derby
Printed and bound in the Great Britain by Marston Book Services Limited, Oxford

Contents

Contributors

Palitha Abeykoon Ministry of Health, Colombo, Sri Lanka

Peter Brooks Faculty of Health Sciences, University of Queensland, Brisbane, Australia

Charles W Callahan De Witt Army Community Hospital, Ft Belvoir, Virginia, USA

Rithy Chau Sihanouk Hospital Center for HOPE, Phnom Penh, Cambodia

Jie Chen Key Laboratory of Health Technology Assessment, Ministry of Health; School of Public Health, Fudan University, Shanghai, China

Michael Clarke International Development Research Centre, Ottawa, Canada

Stephen Cone Virginia Commonwealth University Medical Center, Richmond, Virginia, USA

Gianfranco Costanzo Ministry of Labour, Health and Social Policies, Alliance of the Italian Hospitals Worldwide – Secretariat for Technical Assistance, Rome, Italy

Sangeeta Desai Department of Pathology, Tata Memorial Hospital, Mumbai, India

Vajira H W Dissanayake Human Genetics Unit, Faculty of Medicine, University of Colombo, Colombo, Sri Lanka

Joan Dzenowagis World Health Organization, Geneva, Switzerland

Sisira Edirippulige Centre for Online Health, University of Queensland, Brisbane, Australia

Laurent Elder International Development Research Centre, Ottawa, Canada

Luiz A Facchini Department of Social Medicine, University Federal of Pelotas, Pelotas, Brazil

Gerald Gabler Department of IT and Telecommunications, Graz University Clinics and General Hospital, Graz, Austria

Irfan Hayee COMSATS Headquarters, Islamabad, Pakistan

Paul Heinzelmann Center for Connected Health, Partners HealthCare; Department of Medicine, Massachusetts General Hospital, Harvard Medical School, Boston, Massachusetts, USA

Kendall Ho Faculty of Medicine, University of British Columbia, Vancouver, Canada

Adesina Iluyemi Centre for Healthcare Modelling and Informatics, School of Computing, University of Portsmouth, UK

Steven Kaddu Department of Dermatology, Medical University of Graz, Graz, Austria

Jayantee Kalita Department of Neurology, Sanjay Gandhi Postgraduate Institute of Medical Sciences, Lucknow, India

Hameed A Khan Pakistan Atomic Energy Commission, Islamabad, Pakistan

Shariq Khoja Faculty of Health Sciences, Aga Khan University, Karachi, Pakistan

Boris A Kobrinskiy Moscow Research Institute of Paediatrics and Children's Surgery, Moscow, Russia

Olivier Koole Institute of Tropical Medicine, Department of Clinical Sciences, Antwerp, Belgium

Carrie Kovarik Department of Dermatology, Dermatopathology, and Infectious Diseases, University of Pennsylvania, Philadelphia, USA

Joseph Kvedar Center for Connected Health, Partners HealthCare; Department of Dermatology, Massachusetts General Hospital, Harvard Medical School, Boston, Massachusetts, USA

Daniel Liu Sihanouk Hospital Center for HOPE, Phnom Penh, Cambodia

Lut Lynen Institute of Tropical Medicine, Department of Clinical Sciences, Antwerp, Belgium

C Becket Mahnke Tripler Army Medical Center, Honolulu, USA

Maria F S Maia University Federal of Pelotas, Pelotas, Brazil

Rohana B Marasinghe Centre for Online Health, University of Queensland, Brisbane, Australia

Alvin B Marcelo National Telehealth Center, University of the Philippines, Philippines

Maurice Mars Nelson R Mandela School of Medicine, University of KwaZulu-Natal, South Africa

Ronald C Merrell Virginia Commonwealth University Medical Center, Richmond, Virginia, USA

Anjali Mishra Sanjay Gandhi Postgraduate Institute of Medical Sciences, Lucknow, India

Saroj K Mishra Sanjay Gandhi Postgraduate Institute of Medical Sciences, Lucknow, India

Usha K Misra Department of Neurology, Sanjay Gandhi Postgraduate Institute of Medical Sciences, Lucknow, India

Paola Monari Alliance of the Italian Hospitals Worldwide – Secretariat for Technical Assistance, Rome, Italy

Azra Naseem Institute of Educational Development, Aga Khan University, Karachi, Pakistan

Andre Nebel de Mello Laboratorio de Sistemas Integraveis da Escola Polictecnica da Universidade de São Paulo, São Paulo, Brazil

Alessander Osorio University Federal of Pelotas, Pelotas, Brazil

Philip O Ozuah Children's Hospital at Montefiore, Albert Einstein College of Medicine, New York, USA

Nivritti G Patil University of Hong Kong, Hong Kong, China

Donald A Person Tripler Army Medical Center, Honolulu, USA

Vladimir I Petlakh Moscow Research Institute of Paediatrics and Children's Surgery, Moscow, Russia

Puthen V Pradeep Sanjay Gandhi Postgraduate Institute of Medical Sciences, Lucknow, India

Mohan R Pradhan Health Net, Kathmandhu, Nepal

Verena Renggli Institute of Tropical Medicine, Department of Clinical Sciences, Antwerp, Belgium

Marina Reznik Children's Hospital at Montefiore, Albert Einstein College of Medicine, New York, USA

Edgar J Rodas University of Azuay, Cuenca, Ecuador

Richard E Scott Health Innovation and Information Technology Centre (HiiTeC), University of Calgary, Calgary, Canada

H Peter Soyer Dermatology Group, School of Medicine, University of Queensland, Brisbane, Australia

Pat Swinfen Swinfen Charitable Trust, Canterbury, UK

Roger Swinfen Swinfen Charitable Trust, Canterbury, UK

Elaine Thumé Department of Nursing, University Federal of Pelotas, Pelotas, Brazil

Elaine Tomasi Department of Psychology, University Catholic of Pelotas, Pelotas, Brazil

Richard Wootton Scottish Centre for Telehealth, Aberdeen, UK; University of Queensland, Brisbane, Australia

Zhiyuan Xia Telemedicine Centre, Fudan University, Shanghai, China

Maria Zolfo Institute of Tropical Medicine, Department of Clinical Sciences, Antwerp, Belgium

Foreword

Telehealth in the Developing World is a very wide-ranging book, rich in practical experience, which will be of interest both to those who want to learn about the developing world and to those who want to learn from developing countries. It is full of real-life stories. Telemedicine, rightly in my view, is seen as central to the improvement of health and life in developing countries. Much has been said and written about telemedicine and its potential to transform life, but these are still early days. A great deal of what has been written and said has been theoretical. This book reflects the reality.

All the projects described here have been driven by people of vision and passion. All have had to confront the problems of the real world, whether these have been the realities of desperate poverty or the, equally real, obstacles of clinical, technical and governmental politics. All the pioneers have been on journeys of discovery, working out how to be effective in the particular environment where they are operating. Who can fail to be impressed by the Swinfen Charitable Trust and its journey? It has pioneered the use of the simplest of modern electronic technology to ensure that people working in isolation in poor countries can benefit from the opinions of specialists in the richest countries.

Other impressive pioneering work in particular specialities – such as teledermatology, telepaediatrics, telepathology, telepsychiatry and e-mental health – is described here. There are also descriptions of progress in developing countries, such as China, Pakistan, Chechnya and Ecuador, as well as accounts of linking with Italian expatriates and cross-cultural experiences between the USA and Cambodia.

Importantly, these accounts show how telemedicine enables professionals to be put in touch with other professionals. Individual clinicians in remote areas are able to tap into advice from their peers and, very motivationally, to feel part of their profession and of an international group of colleagues. This by-product of telemedicine must not be underestimated. It has sustained human beings when other resources have failed.

Underpinning all this are accounts of public and technical policy that attempt to answer the question of how the enthusiasm of the pioneers can be turned into sustainable mainstream activity. This is, of course, the vital question.

Health care, as we know, is primarily about people-to-people interactions. It is about understanding, diagnosis, physical contact, communication and, ultimately, providing care. All of this is facilitated by the technical processes of imaging, pathological testing, information gathering, research and so forth. The task for every health care system is how to maximize the personal contact at the same time as maximizing the technical input, while all the time operating within a sustainable financial framework.

People working in developing countries have had to think about this task with even more urgency than those of us working in richer countries. They have had to think about how to obtain an expert opinion in remote places, how to support local clinicians who may not have all the skills they need, how to make sure technical information is interpreted wisely in very difficult circumstances and how best to use very scarce resources. Telemedicine offers help in meeting these conflicting needs by improving access to data and to individuals, while driving down the costs of doing so.

We in the developed world have large and industrialized health systems that grow costlier by the day as we absorb new technologies. At some point, as costs and demand both rise, we too will need to learn some of the lessons that our colleagues are learning in Africa, South America and Asia. The pioneers in this book are learning lessons for developing countries. They are learning lessons for us all.

LORD CRISP
Honorary Professor at the London School of Hygiene and Tropical Medicine

Preface

This is the ninth book in the Royal Society of Medicine's series of multi-author books on telemedicine topics. The series aims to provide examples of best practice. This book's predecessors are:

- *The Legal and Ethical Aspects of Telemedicine*, BA Stanberry, 1998
- *Introduction to Telemedicine*, R Wootton and J Craig (eds), 1999
- *Teledermatology*, R Wootton and AMM Oakley (eds), 2002
- *Telepsychiatry and e-Mental Health*, R Wootton, P Yellowlees and P McLaren (eds), 2003
- *Telepediatrics: Telemedicine and Child Health*, R Wootton and J Batch (eds), 2004
- *Teleneurology*, R Wootton and V Patterson (eds), 2005
- *Introduction to Telemedicine*, 2nd edition, R Wootton, J Craig and V Patterson (eds), 2006
- *Home Telehealth: Connecting Care Within the Community*, R Wootton, SL Dimmick and JC Kvedar (eds), 2006

Much has been written about the potential use of telemedicine in developing countries, but equally much of it has been criticized as little more than wishful thinking. While it is sometimes said that there are relatively few cost-effective and sustainable telemedicine projects in the industrialized world, there are even fewer in developing countries. The present volume therefore aims to summarize the experience of starting and sustaining telehealth projects in the developing world. It represents a description of how telemedicine in the broadest sense can be applied to improve the delivery of health care in developing countries.

The book's contributors have substantial practical experience across a wide range of application areas, and most have published previous reports of their work in the peer-reviewed literature.

It is a pleasure to acknowledge the support of Canada's International Research and Development Centre, the Li Ka Shing Faculty of Medicine at the University of Hong Kong, the Health Innovation and Information Technology Centre (HiiTeC) of the University of Calgary, and the U21 Health Sciences Group in the production of the book. We have divided the material into sections:

- background and introductory material
- a section on policy matters

- a section describing educational applications
- a section about clinical applications
- a view of the future.

We hope that within the broad spectrum of ideas expressed in this book everyone will find something of relevance. We also hope that you enjoy reading it.

RICHARD WOOTTON
Edinburgh, UK

KENDALL HO
Vancouver, Canada

NIVRITTI G PATIL
Hong Kong, China

RICHARD E SCOTT
Calgary, Canada

SECTION 1

BACKGROUND

1 Introduction

Richard Wootton, Kendall Ho, Nivritti G Patil and Richard E Scott

What is telemedicine?

There is no generally accepted definition of telemedicine. The literal meaning is 'health[care] at a distance'. Thus, telemedicine may represent health care practised in real time, using a video link for example, or asynchronously, perhaps by email. The type of health care interaction is perfectly general, and may encompass diagnosis and management, education – of staff, patients and the general population – and administrative meetings.

The history of telemedicine has been bedevilled by loose terminology, which, some observers feel, has not assisted its cause.[1] What began originally as 'telemedicine' has become successively 'telehealth', 'online health', 'e-health', 'connected health', etc. In this book, different contributors use slightly different terms to describe their telemedicine experience, depending on their local environment. While the editors have tried to reduce the number of terms used, we have deliberately not enforced a uniform terminology throughout, in recognition of these local differences.

Scope of the problem

Telemedicine is one aspect of the use of information and communication technology (ICT) in health care. It is widely believed that ICT generally has the potential to improve clinical care and public health. In addition to facilitating medical education, administration and research, appropriate use of ICT may:

- improve access to health care;
- enhance the quality of service delivery;
- improve the effectiveness of public health and primary care interventions;
- improve the global shortage of health professionals through collaboration and training.

However, many questions remain about the potential value to people in resource-constrained settings such as the developing world.

There are major problems of inequity of access to health care in developing countries, to which telemedicine offers a potential solution. It may be valuable in other ways as well.

Crisp report

In 2007, Lord Crisp reported about how UK experience and expertise in health could best be used to help improve health in developing countries.[2] He concluded that sufficient progress towards the United Nations' Millennium Development Goals (e.g. in reducing child and maternal deaths, and tackling HIV/AIDS, tuberculosis and malaria) would not occur unless:

- developing countries are able to take the lead and own the solutions – and are supported by international, national and local partnerships based on mutual respect;
- the UK and other industrialized countries grasp the opportunity – and see themselves as having a responsibility as global employers – to support a massive scaling-up of training, education and employment of health workers in developing countries;
- there is much more rigorous research and evaluation of what works, systematic spreading of good practice, greater use of new information, communication and biomedical technologies, closer links with economic development, and an accompanying reduction in wasted effort.

Clearly, telemedicine could play a major part in facilitating all of these activities. Furthermore, one can imagine the consequences if every hospital in the richer countries were to be linked up on a formal basis with a small group of hospitals or health centres in developing countries. Through mutual learning and collaboration in health service provision, such health partnerships could ultimately change health-care delivery at the national level; they might also change how the industrialized nations perceive the world. Telemedicine and ICT would be essential to maximizing the potential of these health partnerships.

Aim of the book

Any discussion of telemedicine in the developing world raises difficult questions about resource use, sustainability and global equity in access to health care. Despite the large number of published articles on the *concept* of telemedicine in the developing world, there are remarkably few examples of successful implementation.[3] In this book, we have attempted to assemble a representative cross-section of the very wide range of work that has been carried out to date. Thus, the book offers a state-of-the-art review of telemedicine in the developing world, and should also provide the basis for a high-level operations manual. It could be considered unethical, after all, not to learn from the experience of others and to squander scarce resources on an idea that may have already been proved to be unfeasible.

The major sections of the book cover policy, clinical and educational matters. We hope that you enjoy reading it.

References

1   Wootton R. Telemedicine and isolated communities: a UK perspective. *J Telemed Telecare* 1999; **5**(Suppl 2): 27–34.
2   Crisp N. *Global Health Partnerships. The UK Contribution to Health in Developing Countries.* London: COI, 2007. Available at: www.dh.gov.uk/en/Publicationsandstatistics/Publications/PublicationsPolicy-AndGuidance/DH_065374.
3   Wootton R. Telemedicine support for the developing world. *J Telemed Telecare* 2008; **14**: 109–14.

SECTION 2

POLICY

2 Bridging the digital divide: Linking health and ICT policy

Joan Dzenowagis

Introduction

The past decade has seen a remarkable growth in the diffusion of information and communication technology (ICT) across the world. This growth has been fuelled by technological advances, economic investment, and social and cultural changes that have facilitated the integration of ICT into everyday life. The general public – consumers – as well as a range of new stakeholders have had a significant impact on shaping this growth, for example by demanding better products, services and value for money. As these technologies enter the mainstream of business and cultural life, there is also a greater awareness of their potential as economic and social tools and, with it, new social and political pressure to re-frame ICT as a public good to be made accessible and available to all. This shift has had important ramifications in countries and at the international level as well.

Despite this encouraging progress, however, the uptake of ICT globally continues at an uneven pace, and the 'digital divide' remains a significant obstacle to achieving global development goals. The digital divide is understood broadly to be the gap between those with access to ICT and its benefits and those without. It is specifically acknowledged in the United Nations Millennium Development Goals (MDGs). Goal 8, Target 18 of the MDGs proposes 'a global partnership for development to make available the benefits of new technologies, especially information and communication technologies'.[1]

Recent events such as the G8 Summits and the World Summit on the Information Society[2] have continued to promote this target and to highlight the striking gaps in access to ICT worldwide. In some countries, both urban and rural regions remain isolated from the knowledge society: infrastructure is non-existent, costs for basic services are beyond average income levels and well-intentioned ICT pilot projects end without ever scaling-up. While this can be disastrous for national economies competing in a global environment, it is also a tragedy for the health sector, where ICT is essential to improve health and help alleviate inequalities.

ICT in the health sector

In the health sector, ICT is a cornerstone of efficient and effective services. In many countries, use of ICT within the sector continues to grow, and the Internet in particular is driving significant change. For example, in middle- and high-income countries, the Internet is dramatically changing the way in which consumers interact with health services, including access to health information and the ability to purchase pharmaceuticals and other health products. The Internet also plays a key role in expanding the reach of health services to remote areas. The spread of broadband networks and the development of new e-health applications, defined as the use of ICT for health, have a mutually stimulating effect on further developments. However, it is clear that, despite the numerous creative and sometimes quite costly efforts to improve the situation, access to these developments is not universal, and many countries do not benefit as they might from advances in ICT in health.

For policy makers committed to improving national health systems, working with ICT policy makers and participating in the national policy-making process is essential to ensure that national ICT policy, when implemented, will meet the interests of the health sector in the years to come.

Measuring the digital divide

It has only been within the past few years that meaningful measures of the digital divide have been developed. The potential choice of indicators is enormous and the continuing evolution of technology shortens the useful lifespan of established indicators, creating the need for their regular revision. However, whether measured by ICT diffusion, technology investment or other related measures, the digital divide is manifest within and between countries in a variety of ways.

The digital divide is evident in low-income countries, where technology is unaffordable for private enterprise as well as for individuals, and where government policies and regulations do not encourage or support ICT business development. It is evident in the contrast between urban and rural areas, where investment in basic ICT infrastructure and services is chronically inadequate. It is also evident in communities and households, where literacy rates, educational levels and incomes are low and where content imported from abroad does not suit local needs or transmit in local languages. Most of these aspects are captured by the ICT Diffusion Index,[3] which takes into account the complex dimensions of access, connectivity and policy in countries. The index results in a composite score between 0 and 1, giving a picture of ICT status in general but not addressing ICT diffusion by sector. The link between ICT, health and development is clear in Figure 2.1, showing country ICT diffusion and mortality strata, by WHO region.[4,5]

Following the World Summit on the Information Society in 2003 and 2005, many countries undertook the development of national strategies that aimed to increase the use of ICT. Such strategies sought to increase investment and stimulate innovation, particularly in small and medium enterprises in the private sector, and to improve

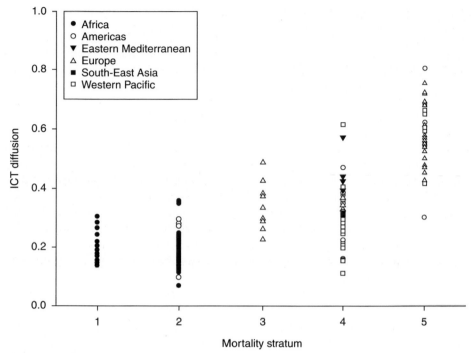

Figure 2.1 ICT diffusion and mortality. (Stratum 1 = very high adult and very high child mortality; stratum 5 = low adult and low child mortality.)

efficiency and effectiveness in the public sector (e.g. in government and education). For both the public and private sectors, the use of ICT in health, or e-health, is considered to represent a key instrument for health care delivery and public health action,[6] and a number of governments have supported specific investments and policy instruments towards this end.

In high- and low-income countries, e-health has already demonstrated its value, particularly in containing cross-border threats to health and safety. However despite the documented value of ICT in terms of improving quality, cost and access to health care, the picture globally remains mixed. In particular, the ability to plan and implement e-health on a large scale, while adapting it to local health problems, presents a huge challenge for countries and institutions.

Despite the difficulties, there have been major ICT investments, particularly in countries such as those in Eastern Europe. These economies are growing rapidly, and large-scale infrastructure investments supported by the European Union include ICT for health institutions and universities. In higher-income countries, there is spending in the areas of information systems, electronic health records, e-prescribing systems, diagnostic tools and medical imaging. In developing countries, ICT pilot projects are being funded by international donors, leading to uncoordinated deployment of ICT in health service delivery and incompatible systems at many levels. In addition, investments are being made in applications that support 'vertical' health programmes such as disease surveillance, management of drug supply, and planning and monitoring human resources for health.

Driving forces for ICT in health

Challenges in global public health

Despite significant progress in public health over the past 50 years, the fundamental conditions for health have not been achieved in many countries. Most of the burden of premature death and illness among the poor is due to problems for which solutions are known and prevention is possible, yet the health of populations in developing countries continues to be at risk. Today, the gap in health between the wealthy and the poor, both within and between countries, continues to grow.

The health divide is evident especially in low-income countries, which face a high burden of endemic and epidemic-prone infectious diseases, unacceptably high levels of child and maternal mortality, a continuing HIV/AIDS pandemic and the rapid spread of chronic conditions accelerated by poverty. In many countries, there is a deepening crisis in access to basic health services, linked to a shortage of essential health workers.[7] In the face of these and numerous other challenges, governments are attempting to build and sustain their health systems.

Over the last decade, the need to develop and organize new ways of providing health services has been accompanied by major advances in ICT, enabling better support for health services and systems, and improving global awareness of health issues. These technologies hold great promise for the health sector in both low- and high-income countries, and some countries are realizing the benefits today. This is true not only for the delivery of health services, but also for health-related markets more generally. As the use of ICT grows, it is vital that the health sector participates in key international forums and helps to shape national policy to ensure that ICT improves outcomes for health, particularly for the most vulnerable populations.

Forces for change

In all countries, including developing countries, forces from health care and the ICT industry are spurring the growth of e-health. These forces include industry developments in wireless and satellite systems, the spread of broadband communications, better access to applications and services, and increasing digital processing power and storage capacity. This growth has led to significant regulatory change, advances in consumer protection, greater patient mobility, and new opportunities for trade and cross-border services in health.[8] In the health sector, driving forces for adoption of ICT include such factors as government pressures to control costs, chronic and ever-increasing health work force shortages, greater expectations by consumers for higher quality and safer care, and changing models of health care delivery.

From the micro-level to the macro-level, from basic human genetics research to the provision of humanitarian aid and disaster relief to populations at risk, ICT supports the health sector in addressing a vast range of immediate and long-term challenges to human life and health, through the functions outlined in Table 2.1.

Table 2.1 Examples of the use of ICT in health systems and services

Broad area	Examples
Access to information and knowledge	1. Improved access to health information, research, literature and training materials, such as access to biomedical and social sciences research. This supports the health research enterprise and enables comprehensive, evidence-based management of acute and chronic conditions
	2. Improved access to resources on prevention, awareness and education, for the general public as well as for health professionals, researchers and policy makers
Networking and collaboration	1. Collaboration for the management and coordination of care across different health providers, community health services and health institutions
	2. Better exchange of knowledge among policy makers, practitioners and advocacy groups
	3. Rapid and coordinated response to disasters and disease events
Information for policy and action: measuring progress, tracking quality and trend analysis	1. ICT for collecting, organizing and disseminating public health evidence and information for advocacy, practice and policy
	2. Improved ability to describe, model, analyze and monitor trends on health status, income, employment and service coverage, and disaggregate by gender
	3. Support for research on policy effectiveness
Health education and training	1. Direct support to education and training for health professionals and workers, including both pre-service education and in-service training and resources
	2. Improved efficiency and effectiveness of education delivery through strategic application of ICT and ICT-enabled skill development
	3. Improved availability of quality educational resources through ICT
	4. Outreach to special populations (girls and women) using appropriate technologies
	5. Enhanced delivery of basic and in-service education
Public accountability through greater flow of information	1. Greater transparency, accountability and accessibility in delivery of public services
	2. Improved enforcement of regulations and performance monitoring of decentralized services
Delivery of health services	1. Prevention of disease, health education and promotion, and support for diagnosis and treatment
	2. Establishment of health registries and health information systems
	3. Extension of care to rural and remote areas through telemedicine applications; increased access of rural health workers to specialist support and consultation

A number of these uses of ICT promise particular benefits for developing countries. For example, decreasing the isolation of the health community is seen as a major benefit, and is thus a driver for adoption. ICT is increasingly well integrated in educational settings in middle- and high-income countries, where communication, collaboration and access to information are at the core of research and teaching. Universities in the developing world need to connect on an equal footing with their counterparts. This access will play an important role in advancing locally relevant research, and will improve capacity by enabling participation in the peer-review process required for publishing and participation in research conferences.

Improved access to care is an important benefit of ICT, particularly for countries tackling the challenge of providing health care to people over a broad geographical area. One of the main drivers behind public investment in e-health systems is the expectation that ICT will improve access to services and reduce the inequities experienced by people in remote locations. This is a serious matter in countries that have chronic shortages of physicians, nurses and health technicians. The problem of shortages is often coupled with public concern over access and demographic shifts with concomitant major health resource implications, such as ageing populations and rapid population growth in native or aboriginal communities.[9] In contexts such as these, the goal of access to health care has driven the adoption of ICT for remote diagnosis, monitoring and consultation.

Quality of care is another important driver for ICT adoption. Health service providers are not only attempting to deliver more effective care, they are also attempting to deliver care that is safe. Both goals require the use of ICT to measure, monitor and report on quality improvement initiatives, as well as the use of information systems – such as pharmaceutical ordering systems – that are proven to reduce errors.[10] Developments such as e-prescription and computer-assisted imaging are part of this. With respect to technology-assisted care, it is critical to ensure that the care and information provided through e-health meet appropriate standards, relating to the quality of information transmitted as well as to the overall reliability of the system and the satisfaction of users, both professionals and patients.

To date, e-health has mainly been used to improve productivity in delivery systems focused on patients and hospitals. In the future, it can be expected that ICT will be used to facilitate personalized and home-centred care. To this end, there has been significant investment in research and development, such as in the European Union (EU) Framework Programmes, which have invested over 500 million euros in establishing a European health area, e-health conferences and an e-health action plan.[11]

The concept of citizen-centred care has become the basis of programmes designed to empower consumers in part by improving the health information environment. Many observers expect that the Internet and the web will become the place to obtain health advice for citizens. In 2007, the worldwide Internet population was estimated at 15.8 users per 100 inhabitants, up from 5.3 users per 100 in 1999.[4] Health is consistently among the most sought-after types of Internet information.[12] Some governments, worried that the volume and quality of health information on the Internet might pose a risk to citizens, have responded by creating or sponsoring health information portals. Others have provided guidelines for website quality and promoted consumer education as a protection against the growing problem of Internet fraud and spam.

Economy and efficiency of care is another important driver for the adoption of ICT in health. Key areas aimed at controlling costs over the long term include hospital information systems, regional networks, secure reimbursement and procurement systems, and patient 'smart cards' carrying personal medical data. The electronic health record is central to the ability to improve quality, access and economy of care. It is also fundamental to realizing the concept of an expanded, digitized health care network that enables more effective public health services.

Just as ICT is at the core of much of the improvement in national health systems, global health security is also critically dependent on ICT. Reliable and secure ICT systems enable tracking of diseases and monitoring of populations at risk, and provide the basis for global defence against bioterrorism as well as early response to natural and man-made disasters. For example, the best way to prevent international spread of diseases is by detecting public health risks early and mounting an effective response while the problem is still localized. Rapid reporting, enabled and validated through global electronic communication, was a critical factor in the containment of the SARS epidemic in 2003 and is a key aspect of preparedness for pandemics such as that anticipated with avian influenza. Fortunately, steady improvements in satellite technology, and particularly its more widespread use, have enabled a faster, more coordinated response globally and nationally to disease events and natural disasters.[13]

An overview of ICT policy

It is important for health policy makers to have an overview of the forces and policies that shape the availability and cost of ICT, and to understand potential points of influence. This will ensure that the health sector benefits from ICT to the greatest extent possible. Globally, the ICT policy picture is complex and changing, and is not easily governed by traditional forms of national and international public authority. Beyond this, the Internet in particular has given rise to new patterns of international cooperation. Whereas the technical management of the Internet is dominated by companies working in industry forums to devise private systems of rules, in parallel governments and firms are collaborating to devise shared rules on communications behaviour and global electronic commerce conducted over that infrastructure.[14] This is not a trivial matter for the health sector, as decisions made in this unwieldy international system will have a direct effect on the future development of e-health, such as patient mobility and the viability of cross-border services in health.

Interested parties

In addition to governments, other major stakeholders in the ICT policy-making process include a wide range of organizations and firms, such as international organizations (e.g. the United Nations, the International Telecommunication Union and the World Trade Organization), consumer rights organizations (e.g. Consumers International), regional Internet registries, private businesses (e.g. ICT systems and equipment vendors, telecommunications operators, Internet service providers, and financial and certification companies), business forums (e.g. the International Chamber of Commerce) and civil society organizations (e.g. Privacy International and the Association for Progressive Communications). A wide variety of civil society organizations are increasingly engaged in ICT forums in order to have their perspective reflected in ICT debates.

Pivotal role of governments

While the above groups are active in seeking influence at the international level, government policy at the national level can have a dramatic effect on the diffusion of

ICT.[15] It is governments that create the policy environment that will foster technology use and encourage national and international investment in ICT infrastructure, development and a skilled workforce. Government action is also important in extending the benefits of technology to all social groups, as governments have the power and mandate to balance the needs of their citizens for long-term economic growth and social prosperity. Ultimately, how and what users have access to depend on specific legal, economic, political and social conditions. Not least, national systems of innovation strongly influence the diffusion process in a country.[16]

Linking health goals to ICT policy

ICT represents not a single innovation but rather a cluster of related technologies that must be present together to support adoption by users, such as servers, communication links, software and user devices. In the simple model shown in Figure 2.2 there are three levels. At the bottom, is the connectivity level or underlying telecommunications and network infrastructure level, without which there can be no ICT. In the middle, a services level consists of organizations providing ICT applications and services, reflecting the extent to which ICT services are available in a country. At the top, is the individual and organizational user level, where ICT adoption is typically measured by the overall number of users in a country.[17]

Policy implemented at each level affects meaningful access to ICT in a country and therefore in the health sector. Policies on the infrastructure level provide the basis for expanding physical infrastructure such as satellite, wireless and broadband by shaping market conditions and competition. Providing access to technology is critical, but more than physical access is necessary. Networks and services are insufficient if ICT

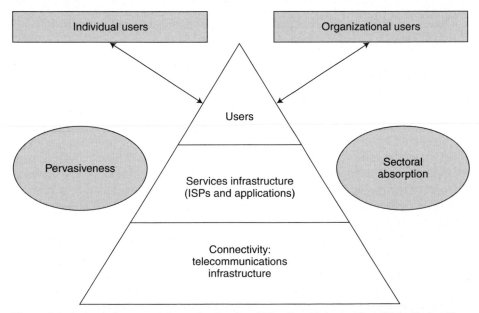

Figure 2.2 A simple framework for understanding ICT policy. (Adapted from Wolcott et al.[17])

is not used because it is not affordable, people cannot understand how to use it or the local economy cannot sustain its use. Policies at the services level therefore shape the legal and regulatory framework that creates conditions for a viable, secure online environment, promotes diffusion and uptake of services, and supports minimum levels of consumer protection. At the user level, a wide range of government and organizational policies affect user adoption and conditions of use. For example, a United Nations group has developed an index of ICT diffusion.[18] This considers the indicators for Internet access in a country as including Internet users per 1000 inhabitants, adult literacy rate, cost of a 3-minute fixed-line telephone call and gross domestic product (GDP) per capita. Seen from this broad perspective, government investment and policies to boost literacy – as much as direct involvement in ICT policy – are important in ensuring that all citizens can benefit from ICT.

Health policy makers in the process of developing or implementing national e-health strategies need to be able to work effectively with ICT policy makers. However, there are few precedents for cooperation between the sectors and little experience to draw on to align policy interests.

Linking health and ICT policy

The potential points of influence, or entry points, in a complex environment such as ICT policy are not necessarily obvious. At a minimum, national health policy makers need to know the basics of ICT policy objectives and approaches in order to be effective advocates for improving infrastructure, access and affordability, or for obtaining concessions or aid for the health sector. While every country is unique, national policies generally set out goals and objectives for the development of the ICT industry, development of the economy and support for key sectors of the economy. The list below highlights core elements included in national ICT policy.

Core content of ICT policy

The core content of any ICT policy must include five factors:

1. *Infrastructure development.* These policies promote the development, expansion, operation and increased efficiency of ICT networks at the infrastructure level. This is an area of great interest to the health sector, but not traditionally one where the sector has much influence. Those involved include governments (ministries of information technology and telecommunications), the private sector (multinational corporations), independent bodies (regulators) and international organizations (International Telecommunication Union).

2. *Universal and equitable access to ICT services.* These policies, implemented primarily at the infrastructure and services level, aim to improve the availability and affordability of ICT services. They are designed to facilitate access to ICT networks and services for all citizens, as well as for under-served groups such as the disabled and women. This area is of vital interest to the health sector, and is

becoming more open to influence as policy-makers strive for more transparent and inclusive policy-making processes.

3. *Promotion of market competition.* Policies in this area aim to stimulate ICT development and adoption by creating an environment for fair competition between providers of infrastructure and services, corresponding to the infrastructure and service levels of the model. Outcomes are of great interest to the health sector, but this is not typically an area of direct influence.

4. *ICT as a means of achieving national social and economic goals.* These policies are designed to exploit ICT in achieving national social and economic goals, such as health, education and economic development. Policies in this area correspond to the service and user levels of the model. This is a natural and realistic entry point for the health sector in policy discussions.

5. *Encouraging private sector investment.* Policies aim to promote private enterprise development of ICT infrastructure and services. Policies in this area correspond to the infrastructure and services levels of the model, and are also related to overall government policies for transparency, accountability, anti-corruption and so on. Robust and sustainable private sector investment in ICT benefits the health sector, and this policy area is increasingly open to sectoral advocacy and influence. There are significant variations in telecommunications investment across the world.[4]

Countries place different emphasis on the above elements, depending on factors such as their level of economic development, the strength and maturity of the private sector, the orientation of development partners and existing policy capacity. For example, one country may see a need for stronger emphasis on competition in services rather than on expansion of ICT infrastructure. Examples of ICT policy and potential impact on the health sector are highlighted in Table 2.2.

Factors affecting ICT use in the health sector

There are several factors that affect the use of ICT in the health sector. These include costs, access speed, education and collaboration between stakeholders.

Costs for ICT

These influence uptake in all sectors. They are normally reflected at the service level, and incorporate the costs passed on to the user from the infrastructure level. In general, two basic disparities exist in the affordability of ICT: in the basic cost of the technology and in the cost relative to per capita income. Access costs such as high Internet service provider and telephone call fees can be two to four times as high in developing countries as in developed market economies.[19] When the monthly cost for Internet access exceeds the monthly income of a significant proportion of the population, its level of use will remain low.

Access speed

This directly affects cost. In nearly all countries, telephone calls are charged on a per-minute basis for telephone mainlines, with an additional access charge. Where Internet access is through a dial-up connection, download times are long, and costs therefore

Table 2.2 Policy areas related to ICT

Level	Description	Examples
Infrastructure	Telecommunications and related systems	Policies that affect basic ICT infrastructure: 1. Telecommunications licensing system 2. Telecommunications operator privatization and market liberalization 3. Spectrum allocation 4. Internet domain management 5. Banking and financial sector regulation 6. Standard setting 7. Customs standardization 8. Rules on taxation, tariffs, foreign ownership of ICT infrastructure
Services level	Trust and security – transactions that affect use of services and applications	Policies that affect business, government and consumer trust towards ICT and others online, including: 1. Electronic signatures 2. Data security 3. Cybercrime, fraud and spam 4. Privacy 5. Intellectual property 6. Regulation of content and freedom of speech 7. Consumer protection
Service level	Technology diffusion	Service and access fees, universal service provisions, and private sector and civil society access
User level	Capacity building	Policies that build the capacity to use ICT, including curriculum and materials, and technical education. For the general public, this also includes policies to ensure basic literacy, without gender difference
Overall environment	General government environment	Government structure (transparency, independence of judiciary and regulatory authorities), discrimination policy

increase. The trend to using large web pages and files is not an obstacle in countries where bandwidth is increasing, but in low-income countries the long download time further increases the cost. Although telemedicine can be successfully practised via low-bandwidth connections, lack of affordable broadband infrastructure significantly hampers the ability to conduct telemedicine applications where transfer of high-resolution images is required (see Chapters 13 and 19).

Education
This clearly affects ICT use, and international disparities are evident at the user level. The degree of technical capacity at this level is a result of long-standing government investment or under-investment in education and training, not only through initiatives such as staff development programmes and technical training in schools, but also including investment in secondary and tertiary education.

Collaboration between stakeholders

At the infrastructure and service levels, regulations such as those for importation of telecommunications equipment in emergency situations show the need for cross-border collaboration in ICT and health. Clearly, ICT is central to an effective health sector response in disaster situations, whether natural disasters or man-made (e.g. armed conflict). In the absence of formally established procedures covering disasters and emergencies, customs clearance and type-approval procedures for telecommunications equipment, allocation of radiofrequencies and authorization for radio communications can delay installation of urgently needed communications systems. For example, regulations on telecommunications equipment importation and type approval delayed help when a non-governmental organization arrived to install radio communications in Bam, Iran after a major earthquake in 2004. Lengthy national and local customs and telecommunications regulatory clearance resulted in an unnecessary and costly delay before the equipment could be installed where needed.

Legal framework, skills and protections for a network economy

Trends in the uptake of advanced applications of ICT such as e-commerce show even greater disparities than trends in basic access to computers. Many countries still lack the infrastructure, capacity and resources to develop and manage health applications, including those emerging from e-commerce and e-government. Without these prerequisites, ICT in health will not grow significantly in developing countries. Furthermore, countries must have the skills of a networked society in order to deal with common challenges and threats. For example, security threats are growing and are becoming more malicious, damaging and widespread, with serious implications for countries. Threats to a networked economy include spam and security violations. These are increasingly propagated from developing countries with weak laws, weak policies and inadequate security. The consequences can be severe for developing countries, where awareness, protection tools, legislation and enforcement are still underdeveloped.[20] Basic measures are required to ensure that security threats emanating from developing countries do not pose a threat to the Internet. Collaboration is essential in this respect, to ensure that technology resources are not diverted from the health area to deal with these security concerns.

ICT policy orientation in middle- and high-income countries

At the policy level, most high-income countries maintain a separation between government ministries in charge of telecommunications and information technology.[21] However, telecommunications policy makers and regulators are increasingly attempting to incorporate the entire range of ICT in their policy domains. While health is often mentioned in the list of general benefits of ICT to society, the specific benefits of ICT for the health sector are rarely mentioned in ICT policy statements. It is also rare to find specific actions or commitments by ICT policy makers to improve health, which is often viewed as a sector that would benefit from the latest developments in ICT. In this context, health applications often appear in policy programmes mainly to justify the importance of broadband technologies.

While the interests of the health and ICT sectors appear to be shared at conceptual levels, they are not in practice implemented to the extent that might be desired. For example, policy makers may view the health sector as a test bed for the application of high-speed telecommunications systems. The health sector would certainly benefit from the network technologies that enable transmission of the images used in medical diagnosis. It is questionable, however, whether ICT policy makers recognize these benefits and subsequently afford high priority to the health community.

Private sector ICT vendors naturally have technology-centred views and are concerned with health as a business. They are interested in digital opportunity, rather than the digital divide. They explore business opportunities to sell ICT equipment and systems. The lack of telecommunications infrastructure in rural areas may be perceived as a business opportunity for a vendor to prove the benefits of wireless broadband systems, but unless this can be profitable, it will not be sustained or implemented on a large scale.

ICT policy orientation in low- and middle-income countries

Lack of reliable infrastructure is a severe constraint for low- and middle-income countries. The lack of adequate infrastructure to support high-quality, high-speed Internet connections is a major obstacle for economic and social development, and lack of bandwidth excludes countries from taking part in the global information society. A fundamental challenge is the cost of bandwidth, which, because of policy, regulation and technology challenges, can be up to 50 times as high as the cost of bandwidth in industrialized countries.[19] Operational costs on this scale put ICT out of reach for the health sector, and represent a difficult trade-off for government decision makers when considering how best to allocate health and social welfare budgets.

Provision of basic ICT services to the general public is becoming a high priority as donor-financed initiatives are beginning to stress core policy reform, incentives for private sector investment towards providing access to rural and underserved areas, development of national backbone links, and deployment of broadband and government networks.[22] This long-term perspective represents a significant shift from the previous decade of project-based ICT development initiatives such as tele-centres, where the benefits to the health sector were often mentioned in the rationale for their construction but where in reality the benefits were rarely realized.

Opportunities presented by policy reform processes

Policy reform processes in countries can provide an opportunity for the health sector to participate in consultations when ICT policy is being developed or revised. Countries trying to improve policy making may also require training or guidelines for the public sector policy process that specifically mandate broad consultation with stakeholder groups. For example, it is evident that ICT policy makers would benefit from understanding how policy affects the technology users in all sectors. This can be achieved by means of evaluation, consultation mechanisms or a combination of the two. A government mandate for input, dialogue and better information flow provides a good starting point. At the least, the sectors can acknowledge each other's interests and responsibilities, although they may not share the same perspective or priorities.

Policy adjustment to meet local needs

It would seem obvious that policy directions must reflect and be adapted to the local context, but this is not always the case in ICT policy. Often, basic ICT policy principles are agreed at the international level, or policies of high-income countries are simply transferred to low- and middle-income countries. However, the local context – in terms of local needs, skills and political issues – has a significant effect on whether generally accepted policy reforms are adopted and put into practice. Even national governments with the political will to drive change often face challenges in putting policies into effect, particularly where the necessary legal framework and human resources are lacking.

Opportunities for action

There is much that the health sector can achieve by becoming actively involved in ICT policy making, particularly in the long term. But the health sector may first need to build its own capacity to use evidence and information for policy and planning. A country's level of ICT diffusion and general policy-making capacity will show the potential areas for focus and action. The following are some examples.

A holistic approach to ICT development

ICT is an enabler, not an end in itself, and national ICT strategy should be 'outward looking' and designed to ensure effective fulfilment of national development activities. ICT strategy should ensure that there is compatibility across government sectors (e.g. access and security protocols, and user interfaces). Resources should be provided for initiatives that produce significant cost savings and improve services to users.

A growing number of countries are seeking assistance to develop sector-based ICT programmes, including e-education, e-health and e-government. However, without an overall coordination mechanism at the country level, these ICT programmes may lead to sector-specific ICT infrastructure owned and operated by the relevant ministry, thereby duplicating private sector or other infrastructure. A holistic approach is required, with governments ensuring that investment in ICT is coherent and sufficient to meet common needs across the sectors. The health sector may need to lobby for a more active role in policy formulation. This is possible by highlighting existing policies that show their investment and commitment to benefiting from ICT. For example, a coordinated framework may have been developed for the integration of ICT services in district health settings. There may already be arrangements for improving managerial and technical competence to oversee e-health projects. Or projects may already be planned and funded, thereby ensuring that the health sector will obtain a substantial benefit when ICT becomes more readily available. Not least, health policy makers should be aware of the relevant policy trends in other countries and build on documented experience.

Making the case for health

ICT infrastructure, costs, human resources and telecommunications regulations are four major factors that shape the development and uptake of ICT. Health policy makers must work to ensure that policies in these four areas align with health interests wherever possible. Policy makers should therefore anticipate their needs and requirements for infrastructure and bandwidth. They should propose benchmark targets for access to basic services, cost of basic services and establishment of new services for the sector. This requires more than awareness: it requires understanding and planning for what ICT can bring on a medium- to long-term basis. Policy makers should be able to articulate the drivers for access to ICT, and the potential effects of ICT policy change. High-level need and justification are important factors in ICT allocation and policy change.

Health policy makers should have an understanding of ICT solutions that can potentially be provided at low cost to meet the sector's needs. They must also be aware of new solutions (e.g. low-cost voice communication over the Internet) that may be prohibited by telecommunications regulations in some countries. Such knowledge will provide health policy makers with alternatives in the choice of appropriate ICT policy mechanisms.

The costs of ICT services can be expected to be an important factor for some time to come. To improve rates and services, health policy makers must be able to indicate at what level they would consider operating costs to be reasonable and sustainable. This should be based on the funding model and resources of the health sector. Across a country or set of countries, it should be possible to calculate what percentage of gross income of the subsectors could be reasonably spent on ICT services and systems and what potential funding mechanisms might be considered.

Participation in a networked economy requires expertise and resources for dealing with global technical security threats, including viruses and email spam. The sector must be able to show adequate capacity to respond to threats in a networked environment, not only to protect the sector but also so as not to pose a threat to others. Where ICT is relatively new, planning is required to develop the necessary human resources capacity, and in this the health sector must be proactive. Gaps in skills should be identified and a plan developed for training and long-term staff development and retention.

Outlook for the future

Developing countries must boost their capacity in ICT and policy making. Basic ICT access indicators cannot demonstrate the full extent of ICT divides. Countries that are crippled by poverty, disease, foreign debt and corruption may not have the resources or the political will to invest in ICT or be considered good markets for foreign ICT investment. Countries must boost their policy-making capacity in order to ensure that their ICT policy addresses the concerns of multiple stakeholders. Even as the use of basic ICT increases, the control of advanced technology will require an environment based on a comprehensive ICT policy that reflects domestic as well as international interests.

Table 2.3 Examples of ICT trends and their application to health

Technology trends	Applications to health	ICT policy issues
Broadband Internet	Distance delivery of health care services: consultations, transmission of prescription and purchase of medicines, using text, still and mobile pictures, and voice	• Technology standards • Privacy protection • Costs • Geographical availability of broadband Internet
Digitization	Video and pictures Electronic databases and memory chips as patient record archive	• Technology standards • Privacy protection
Wireless communication technologies	Mobile communications: health anywhere from everywhere	• Costs • Geographical availability of wireless communications

For the future, international and domestic divisions in ICT use will be shaped by a number of factors that have the potential to widen or close the gap. These include the following:

- new technology solutions, such as automatic translation services and inexpensive wireless phone-based Internet;
- increasing global coverage of satellite systems and lower costs for access;
- concerted action to diffuse ICT and help people use it effectively;
- broad economic and trade policies that will spur integration of ICT into the global economy as a key engine for growth;
- improved governance and standards setting and the need for evolving models to improve inclusion and representation of stakeholders.

Boosting government awareness and capacity is central to achieving equitable, affordable ICT for the health sector in all countries. The health sector has an important role. Those involved can take concrete action as follows:

- actively participate in the ICT policy debate to improve awareness and understanding of the needs of the sector;
- emphasize that benefits to the health community also benefit the public at large;
- educate ICT vendors to develop equipment and systems that meet the needs of developing countries, i.e. low cost, durable and easy maintenance;
- work with non-governmental organizations and civil society, who have an interest in improving ICT access for the public;
- learn from each other, in order to improve input and participation in ICT policy debate on such issues as costs, infrastructure development, access to the Internet, content in local languages and privacy protection.

Conclusion

ICT is fundamental to providing effective and efficient health services and systems. These technologies can improve workforce and workplace efficiency and boost quality of care by reducing medical errors, reducing costs and improving safety. They provide networks and tools for learning, research and practice. They enable access to information, products and advice for disease prevention and management, and will be essential to the move to personalized health and care in the future.

There are many opportunities for health policy makers to influence the ICT policy process. Their chances of success will be improved by understanding how ICT can benefit health. Health policy makers must be effective advocates for health concerns and must be able to enumerate the effects of ICT policies on health. For policy makers committed to improving national health systems, participating in the national ICT policy-making process is essential to ensure that national ICT policy, when implemented, will meet the interests of the health sector.

Acknowledgements

I thank Ms Yoshiko Kurisaki, SITA, Geneva, Switzerland for preliminary discussions and Mr Shubhabrata Roy, Microsoft, UK, for his assistance with data and graphics.

Further reading

World Health Organization. World Health Assembly Resolution WHA58.1: Health action in relation to crises and disasters, with particular emphasis on the earthquakes and tsunamis of 26 December 2004. Available at: www.who.int/gb/ebwha/pdf_files/WHA58-REC1/english/Resolutions.pdf.

World Health Organization. *Connecting for Health: Global Vision, Local Insight. Report for the World Summit on the Information Society. Country Profiles 2006.* Available at: www.who.int/kms/resources/wsis_country_profiles.pdf.

European Commission. *E-health: Better Healthcare for Europe.* Available at: ec.europa.eu/information_society/activities/health/index_en.htm.

References

1. United Nations Statistical Division. *Millennium Development Goals and Targets.* Available at: unstats.un.org/unsd/mi/pdf/mdglist.pdf.
2. International Telecommunication Union. *World Summit on the Information Society Tunis Commitment.* Available at: www.itu.int/wsis/docs2/tunis/off/7.html.
3. United Nations Conference on Trade and Development. *The Digital Divide: ICT Development Indices 2004.* Available at: www.unctad.org/en/docs/iteipc20054_en.pdf.
4. International Telecommunication Union. *World Telecommunication Indicators Database 2006.* Available at: www.itu.int/publ/D-IND-WTID-2006/en.

5. World Health Organization. *The World Health Report 2004 – Changing History*. Available at: www.who. int/whr/2004/en/index.html.

6. Council of the European Union. *Legislative Acts and Other Instruments. Council Resolution on the Implementation of the eEurope 2005 Action Plan* (Document 5197/03). Brussels: European Union, 2003.

7. World Health Organization. *The World Health Report 2006 – Working Together for Health*. Available at: www.who.int/whr/2006/en/index.html.

8. European Commission, Information Society and Media. *The Networked Future: Living in a World of Converging Information and Communication Technologies*. Luxembourg: European Communities, 2005.

9. Picot J. *MBTelemedicine Evaluation Final Report. Volume 1: Information and Findings*. Report to the Canadian Health Infostructure Partnership Program, Government of Canada, 2003.

10. Ball MJ, Garets DE, Handler TJ. Leveraging IT to improve patient safety. In: *Yearbook of Medical Informatics 2003*. Stuttgart: International Medical Informatics Association/Schattauer, 2003: 1–6.

11. Commission of the European Communities. *Communication from the Commission to the Council, the European Parliament, the European Economic and Social Committee and the Committee of the Regions, June 2005*. Brussels, European Union, 2005

12. Fox S. *Health Information Online*. Available at: www.pewInternet.org/pdfs/PIP_Healthtopics_May05.pdf.

13. World Health Organization. *World Health Report 2007 – A Safer Future: Global Public Health Security in the 21st Century*. Available at: www.who.int/whr/2007/en/index.html.

14. Kamal A. *The Law of Cyber-space*. Geneva: United Nations Institute of Training and Research, 2005.

15. Dzidonu CK. Demand and supply for access and connectivity: the case of Ghana. In: *Low Cost Access and Connectivity: Local Solutions*. New York: United Nations ICT Task Force, 2003: 1–20.

16. United Nations Economic and Social Council, Economic Commission for Africa. National knowledge systems and the status of information access policies in Africa (E/ECA/CODI/4/50). Paper presented at the Fourth Meeting of the Committee on Development Information, Addis Ababa, Ethiopia, April 2005.

17. Wolcott P, Press L, McHenry W et al. A framework for assessing the global diffusion of the Internet. *J Assoc Inform Syst* 2001; **2**: 1–50.

18. United Nations Conference on Trade and Development. *The Digital Divide: ICT Development Indices 2004*. New York: United Nations, 2005.

19. Jensen M. *Interconnection Costs*. Available at: www.apc.org/en/pubs/issue/accessibility/all/interconnection-costs.

20. International Telecommunication Union. *ITU Activities Related to Cybersecurity*. Available at: www.itu.int/cybersecurity.

21. Organisation for Economic Co-operation and Development. *Regulatory Reform as a Tool for Bridging the Digital Divide*. Paris: OECD, 2004.

22. Hamilton P. *Identifying Key Regulatory and Policy Issues to Ensure Open Access to Regional Backbone Infrastructure Initiatives in Africa*. Washington, DC: World Bank, 2004.

3 Telemedicine in developing countries: Perspectives from the Philippines

Alvin B Marcelo

Introduction

The University of the Philippines Manila National Telemedicine Center was established in 1998 to investigate the use of information and communications technology (ICT) to improve health care delivery for all Filipinos. The Center is based at the Philippine General Hospital. It manages referrals from more than 40 doctors in remote areas around the country, connecting them to more than 600 experts at the Philippine General Hospital. In implementing e-health and telemedicine, the National Telemedicine Center chose an approach based on community involvement as well as technology. Three different case studies are described below that demonstrate different aspects of this strategy. The case studies are CHITS, the E-Learning for Health Project and the SMS Telemedicine Project.

The approach to implementation consisted of three distinct steps:

1. The human experience: start from where the people are.
2. The technological opportunity: identify appropriate, available, accessible and culturally acceptable technologies.
3. The sustenance factor: embed the technology into the local fabric.

The human experience

Although technology offers benefits in terms of applying new processes and approaches to problem-solving, the fact is that most health interventions are only as effective as their ability to become embedded in routine activity. This means that if e-health implementations are approached from a purely technical standpoint it will invariably fail to realize their full potential.

The essence of the human experience is communication and interaction. The National Telemedicine Center has observed that the benefits for communities of e-health and telemedicine occur when the technology presents itself (a) as an enhancement to existing human relationships that have been established through conventional routes or (b) as a solution to a long-felt community need. In either case, the Center's experience has shown that technology has higher chances of sustaining itself in areas where mature human relationships and interactions already exist.

My experience with the Community Health Information Tracking System[1] (CHITS) has allowed me to observe a highly technical training programme evolving into one that is less technology based and more community oriented and dialectical. During the initial CHITS training, much time was wasted in teaching elderly health workers how to use a mouse and to type on a keyboard. At the end of the training sessions, participants still appeared to be afraid of accidentally damaging the computer. Post-training interviews revealed that the health workers never became comfortable with the technologies that were being introduced (the PC and the electronic medical record application).

Community Health Information Tracking System

CHITS was funded in 2004 by the International Development Research Centre of Canada and subsequently by the United Nations Development Programme (UNDP). The aim was to develop an integrated disease surveillance system. CHITS was developed in close consultation with village health workers to best identify their needs. The result was an open-source application for the village health centre that combined the features of an electronic health record and clinic appointment system while also integrating modules for national health programmes.

CHITS was a starting point for the integration of information systems. Through CHITS, community-based health information was made available not only to public health agencies requiring community level information but also to the community that generated the information. It enabled the community to use this information for local decision-making.

Currently, CHITS is in use in 12 health centres in two cities and two provinces in the Philippines. It has made the work of village health workers easier, since information is entered only once during a patient consultation and can then be used to generate the different reports that need to be submitted to the Department of Health. Since data are stored electronically, it is now easier to access and consolidate information, and there is less risk of data loss. More timely reports allow community leaders to make better decisions for their people.

There are approximately 100 000 transaction records from the 12 health centres presently using CHITS. The information is stored in databases using simple data elements patterned after the Department of Health. Access is limited to authorized personnel, who undergo a two-day electronic health record training prior to using the system. In this training programme, the ethics of health information management are taught with special attention to the responsibility and security required for digital data. All data are owned by the relevant health centre, which also controls access. The data can be extracted using open-source software tools.

In the light of early experience, revisions in the training programme were made. Foremost among the changes was the shift from a highly structured training programme on how to use the keyboard and mouse to a less strict, more fun approach to using the interfaces by allowing the health workers to play games on the computer.

The trainers discovered that health workers were often afraid of the new 'formal' skills that they needed to acquire, but were more relaxed (albeit sometimes fiercely competitive) when asked to beat each other in a game of solitaire. So, instead of coercing the participants into a strict regimen of clicking and copy-pasting, they are given time to develop confidence in the use of the keyboard and the mouse through simple games. The game orientation removes the fear that they have to perform well in a short period of time. This is what is meant by starting from where the people are. A recognition of the cultural aspects of community life is important in starting them off into a new direction such as computerization and automation.

In 2006, CHITS was chosen as one of the key e-government projects by the APEC Digital Opportunity Center in Taiwan.[2] It was also a finalist in the 2006 Stockholm Challenge.[3]

The technological opportunity

The process of understanding local cultures and processes, respecting the local experts, and analyzing their thought processes can often be frustrating. However, it is essential if external technology is to be embedded into the community's way of life. Once the community has been understood, the technologies that are available and appropriate can be determined. The National Telemedicine Center's experience with its E-Learning for Health Project has demonstrated the importance of this step.

E-Learning for Health Project

The migration of health professionals from rural areas in the Philippines has progressed to the point that many municipalities are unable to provide regular training to community health care volunteers. Many of these under-served communities are also in hard-to-reach, remote areas, and travel costs can be high. With support from USAID, the National Telemedicine Center developed four video modules about common topics relevant to the management of disease in the community:

- community management of accidental childhood poisoning
- community management of stroke
- community management of tuberculosis
- community introduction to the avian influenza threat.

These video modules last 7–10 minutes each and are narrated in the vernacular with English subtitles. The audiences are community health care volunteers in remote communities. After the video showing, an interactive question and answer session is established between the expert in Manila and the volunteers using the best available technology (ranging from videoconferencing to mobile phone calls). Various telecommunication media have been employed for the educational sessions which are held in various locations (Figure 3.1):

- childhood poisoning between Manila and Basak Pardo, Cebu, using broadband Internet (Figure 3.2)

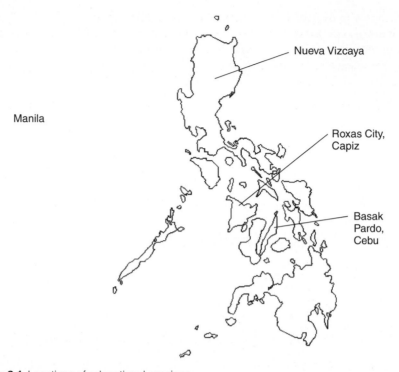

Nueva Vizcaya

Manila

Roxas City,
Capiz

Basak
Pardo,
Cebu

Figure 3.1 Locations of educational sessions

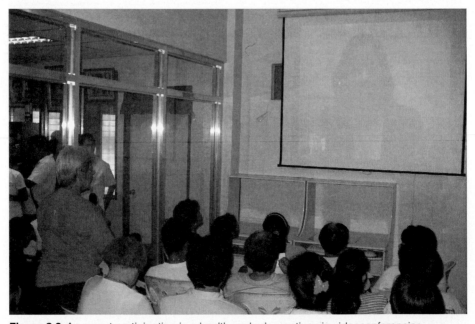

Figure 3.2 An expert participating in a health worker's meeting via videoconferencing

- stroke between Manila and Nueva Vizcaya, using cellphones
- avian influenza and tuberculosis between Manila and Roxas City and Tapaz, Capiz Province, using Internet videoconferencing.

One reason for the success of this teaching model was the familiarity of the audience with the lecture format. We were able to elicit participation from the audience by providing them with access to an expert in Manila. There were several benefits. First, there were cost and time savings from travel by not having to transport the expert to a remote area. Second, the expert could serve several communities in a single session. The audience were able to receive updates using a novel method that did not require them to establish new skills. In all cases, the local participants were given the opportunity to participate and ask questions directly of the expert using the vernacular.

In the Philippines, massive migration of doctors and nurses has resulted in a lack of trainers in the public health sector. Even where there are many community health volunteers, there are not enough trainers and leaders to provide them with the requisite knowledge.

Visiting the under-served communities has made the staff of the Center aware of what technologies are available. Televisions and video CD players can be found in almost all communities. In populated areas, there is invariably mobile phone coverage, so that voice calls and/or a short-message service (SMS) are also available.

The E-Learning for Health Project has shown that, by using locally available technology and the best available bandwidth, it is possible to establish interaction between a group of health care volunteers (in a remote community) and an expert (in an urban area). Voice calls were found to be most effective, although participants also appreciated videoconferencing. The community members were keen to accept the new modality, because it employed technologies that were already familiar to them. Pretests and post-tests given to participants revealed that they were able to gain knowledge from the e-learning activity.

The sustenance factor

Stand-alone, intermittent, expert-driven events (such as the E-Learning for Health Project and CHITS) are easy to implement, but are they sustainable? In order to achieve permanence, e-health and telemedicine applications must be embedded into the local fabric of the community.

How, then, do we overlay the technologies (step 2) over the local issues (step 1) to ensure that the technical solution finds a home in the heart of the community? E-health should be considered as another community activity that will need to involve discussions, arguments and deliberations. E-health should thus become the vehicle for more rapid and more structured community development through enhanced communications and process documentation. This becomes more apparent with the use of mobile phones for health-related concerns such as announcements for community meetings, reminders for vaccinations and prenatal check-ups. It also involves gathering the health volunteers and workers regularly to attend e-learning sessions on community health development.

In one high-profile government-funded project, the BuddyWorks Community Partnership in Delivering Telemedicine Services, remote sites were provided with workstations and broadband Internet connections to allow them to refer difficult cases to experts in a central facility. A total of 10 facilities in four provinces was involved. However, despite the substantial investment, referrals from the remote sites did not occur. Analysis revealed a workflow that prevented the users from assimilating desktop Internet technologies for communicating clinical dilemmas. In the proposed system, the remote physician needed to log on to a computer with Internet access, go to the agreed website portal, enter the relevant clinical data and wait for the response of an expert – who would probably be busy with his or her own patients at the time. The process had so many steps that the risk of a failed transaction was very high.

SMS Telemedicine Project

In response, the workflow was revised to allow the doctors to communicate via SMS. Most doctors already owned a mobile phone. Using SMS, they were able to communicate more effectively. It was then decided to supplement the existing network by providing modest prepaid SMS allowances to the doctors and offering them free conference call services for voice-based referrals. This system has proved to be sustainable and effective. During a 6-month period, over 300 referrals were received from 44 doctors in remote areas.

Conclusion

It is widely accepted that all societies, especially those of developing countries, can build more cohesive communities through the primary health care approach. Telemedicine and e-health have a great potential to facilitate service delivery in primary care. For example, rural health workers commonly suffer from inefficient, paper-based recording systems. CHITS, based on free and/or open source software and SMS, provided a more effective alternative.

At the core of any telemedicine service is an electronic health record. This is how CHITS plays a role in telemedicine – by providing a consistent view of the patient's records. The current telemedicine services in the Philippines are simple enhancements to existing trust structures. By using SMS and mobile phones, the National Telemedicine Center is able to provide access to experts for patients who would not otherwise have been able to consult them. The use of SMS technology has increased the area of coverage of the Center.

The challenges that plague the Philippine system are the continuing loss of health professionals from internal and external migration. As more and more health workers seek work in other countries and rural physicians move from rural to urban practices, the number of municipalities without doctors will increase. Establishment of an efficient and effective referral network, based on mobile phone technology, is a key component in mitigating the effects of this migration. The faster the trust relationships between the remote doctors and physicians are established, the quicker telemedicine services can take hold in the relevant communities.

Further reading

International Medical Informatics Association. *IMIA Code of Ethics for Health Information Professionals*. Available at: www.imia.org/ethics.lasso.

Declaration of Alma-Ata. International Conference on Primary Health Care, Alma-Ata, 6–12 September 1978. Available at: www.who.int/hpr/NPH/docs/declaration_almaata.pdf.

Heeks R, Mundy D, Salazar A. *Why Health Care Information Systems Succeed or Fail*. Institute for Development Policy and Management, 1999. Available at: unpan1.un.org/intradoc/groups/public/documents/NISPAcee/UNPAN015482.pdf.

University of Texas Medical Branch Web Education Courses. *Telemedicine 101: Basic Principles of Telemedicine*. Available at: www.utmb.edu/teletraining/th101/index.html.

World Health Organization. Executive Board. *eHealth: Proposed Tools and Services*. Available at: www.who.int/gb/ebwha/pdf_files/EB117/B117_15-en.pdf.

References

1. Tolentino H, Marcelo A, Marcelo P, Maramba I. Linking primary care information systems and public health information networks: lessons from the Philippines. *Stud Health Technol Inform* 2005; **116**: 955–60.
2. APEC Digital Opportunity Center. Available at: www.apecdoc.org.
3. Stockholm Challenge. Available at: www.stockholmchallenge.se,

4 Information technology for primary health care in Brazil

Elaine Tomasi, Luiz A Facchini,
Elaine Thumé, Maria FS Maia and
Alessander Osorio

Introduction

Decision making in public health depends on the availability of reliable information, which is generated, analyzed and disseminated by information systems.[1,2] However, most national health information systems lack the information needed to address health inequities, namely, reliable, longitudinal data that links measures of health with measures of social status at the individual or small-area level.

At all levels of health care, particularly in primary care, there is a consensus concerning the usefulness of information technology, especially for promoting greater efficiency in management processes.[3,4] Although studies evaluating the impact of such technologies on health are still rare,[5,6] most authors agree that there are positive effects from these systems and that they can be improved further through regular monitoring.

Low levels of computerization in primary health care are very common. Furthermore, many papers stress the need for continued motivation and training for all team members as a prerequisite for the success of any initiative in this area.[7,8] It may be pertinent here to quote the reflections by Branco[9] on the significance of training, that is, the amplification of knowledge:

> ... knowledge of the logic behind health information production and flux must be provided to all persons involved, and should include an understanding of the goals of the systems to which they have access, and of the possibilities for use of the information produced ...

Martinez et al[10] analyzed communication and information needs in primary health care in rural areas from Peru and Nicaragua. They found three main factors related to the inefficiency of the health systems: poor infrastructure, a lack of information systems and deficiencies in the training of health professionals. Other authors have emphasized the need to incorporate good-quality health care data from local levels into national databases.[11-14] Similarly, Gething et al[15] stated that the value of information systems in health is to point out the needs and priorities at both national and local levels, but the process of feeding data into the systems often fails.

Another source of problems is the contrast between the availability of information technology (IT) at the central level of health system management and its shortage elsewhere, particularly in primary care. There is often pressure for new data, increasing the time required for collection, with no assurance about its analysis, dissemination and usefulness in decision making. The great quantity of data about each patient, recorded by health professionals, seems to have little meaning in their daily activities.[16] We believe that all of these factors contribute to the current situation – but especially the lack of motivation of most health care staff and the poor integration between health care and IT professionals.

Establishing IT in the health services, especially in primary care, is a challenge for the advance of information systems, not only in the smaller and poorer towns. In bigger cities, the central levels of the health system generally have good access to IT resources, but the recording of the actions of the major part of the health services is still performed manually.[16]

There are few reports in the literature about the experience with the development and use of computerized systems in primary care. Herman et al[17] described the Community Health Information Tracking System (CHITS) in the Philippines, which has the objective of integrating local and national level information and pointing out 'islands' in the information systems and a great amount of repeated work in the management of such systems (see also Chapter 3). Aspects related to access to data from different information systems, and their use and control, should be considered, including their creation, implementation, monitoring and evaluation.[18]

IT in primary care in Brazil

Two recent initiatives from the Brazilian government are the National Information Policy on Informatics in Health (NIPIH/PNIIS)[19] and the National Telemedicine Programme in 2006.[20] The NIPIH focuses on health work, on the user and on the electronic health record. The proposals are underpinned by standards to represent and share health information, the connectivity structure, the training of human resources in the information systems in health, and, above all, the guarantee of privacy and confidentiality of the information.

National Telemedicine Programme

Telemedicine activity currently involves about 30 universities and research institutes in 9 of the 27 Brazilian states. The pilot project in telemedicine for primary care involves the installation of 900 PCs, mainly for decision support. These PCs are connected to a wide area network, and can also be used for videoconferencing. They have an electronic medical record, which can be shared with other units. Priority is being given to cities where there is a family health programme, a population of less than 100 000 and geographical barriers to health care. The Ministry of Health, together with the Ministry of Education, has been investing in distance learning for training and continuing education of health professionals.

National information systems

The information systems available in Brazil consist of large databases of statistics. These include births, deaths and a disease surveillance system. There are also tools for the management of outpatient and hospital services.

The only computerized health information system used in family health centres is the Primary Care Information System. This is the source of information, and provides most of the tools and the forms completed by the primary care team. Most health professionals recognize it as a tool for improving the epidemiological profile, but it is underutilized. According to the staff concerned, this underutilization is due to various limitations of the system, to a lack of knowledge and lack of preparation for exploring its full capacity, to a lack of training and to a lack of incentive to use it for data analysis. The system has weaknesses, but some professionals also have difficulties in manipulating it both regarding the input of data and in producing reports.

Data collection is fragmented, with no connection with health policies to facilitate the planning and decision making. The data collection and transfer mechanisms generate repeated work and reduce efficiency in the management of information.[19] The system does not allow integration with other systems, and cannot identify users and show their links to health services. For this, a National Health Card is being implemented. However, because of the magnitude of the investment required, progress has been slow.

The proliferation of information systems should be highlighted. For each need, sector, disease or event, new software is created, implying high costs for development and maintenance, and a lack of standardization and interoperability. According to Cohn et al,[12] there is little use of information from the large databases in Brazil, especially in small towns. The full potential of the information has yet to be realized.[12,21]

Telemedicine

Separate from the National Telemedicine Programme, the BH Telemedicine Project was implemented in 2003. The aim was to promote the continuing education of health workers in primary care units, as well as contributing to the modernization of the public health system. The BH Telemedicine network connects primary care centres to the Federal University of Minas Gerais teaching units, with activities in the fields of medicine, nursing and dentistry. The network uses videoconferences for continuing education, and teleconsulting between specialists and staff at the primary care centres for second opinions and for discussion of clinical cases. The videoconferencing network operates at 128 kbit/s.

The telemedicine network has been implemented in 121 primary care centres. About 1500 teleconsultations per year occur between specialists and staff at the primary care centres. In 2006, there were 75 educational videoconferences, including medical, nursing and dentistry areas, involving more than 5000 participants. The activities have resulted in more effective participation of the oral health group, followed by nurses and finally by the physicians.

The project has been evaluated by two groups. The results showed better outcomes for the cases discussed, with about 70% of patients staying in basic units, with no need for referral to a specialist. There was also a reduction of 71% in the number of patients who needed to travel to the Clinics Hospital of Belo Horizonte to be seen.

Computerized tools

In 2005, a survey was conducted to characterize primary care and evaluate differences in the effectiveness of services according to the model of care – family health or traditional.[16] Under the Family Health Programmes (FHP), teams are composed of a doctor, a nurse, a nurse technician and about five community health agents. These teams are responsible for supervising a set number of families (about 1000) living in a particular area. The teams undertake work involving health promotion, prevention, recovery and rehabilitation. In the traditional model, teams do not include community health agents and do not have their activities focused on health promotion and disease prevention.

The survey enrolled 41 municipalities of more than 100 000 inhabitants in the south and north-east regions of Brazil, which represented approximately 20% of these size municipalities in the country. There were systematic differences between the demographic and socioeconomic indicators from the south and north-east of the country. In the south, the average human development index (HDI), life expectancy, number of literate people and homes with tap water supply were higher than in the north-east. North-east municipalities showed a higher proportion of poor people (41% vs 17%), while the southern municipalities showed a higher proportion of elderly citizens (9% vs 7%).

Information about the 236 primary care centres was obtained by questionnaire: 4749 health workers were studied. Among these, 11% were physicians, 7% nurses, 8% professionals with another college degree, 18% nursing assistants, 23% other professionals with a high school degree and 33% community health agents. One-third of the primary care centres had a computer (35%): 40% in the south and 29% in the north-east. Considering the care model, 39% of the family health services had a computer, as opposed to only 25% of the traditional services (Table 4.1). Only 11% of the primary care centres had Internet access: 17% in the south region and 5% in the north-east region. The traditional services had more Internet access (14%) than the family health services (9%) (Table 4.2).

About 20% of the health workers mentioned their use of computers for professional activities. This use was almost 50% among physicians, nurses and other professionals with a college degree, and a little more than 10% among nursing technicians, community health agents and other members of the teams who had a high school education. The use of computers in the primary care centres was even less frequent, being mentioned only by 8% of the professionals (Table 4.3).

Depending upon the region, the use of computers in health centres was 14% in the south and 5% in the north-east. Depending upon the care model, it was 10% in family health services and 6% in the traditional centres (Table 4.4).

Table 4.1 Microcomputers in primary care services according to the model of health care and geographical region (*n* = 236)

	South (%)	North-east (%)	Total (%)
Family health	46	33	39
Traditional	30	16	25
Total	**40**	**29**	**35**

Table 4.2 Access to the Internet in primary care services according to the model of health care and geographical region (*n* = 236)

	South (%)	North-east (%)	Total (%)
Family health	16	4	9
Traditional	17	10	14
Total	**17**	**5**	**11**

Table 4.3 IT use by primary care workers according to location of access (*n* = 4749)

	In home or primary health care unit (%)	Only in primary health care unit (%)
Community health agents	3	6
Other assistants	4	10
Nurse assistants	6	7
Nurses	34	16
Other professionals	35	11
Doctors	47	8
All	**14**	**8**

Table 4.4 Use of computers by primary care health workers according to model of health care and geographical region (*n* = 4749)

	South (%)	North-east (%)	Total (%)
Family health	15	6	10
Traditional	12	3	6
Total	**14**	**5**	**8**

PACOTAPS

PACOTAPS is a tool for decision making. The objective of the PACOTAPS software is to assist health managers and teams with information about population characteristics and health demands.[22] The software provides a structure to receive data about the contacts and procedures performed at primary care centres. The origin document is the Outpatient Contact Form, which is completed by the health team and signed by the user. Once the form has been completed, the data are typed in using a module called *users contact with the services*.

PACOTAPS includes lists of professionals, groups and procedures that are standardized by the Outpatient Information System. For the identification of the diagnosis, PACOTAPS provides the application PESQCID,[23] which allows a guided consultancy to the *International Classification of Diseases (ICD-10)*.[24] Thus, using the system it is possible to find out, for a certain period of time, the distribution of patients by age and gender, the main diagnosis and the proportion of referrals.

Training

About 400 primary care workers from the 41 cities under study were trained in monitoring and evaluation through practice exercises in a computer laboratory, in two regional workshops. The participants could install, become familiar with and use PACOTAPS, with emphasis on the module *users contact with the services*. Thus, they were able to understand its usefulness for the daily activities of primary care centres, and in municipal health management. The simplified data entry and the immediate availability of reports were very attractive, as these are requirements often mentioned by health workers. The training aims to make health workers aware of the need to produce accurate and valid information. At the end of training, each municipality received a CD for installation of the software and the application manual.

Survey results

In the PROESF study, all the 26 019 user contacts with the primary care centres were recorded in PACOTAPS. Information was collected about the users' profiles (age, gender and health problems), the procedures performed and the referrals. One-third of the contacts (35%) were for women between 15 and 49 years old, i.e. of reproductive age. The second largest group was for people 60 years of age or older (19%) and the third largest group was children below 5 years old (15%).

Every user can receive one or more procedures at each contact. For example, a child may receive an immunization and also have a medical consultation for diarrhoea; an elderly person may have his or her blood pressure checked, have a medical consultation for back pain and receive his or her medication; a pregnant woman may have her weight checked, have a medical consultation for urinary infection and be attended to by the social worker for receiving a benefit. Therefore, the number of procedures is usually higher than the number of people attended to. In this sample, more than 37 000 procedures were analysed.

Although nurses and nurses' assistants comprised 25% of the teams, they performed more than half of the procedures (53%). The physicians, who represented 11% of the professionals, accounted for 26% of the procedures. Almost 70% of the procedures were related to factors that influenced the health status and the contact with the services, such as prenatal care and paediatrics, immunization and screening tests. After this, health problems related to the digestive system (7%), circulatory system (4%) and respiratory system (4%) were observed more frequently.

Although 23% of the records did not have information about referrals, it was observed that in 70% of the contacts there was no need to refer the user to other care levels or to request diagnostic tests.

Conclusions

Primary care plays a major role in producing better health care for all people, particularly in developing countries. Efforts are now being directed towards the improvement of different models of care. As in other places, in Brazil, family health care is becoming a successful equity promotion effort, because it is more widely present in poorer regions with a more vulnerable population. Despite limitations that are common to primary care, the family health programme does more for whoever needs more.

The experience of the BH Telemedicine implementation provides guidance for the future:

- potential for innovation in the public network
- standards governing the interaction between teaching and the assisting practice of the health services
- improvements in the assisting structure, with possibilities of reduced costs and better structuring of a multidisciplinary project of telemedicine.

The main challenges regarding IT for primary care are:

1. To improve IT in primary care centres, rather than at the central levels of health system management.
2. To estimate standardization and compatibility between national health information systems, especially through web-based tools rather than the production of local software or information systems.
3. To promote a wide professional training in IT as a strategy to facilitate its use in decision making for clinical practice, and to monitor and evaluate health programmes, focusing on people rather than on technology.

Overall, this will require greater investment in IT and telecommunications directed towards the basic health units. This investment should be made by municipalities, but currently there are other priorities in the country's public health system, and resources are scarce.

Further reading

Araújo Novaes M, Pinto Barbosa AK, Soares de Araújo K et al. Experiences on the use of a second opinion software for the primary care. *AMIA Annu Symp Proc* 2005: 889.

Edworthy SM. Telemedicine in developing countries. *BMJ* 2001; **323**: 524–5.

Goodman KW. Ethics and health informatics: focus on Latin America and the Caribbean. *Acta Bioeth* 2005; **11**: 121–6. Available at: www.scielo.cl/scielo.php?pid=S1726-569X2005000200002&script=sci_arttext&tlng=en.

Hira AY, Lopes TT, de Mello AN et al. Establishment of the Brazilian Telemedicine network for paediatric oncology. *J Telemed Telecare* 2005; **11**(Suppl 2): 51–2.
Rigby M. Impact of telemedicine must be defined in developing countries. *BMJ* 2002; **324**: 47–8.

References

1. AbouZahr C, Boerma T. Health information systems: the foundations of public health. *Bull World Health Organ* 2005; **83**: 578–83.
2. Magruder C, Burke M, Hann NE, Ludovic JA. Using information technology to improve the public health system. *J Public Health Manag Pract* 2005; **11**: 123–30.
3. Kukafka R. Public health informatics: the nature of the field and its relevance to health promotion practice. *Health Promot Pract* 2005; **6**: 23–8.
4. OPS (Organización Panamericana de la Salud). *Sistemas de información y tecnologia de información en salud: desafios y soluciones para América Latina y el Caribe.* [*Information Systems and Information Technology in Health: Challenges and Solutions for Latin America and the Caribbean.*] Washington, DC: OPS, 1998.
5. Macinko J, Guanais FC. *Selected Annotated Bibliography on Primary Health Care in the Americas.* Pan American Health Organization's Primary Health Care Working Group, 2004. Available at: www.opas.org.br/servico/arquivos/Sala5520.pdf.
6. Mitchell E, Sullivan F. A descriptive feast but an evaluative famine: systematic review of published articles on primary care computing during 1980–97. *BMJ* 2001; **322**: 279–82.
7. Magalhães CAS. *Análise da resistência médica à implantação de sistemas de registro eletrônico de saúde.* [*Analysis of Medical Resistance to the Introduction of Systems for Electronic Health Records*]. Rio de Janeiro: Fundação Getúlio Vragas, 2006.
8. Nobel J. Changes in health care: challenges for information system design. *Int J Biomed Comput* 1995; **39**: 35–40.
9. Branco MAF. Informação e tecnologia: desafios para a implantação da Rede Nacional de Informações em Saúde. [Information and technology: challenges to developing a national health information network.] *Physis: Rev Saude Coletiva* 1998; **8**: 95–123.
10. Martinez A, Villarroel V, Seoane J, del Pozo F. Analysis of information and communication needs in rural primary health care in developing countries. *IEEE Trans Inf Technol Biomed* 2005; **9**: 66–72.
11. Ali M, Park JK, von Seidlein L et al. Organizational aspects and implementation of data systems in large-scale epidemiological studies in less developed countries. *BMC Public Health* 2006; **6**: 86.
12. Cohn A, Westphal MF, Elias PE. Data and the process of formulating health policies. *Rev Saude Publica* 2005; **39**: 114–21.
13. Gladwin J, Dixon RA, Wilson TD. Implementing a new health management information system in Uganda. *Health Policy Plan* 2003; **18**: 214–24.
14. Viacava F, Dachs JNW, Travassos C. Os inquéritos domiciliares e o Sistema Nacional de Informações em Saúde. [Household surveys and the National Health Information System.] *Cienc Saúde Coletiva* 2006; **11**: 863–9.
15. Gething PW, Noor AM, Gikandi PW et al. Improving imperfect data from health management information systems in Africa using space–time geostatistics. *PLoS Med* 2006; **3**: e271.
16. Facchini LA, Piccini RX, Tomasi E et al. Monitoramento e avaliação do Projeto de Expansão e Consolidação da Saúde da Família: relatório final. Pelotas: UFPel, 2006. Available at: www.epidemio-ufpel.org.br/proesf/index.htm.
17. Herman T, Marcelo A, Marcelo P, Maramba I. Linking primary care information systems and public health vertical programs in the Philippines: an open-source experience. *AMIA Annu Symp Proc* 2005: 311–15.
18. McGrail KM, Black C. Access to data in health information systems. *Bull World Health Organ* 2005; **83**: 563.
19. Brasil, Ministério da Saúde. PNIIS – Política Nacional de Informação e Informática em Saúde; proposta versão 2.0; inclui deliberações da 12ª Conferencia Nacional de Saúde. Brasília: MS, 2004. Available at: www.datasus.gov.br.

20. Brasil, Ministério da Saúde. Portaria n° 35 de 4 de janeiro de 2007 que institui, no âmbito do Ministério da Saúde, o Programa Nacional de Telessaúde. Brasília: MS, 2007. Available at: dtr2004.saude.gov.br/dab/docs/legislacao/portaria35_04_01_07.pdf.
21. Barbosa AK, de A Novaes M, de Vasconcelos AM. A web application to support telemedicine services in Brazil. *AMIA Annu Symp Proc* 2003: 56–60.
22. Tomasi E, Facchini LA, Osorio A, Fassa AG. Aplicativo para sistematizar informações no planejamento de ações de saúde pública. [Software program to systematize data for planning public health actions.] *Rev Saúde Publica* 2003; **37**: 800–6.
23. MS (Ministério da Saúde). DATASUS: informações em saúde Brasília: MS, 2002. Available at: www.datasus.gov.br.
24. OMS (Organização Mundial da Saúde). *CID 10*. [*International Classification of Diseases*, 10th revision.] São Paulo: EDUSP, 1996.

5 Community-based health workers in developing countries and the role of m-health

Adesina Iluyemi

Introduction

The World Health Organization (WHO) has proposed the use of low-cost information and communication technology (ICT) to improve the quality of service delivery and to build up health workers' capacity especially at the primary health care (PHC) level.[1] This application of ICT in health care has been termed e-health.[2] Mobile e-health, or m-health, involves using wireless technologies such as Bluetooth, GSM/GPRS/3G, WiFi, WiMAX, on to transmit e-health data and facilitate services. Usually, these are accessed by the health worker through devices such as mobile phones, Smartphones, personal digital assistants (PDAs), laptops or tablet PCs. Health data stored on devices such as USB memory sticks and memory storage cards (SDs) can also be regarded as m-health tools.

The International Telecommunication Union (ITU) has been piloting m-health for health system and workers development in developing countries since 2002, especially at the PHC level.[3] Most e-health development has been aimed at employing mobile/wireless ICT for PHC service development in developing countries. However, this is often not grounded within local practices in these countries. Attempts to develop new applications without taking account of local sensibilities have been known to fail.[4] How can m-health be made sustainable for health workers and for PHC delivery in developing countries? To answer this question, case studies on the use of m-health applications by community-based health workers (CBHWs) from four developing countries in three continents are presented in this chapter.

Opportunities in m-health for addressing global health problems

Health systems in developing countries face the double burden of chronic and infectious diseases. Scarce financial resources, coupled with the brain drain, have led to the loss of mostly high- and medium-level health workers. The Millennium Development

Goals (MDGs) set out by the United Nations in 2000 provide targets for tackling the disease burdens in developing countries.[5] The health-related MDGs are to:

- reduce child mortality from childhood diseases
- improve maternal health
- combat HIV/AIDS, tuberculosis and malaria.

These diseases have affected the fabric of society. Timely achievements of the health-related goals of MDGs in developing countries according to WHO can be attained by adopting the principles of the Alma Ata Declaration on Primary Health Care.[6] This implies that the PHC service model could be the best approach to the management of the health-related MDGs in developing countries. However, the shortage of human resources is a major impediment to achieving the MDGs. Recently, there have been calls to focus strategies on the development of 'substitute health workers' for providing health services in developing countries.[7,8] CBHWs are long-standing providers of primary health care in many developing countries, and can be considered as 'substitute health workers' in this context.

These factors all provide a rationale for introducing m-health for CBHWs and making policy changes to produce health system reforms in developing countries.

Primary health care

PHC is operationalized through the district health system (DHS). The DHS is a hierarchical organizational structure for PHC service delivery, and is made up of four or five integrated levels of health service delivery configuration. PHC forms the first level of contact of individuals, the family and community with the national health system. Essential health services are provided through the PHC system using community outreach programmes and facilities. CBHWs are regarded as the lowest cadre within the PHC system.

CBHWs are a variety of health workers who are selected, trained and work within communities. They normally have a shorter education than professional workers. In developing countries, they are usually located in rural and semi-urban settings, but may also operate in urban areas. CBHWs are either paid staff or volunteers, and are trained within the local community in which they are expected to operate. They also perform specialist functions such as providing reproductive health and family planning, nutrition education, and community rehabilitation for convalescing and disabled patients. As well as delivering essential health services, CBHWs are also agents for health promotion in the community in which they live and work. They also act as advocates for socioeconomic development and community empowerment.

Five case studies that illustrate aspects of implementing m-health innovations with CBHWs in developing countries are presented below.

Case study 1

Background
The Ca:sh (Community Access to Sustainable Health) programme was instituted in India in 2001. Large quantities of health data are generated by the PHC system in India. This is used for treatment planning, resource allocation, disease surveillance and management. Moving this information from the lower level to the district level of the PHC system in a timely and accurate manner was difficult because of the size of India's health system. The Ca:sh programme was conceived to provide a cost-effective method of managing and accessing these large volumes of health data. The CBHWs (usually auxiliary nurses or midwives) provide community, maternal and childhood care. The m-health application was developed to support the CBHWs in rural communities where most of the population live.

Case description
The m-health application was piloted in 2001 in a rural community with a population of 70 000. The Ca:sh programme was implemented by local staff in conjunction with the international developers. There was a two-stage implementation process involving a participatory approach in order to engage with the CBHWs. The first stage lasted for five months, and problems that were identified were incorporated into the design process. The second stage lasted for nine months, and culminated in a programme evaluation exercise. During this process, technical support and training for the CBHWs were provided by the local implementers. The training for the CBHWs also followed the two phases of the design process.

The m-health application enables the CBHWs to collect household, demographic, antenatal and prenatal, and childhood immunization data at the point of care in the patients' homes. The data collected by the CBHWs are then transferred at regular intervals to a central repository located at a district health centre. Unfortunately, despite a successful demonstration phase, the project was discontinued owing to lack of support by the national government.[9]

Case study 2

Background
The Hispano-American Health Link (EHAS) programme was instituted in Peru in early 2000. Maternal and childhood diseases such as respiratory and gastrointestinal infections are common in Peru, especially in rural areas. Rural villages have health posts that are usually staffed by CBHWs, who provide PHC services. Usually, CBHWs depend on the bigger health centres for second opinions, case referrals, pharmaceutical deliveries and service administration. However, the execution of these activities was very difficult because of poor communications. Often, the CBHWs spent hours or even days travelling to the health posts. The EHAS m-health system was designed to tackle this problem.

Case description
The EHAS programme commenced with a pilot project involving the deployment of 39 sets of m-health equipment to the health posts and centres within a district health system. This was preceded by a comprehensive assessment of the ICT needs of CBHWs in the region. This indicated that lack of communication facilities hampered the coordination of the CBHWs' activities, sharing and exchange of information, and their education. The contents of the m-health application included e-learning materials such as journals, evidence-based guidelines and local health news, mostly for managing childhood and maternal health care.

An online e-learning test and assessment system was also provided. Access to experts' or second opinions was also provided through a store-and-forward teleconsultation system.

The implementation involved the participation of local authorities and host communities in the development and installation of the m-health equipment. Training was provided for the local implementers, who in turn trained the CBHWs. The training included material on computer literacy, the operation of the m-health communication system and simple maintenance procedures. Two local technicians from the district hospital were trained in equipment maintenance and repair procedures. In addition, training was also provided for the managers at the district hospital on how to configure the m-health application to their local requirements.

At the completion of the nine-month pilot implementation, an evaluation was carried out to measure the impact of m-health on the community, on the CBHWs and on health service delivery. This was compared with the baseline study conducted at the start of the project. Findings from the evaluation were then employed to further improve and develop the m-health application. In the last seven years, the programme has provided valuable lessons on using high-bandwidth wireless ICT for rural m-health. Similar programmes in Columbia and Cuba have been inspired by this success.[10,11]

Case study 3

Background

Cell-Life is a project in South Africa focusing on the management of the HIV/AIDS epidemic. South Africa has one of the highest rates of HIV/AIDS rate in the world. In 2004, there were approximately 3.8 million people infected with the HIV/AIDS virus. In response, the South African government commenced a nationwide programme of antiretroviral (ARV) therapy for people living with HIV/AIDS (PLWHA). PLWHA are usually managed by state and community-based organizations. However, these often lack resources. Most PLWHA are resident in rural areas where there is a lack of basic amenities, and often the supply of ARV drugs to these centres is unreliable, thereby predisposing these patients to secondary infections such as tuberculosis. The South African government also recognized the importance of up-to-date information and access to communication facilities for the support and empowerment of PLWHA.

Case description

Initially, Cell-Life started as a community home-based care system for the direct management of HIV/AIDS patients known as 'Aftercare'. However, it has since been expanded to cover other aspects of the HIV/AIDS management process, such as pharmacy stock control, voluntary counselling and testing. The Aftercare module was designed for volunteer CBHWs known as therapeutic counsellors for the management of PLWHA. Therapeutic counsellors are PLWHA who are also undergoing ARV therapy themselves, but are more in control of their health situation. This represents a kind of peer-to-peer homecare management model. Each CBHW is usually allocated to 15–20 PLHWA. This involves the CBHWs providing care and support to their fellow PLHWA in their homes, and ensuring their compliance with ART treatment regimens. The m-health system supports these CBHWs in their health volunteer activities.

The first pilot was implemented in 2002 at a rural HIV research centre. Training and continuous supervision were provided by a doctor from the local university hospital. The mobile devices were provided for the CBHWs by the clinic for their professional and personal use. The clinic is also responsible for maintenance of the mobile devices.

Basically, the m-health innovation is used by the CBHWs for accessing real-time health and ART records of their fellow PLHWA during home visits. Information collected includes drug dosage and side effects, and relevant socioeconomic indicators. This information is transmitted via a public wireless network to a central database for analysis by a care manager; feedback is then provided for the CBHWs as required. Real-time communication between the care manager and CBHWs is usually by voice communication. The care manager also employs the data for monitoring the CBHWs' activities.

In 2002, there were 6 CBHWs and 250 patients. At present, there are about 46 CBHWs in 4 rural and peri-urban sites, managing about 3500 PLWHA. Recent indications are that the programme may not be sustained because of financial constraints.

Case study 4

Background
In India, traditional health practices serve as alternatives to formal health services, and meet the health needs of the mostly rural and poor population. Ayurveda, a 5000-year-old practice, is an example. Ayurveda uses medicinal plants to create low-cost drugs for managing chronic and acute diseases. These services are delivered by traditional CBHWs, who provide home consultation to clients in rural areas. In 2001, Jiva Health, an Ayurvedic health care provider, decided to develop an m-health system known as Jiva TeleDoc for supporting the homecare activities of its CBHWs. The aim was to develop a sustainable solution that was appropriate for the primary health needs of villagers in India.

Case description
The aim of the Teledoc innovation was to identify health care priorities. The design and development were carried out in India. The first pilot was a feasibility assessment study that lasted for a month in a selected village. This was to determine the contextual sustainability factors for the m-health innovation within the village environment. After a successful pilot study, the m-health programme was then extended to another 15 villages, where further piloting was conducted for another three months.

The m-health application enables CBHWs to update and view medical records in their clients' homes, away from the health centre. A store-and-forward teleconsultation can be carried out by the CBHWs with the urban health centre. At the urban health centres, an Ayuverdic doctor interprets the received data and then prescribes drugs, which are then delivered to the clients by CBHWs. In the pilot trial, CBHWs conducted 800 home visits with the m-health application. The project was then extended to another 30 villages in 2003. By 2006, the m-health application had been employed for the management of nine million homecare visits in about 10 000 villages.[12] The CHITS programme in the Philippines[13] (see also Chapter 3) also began as an m-health project.

Case study 5

Background
In Uganda, the Ministry of Health recognized that the ability to collect and analyze reliable information was vital for providing effective health care to the population. Therefore, a functional health management information system was required. An international coalition led by a university-based organization developed the Uganda Health Information Network (UHIN), an m-health application. The network used low-cost mobile ICT in a computerized health management information system and also provided access to e-health learning materials for all health workers, including CBHWs.

Case description
The m-health work started as a pilot project in two health districts in Uganda in 2003. Pre-implementation planning was carried out through awareness-raising workshops at the pilot sites. Experience from previous m-health projects involving mobile devices without wireless connectivity in other parts of Africa also provided insights. The implementation was carried out by Ugandan workers from local and national health organizations and coordinated by a university-based research and development institution. The information content was developed through a participatory approach with the local health workers who were going to be the eventual users. This process involved the digitization of the existing paper-based health data forms, decision support guidelines and educational materials.

Technical support and training were provided continuously throughout the early phase of the implementation process. Basically, the innovation consisted of two main applications, namely the health management information system and the e-learning contents. The e-learning contents included locally developed and WHO guidelines for managing health-related MDGs.

In 2003, 200 PDAs were distributed to 386 health workers in two health districts. By 2006, 350 mobile devices were in use. A large proportion of these health workers were CBHWs. As there were too few mobile devices to go round, up to six CBHWs in health posts or centres were observed to be sharing one device for their daily PHC activities.[14]

Case study summary

The development and implementation of the m-health applications in the above case studies involved mostly international and not-for-profit academic and research organizations working with local collaborators. These are listed in Table 5.1.

Table 5.1 Stakeholders involved in m-health project development and implementation

	International implementers	Local implementers
Ca:sh	1. Dimagi USA 2. Massachusetts Massachussets Institute of Technology (MIT), USA	1. Media Lab India 2. All India Institute of Medical Sciences (AIIMS), India 3. State Ministry of Health of Haryana, India
EHAS	1. Biomedical Engineering and Telemedicine Group of the Technical University of Madrid (GBT–UPM), Spain 2. Engineering Without Frontiers (ISF), Spain	1. Catholic University of Peru (PUCP) 2. Cayetano Heredia University of Peru (UPCH) 3. Ministry of Health of Peru (MINSA)
Cell-Life	None	1. Cell-Life 2. University of Cape Town (UCF), South Africa 3. Cape Peninsular University of Technology, South Africa 4. Desmond Tutu Institute
Jiva TeleDoc	1. Media Lab MIT	1. Jiva Health, Jiva Institute, India 2. Media Lab India 3. Indian Institute of Technology
UHIN	1. AED/ Satellife	1. Uganda Chartered HealthNet (UCH), Uganda 2. Makerere University Medical School, Uganda 3. District Health Authorities, Uganda

Table 5.2 M-health technology

Case	Technology
Ca:sh	1. PDAs
	2. Compact storage card (SD)
EHAS	1. VHF wireless networks and transceivers
	2. WiFi wireless networks and transceivers
	3. WiFi cards and routers
	4. Laptops
	5. Solar panels
	6. Email
Cell-Life	1. Smartphones and mobile phones
	2. SIM cards
	3. SMS/GSM/GPRS/3G
	4. Mobile web
Jiva TeleDoc	1. Smartphones
	2. GSM/GPRS
	3. Mobile web
UHIN	1. PDAs
	2. Portable wireless servers
	3. GSM/GPRS
	4. Solar panels
	5. Mobile email

Table 5.3 M-health project funding sources

Case	Funding organizations
Ca:sh	1. Media Lab India
	2. Ministry of Information Technology, Government of India
	3. Fogarty International Centre, National Institutes of Health (NIH), USA
	4. Media Lab, Massachusetts Institute of Technology, USA
EHAS	1. Spanish Agency for International Cooperation (AECI)
	2. Spanish Interministerial Commission for Science and Technology (CICYT)
	3. Latin American Program for Science and Technology for Development (CYTED)
	4. Supervisory Organization for Private Investments in Telecommunication in Peru (OSIPTEL)
	5. World Bank InfoDev program
	6. Committee for Solidarity and Development of the UPM, the Council of Madrid
	7. Spanish Association of Engineers of the ICAI and the Official Association of Industrial Engineers of Spain (COIIM)
Cell-Life	1. Vodacom Foundation
	2. National Research Foundation of South Africa
UHIN	1. Connectivity Africa: International Development Research Centre (IDRC), Canada
Jiva TeleDoc	1. George Soros Foundation
	2. Flora Family Foundation
	3. Media Lab Asia

Different low-cost technologies were employed in the m-health work described in the case studies (Table 5.2). The source of funding for these m-health programmes was mostly international not-for-profit organizations (Table 5.3).

The effects of the m-health projects can be considered under four headings: technology interfaces, social, finance, and government.

Technology interfaces

The m-health projects described above were generally employed to extend essential PHC services to mostly rural communities previously without services. Different types of CBHWs were involved. For example, in the Ca:sh project, they performed specialist functions in maternal and childcare.

The importance of engaging users in the development process was a common factor in most of the cases. The participatory design approach[15,16] adopted in the Ca:sh[17] and EHAS[18] projects should be more widely employed, even though it did not result in sustainability for the Ca:sh project. Participatory action research[19] was employed in the design and implementation process of the TeleDoc and EHAS projects. Here, community members, the users of the m-health services, were engaged in the development work. An iterative design approach was employed in all the projects, but most notably in the Ca:sh[17] and EHAS[20] projects.

User interface design was also important. The users were involved in the mobile devices interface design process, especially in the Ca:sh project. Of particular importance is engaging users in the adaptation process of fitting paper-based content to device screens. User engagement in interface design has a role to play in successful mobile device usability and eventual adoption.[15] However, this cannot be carried out in isolation. In a failed innovation, CBHWs abandoned their devices, despite an intensive long-term action, research-oriented design process, because other contextual factors were not appropriated into the planning process.[21]

The prior exposure of the CBHWs to mobile devices in the Cell-Life project and their exposure to desktop computers in the Ca:sh project were reported as being important to rapid adoption. Another factor was the training provided to the CBHWs. Training for users has been identified as important to the successful adoption of e-health in developing countries.[22] In the Cell-Life project, there was an increased health care workload on the CBHWs.[23] However, the health care competence of the CBHWs was observed to be enhanced by m-health in both the Cell-Life and UHIN projects.[14,23]

Social

Personal security concerns may be a barrier to the adoption of m-health. In the Cell-Life project, some CBHWs were observed to leave their mobile devices at home because of fear of armed robbery while working in the community.[23] There were also social effects of m-health on the work of the CBHWs. Some CBHWs complained about intrusion into their private lives in the Cell-Life project.[23] This perceived intrusion was identified as a limiting factor in the adoption of m-health.

A positive social effect observed in the Cell-Life project was that the CBHWs' status within their working and professional community was enhanced by the m-health work.[23] Another social effect, albeit a negative one, was observed in the UHIN project as an outcome of the CBHWs' team-working. As a consequence of the shortage of mobile devices, the CBHWs had to share them.[14] Sharing a mobile device is common in many developing countries.[24] This should not, however, be the case with CBHWs, because of their health care role. Each health worker deserves to have a personal device in order to manage and secure their patients' data, access email and use the device at any time for educational purposes.

Finance

Sustaining m-health projects in developing countries should be important to health policy makers. Most of the cases described above started as pilots, and most have since been expanded beyond their sites of origin. Thus, valuable lessons can be gained from their experiences.

The funding sources for these m-health projects are summarized in Table 5.3. Most were funded from outside the countries of implementation, with the exception of Cell-Life and Jiva TeleDoc. Most of the financiers were non-governmental organizations. It is known that developing countries are replete with abandoned health projects caused by the short-term focus of international implementers.[4,25] This observation is also supported by empirical work on the sustainability of PHC innovations in developing countries.[26] Sustainable PHC innovations were dependent on the degree of integration of local and contextual organizational factors in their planning. Financial sustainability of PHC innovations was observed to be important to local stakeholders.[27]

The financial basis of some of these cases is therefore worth considering. For instance, both the Jiva TeleDoc and Cell-Life innovations were run as social enterprises. Social enterprises are organizations that develop new solutions to social problems.[28] They can be run as a business or as a not-for-profit operation. However, the common goal is to ensure financial sustainability while solving societal issues. They are also known to provide an alternative to inefficient public services.[28] The m-health projects were social enterprises that filled the gap created by underperforming public health services. In future, perhaps, health policy makers should adopt this approach to meet the health-related MDGs of developing countries.

However, taking the social enterprise approach is not without its own problems.[29] Both the TeleDoc and Cell-Life applications were developed with seed funding from their sponsors, but achieving financial sustainability was difficult. The Cell-Life m-health work started as a donor-funded research project in response to government policy on HIV/AIDs care.[30] However, it has since mutated to an 'academic research-based' social enterprise.

Other m-health applications have also struggled to achieve financial sustainability. In the case of the now defunct Ca:sh innovation, long-term sustainability could not be attained owing to withdrawal of funding by its main sponsor, the Indian government.[9]

Indeed, the long-term viability of private funding for m-health innovations in developing countries has been questioned. In an analysis of the financial constraints encountered in scaling up the TeleDoc application, Singh[31] argued for complementary government funding.

Government

Despite some impressive results in the UHIN project, including scaling up from two to five health districts,[14] institutionalization into the national health system has not yet been achieved. The UHIN project started as a commitment made by government leaders on MDGs at the G8 meeting in 2002. It was funded initially by the Canadian government. Substantial buy-in has been achieved with governments at the district level. However, this has not occurred at the national government level. This may jeopardize its future financial security.[32]

Despite these financial concerns, the UHIN project managed to attain international visibility. It has been transferred to neighbouring Mozambique and planning is under way in Rwanda. Information from the Mozambique project indicates that early involvement of the government has contributed immensely to its diffusion.[32]

From the above, it can therefore be surmised that direct or indirect government support affects the financial sustainability of m-health applications in developing countries. Governments at local/district, national and even international levels have a significant role to play.

International governmental and non-governmental financial support is also important. Funding from the Spanish government enabled the implementation of the EHAS project. Non-governmental international financiers may, however, have a different outlook. Engineering professionals, telecommunication companies and international development organizations all contributed to the EHAS project.

Conclusion

Frequent misalignment between international development strategies and local realities in developing countries has been observed as a major cause of failure of initiatives and of wasted resources.[4] There has often been a lack of coherence between micro-level practices and strategic or macro-level policies.[33] The outcomes of the m-health case studies are the results of micro-level practices within the health systems of developing countries. National and international policy initiatives, especially within the sphere of global health, are typical of macro-level practices. National and international grants, and social philanthropy, are important for sustainable m-health. So is institutional support from both national and international organizations. Institutional and financial support from national and district governments is required for long-term, successful m-health.

Further reading

Al-Hakim L, ed. *Web Mobile-Based Applications for Healthcare Management.* Hershey: IRM Press, 2007.

Istepanian R, Laxminarayan S, Pattichis CS, eds. *M-Health: Emerging Mobile Health Systems.* Berlin: Springer, 2005.

Bangert DC, Doktor R, Valdez M, eds. *Human And Organizational Dynamics in E-Health.* Oxford: Radcliffe Publishing, 2005.

Latifi R, ed. *Current Principles and Practices of Telemedicine and e-Health.* IOS Press, 2008.

Spil T, Schuring RW. *E-Health Systems Diffusion and Use: The Innovation, the User and the UseIt Model.* Hershey: Idea Group Publishing, 2005.

Xiao Y, Chen H. *Mobile Telemedicine: A Computing and Networking Perspective.* Boca Raton: Auerbach Publications, 2008.

References

1. World Health Organization. *WHA58.28 e-health.* Geneva: WHO, 2005.
2. World Health Organization. *Strategy 2004–2007. E-health for Health Care Delivery.* Geneva:, WHO, 2004
3. Tomioka Y, Androuchko V, Nakajima I et al. An aspect of the ITU-D activities from a viewpoint of ehealth and human resource development. In: *Proceedings of 8th International Conference on e-Health Networking, Applications and Services,* 2006: 283–6.
4. Heeks R. Information systems and developing countries: failure, success, and local improvisations. *Inf Soc* 2002; **18**: 101–12.
5. United Nations. *Millennium Development Goals.* Available at: www.un.org/millenniumgoals/.
6. Kekki P. *Primary health care and the Millennium Development Goals: issues for discussion.* Geneva: WHO, 2004.
7. Dovlo D. Using mid-level cadres as substitutes for internationally mobile health professionals in Africa. A desk review. *Hum Resour Health* 2004; **2**: 7.
8. Hongoro C, McPake B. How to bridge the gap in human resources for health. *Lancet* 2004; **364**: 1451–6.
9. Keim B. Vikram Kumar. *Nat Med* 2007; **13**: 113.
10. Martínez A, Villarroel A, Puig-Junoy J et al. An economic analysis of the EHAS telemedicine system in Alto Amazonas. *J Telemed Telecare* 2007; **13**: 7-14
11. Martínez A, López DM, Sáez A et al. Improving epidemiologic surveillance and health promoter training in rural Latin America through information and communication technologies. *Telemed J E Health* 2005; **11**: 468–76.
12. Bhattacharyya A. Distance Doc. GPs with GPRS. *BusinessToday India* 2004; 1128–30.
13. Tolentino H, Marcelo A, Marcelo P, Maramba I. Linking primary care information systems and public health information networks: lessons from the Philippines. *Stud Health Technol Inform* 2005; **116**: 955–60.
14. SatelLife. *Uganda Health Information Network Phase II.* Ottawa: IDRC, 2006.
15. Graves M, Grisedale S, Grünsteidl A. Unfamiliar ground: designing technology to support rural health-care workers in India. *ACM SIGCHI Bull* 1998; **30**: 134–43.
16. Graves M, Reddy NK. Electronic support for rural health-care workers. In: Bhatnagar S, Schware R, eds. *Information and Communication Technology in Development: Cases from India.* New Delhi: Sage Publications, 2000: 35–49.
17. Anantraman V, Mikkelsen T, Khilnani R et al. Handheld computers for rural healthcare, experiences in a large scale implementation. In: *Proceedings of the 2nd Development by Design Workshop (DYD02),* 2002.

18. Martínez A, Villarroel V, Seoane J, del Pozo F. Analysis of information and communication needs in rural primary health care in developing countries. *IEEE Trans Inf Technol Biomed* 2005; **9**: 66–72.
19. Byrne E, Gregory J. Co-constructing local meanings for child health indicators in community-based information systems: the UThukela District Child Survival Project in KwaZulu–Natal. *Int J Med Inform* 2007; **76**(Suppl 1): 78–88.
20. Martinez A, Villarroel V, Seoane J, Pozo FD. Rural telemedicine for primary healthcare in developing countries. *IEEE Technol Soc Mag* 2004; **23**: 13–22.
21. Ranjini CR, Sahay S. Computer-based health information systems – projects for computerization or health management? Empirical experience from India. In: Tan J, ed. *Medical Informatics: Concepts, Methodologies, Tools, and Applications.* Hershey: Medical Information Science Reference, 2008.
22. Kimaro HC. Strategies for developing human resource capacity to support sustainability of ICT based health information systems: a case study from Tanzania. *Electron J Inf Syst Dev Countries* 2006; **26**: 1–23.
23. Skinner D, Rivette U, Bloomberg C. Evaluation of use of cellphones to aid compliance with drug therapy for HIV patients. *AIDS Care* 2007; **19**: 605–7.
24. Donner J. The use of mobile phones by microentrepreneurs in Kigali, Rwanda: changes to social and business networks. *Inf Technol Int Dev* 2007; **3**: 3–19.
25. Heeks R, Mundy D, Salazar A. *Why Health Care Information Systems Succeed or Fail.* Manchester: Institute for Development Policy and Management, 1999.
26. Sarriot EG, Winch PJ, Ryan LJ et al. Qualitative research to make practical sense of sustainability in primary health care projects implemented by non-governmental organizations. *Int J Health Plann Manage* 2004; **19**: 3–22.
27. Sarriot EG, Winch PJ, Ryan LJ et al. A methodological approach and framework for sustainability assessment in NGO-implemented primary health care programs. *Int J Health Plann Manage* 2004; **19**: 23–41.
28. Harding R. Social enterprise: the new economic engine? *Business Strategy Review* 2004; **15**: 39–43.
29. Dees JG, Elias J. The challenges of combining social and commercial enterprise. *Business Ethics Quarterly* 1998; **8**: 165–78.
30. Wessels X. Improving the efficiency of monitoring adherence to antiretroviral therapy at primary health care level: a case study of the introduction of electronic technologies in Guguletu, South Africa. *Development Southern Africa* 2007; **24**: 607–21.
31. Singh N. *ICTs and Rural Development in India.* Available at: ssrn.com/abstract=950322.
32. Batchelor S. *Connectivity Africa External Review Report.* Ottawa: IDRC, 2007.
33. Madon S, Sahay S, Sudan R. E-government policy and health information systems implementation in Andhra Pradesh, India: need for articulation of linkages between the macro and the micro. *Inf Soc* 2007; **23**: 327–44.

6 Global e-health policy: From concept to strategy

Richard E Scott

Introduction

It is likely that all aspects of health or health care will be affected by e-health, the broad use of information and communications technology (ICT) in the health sector. No individual, organization, business or government can therefore afford to ignore this development.

The concept of global health has emerged in the past decade. Given that the capabilities of e-health and the health needs of the global and local population are complementary, worldwide provision of the benefits of e-health, i.e. 'global e-health', is also an appropriate concept. But, to accomplish this, e-health must be integrated into domestic and global health care systems at both practical and policy levels. The focus to date has been on addressing matters related to the practical implementation of e-health in the local or domestic context, which is proving difficult enough. With rare exceptions, attention to the issues of integration and broader e-health policy development has been fragmented or non-existent.

The rapid development of e-health is causing many changes, the social outcomes of which will be mixed. Winners will be best placed to take advantage of the changes. Losers will not only be left behind technologically, but also be in danger of losing the expanded services capable of being provided through e-health. In order to maximize the number of winners, many challenges must be addressed. Principal among these is a global e-health policy.

Need for a global policy

Does a need exist for a global e-health policy? Consider the following 'North–South' scenario.

A 55-year-old man has recently returned home to a remote northern community in a Canadian province after a six-week trip to Tanzania and South Africa, during which he travelled and camped extensively in the bush. Upon his return, he has fallen severely ill and is bedridden with an unknown disease, exhibiting fever, extreme debilitating pain in joints and muscles, and a skin eruption. The patient's doctor has identified a specialist in rare tropical diseases who works at the Nelson Mandela School of Medicine in Durban, South Africa. An urgent video consultation is desired for diagnosis and treatment, and for guidance for local management. Can we do this? Both locations have access to video-consultation units, good experience with local use of this equipment and adequate bandwidth. From a technical perspective, therefore, we can do it.

Both clinicians are agreeable and local chief information officers are approached to arrange the logistics of the consultation. Having been alerted, senior administrators in the relevant health region in Canada ask questions. Who is this specialist in Durban, and what training or certification does she have? Is her expertise recognized in Canada? Is this within her scope of practice? Will she expect remuneration? Will this open the flood gate to many similar requests? Since diagnosis and treatment are needed, will she be considered to be practising in Canada? What are the licensing issues? Who will have clinical accountability? What about liability to the hospital and health region? Will there be any ethical, confidentiality or privacy complications? For clinical continuity and appropriate care, will the consultant need to review the patient's electronic health record, or need to enter her opinion in the record after remote patient examination? If so, what about security, and how will access and authorization be achieved since she is not an employee and does not currently have approval? Is any diagnostic equipment licensed and approved for use – and where? How much does this matter?

The health region's risk manager advises against the teleconsultation, and the Provincial Privacy Commissioner says that he will examine the issue and provide a response – probably next month. The outcome is confusion and uncertainty about what to do or how to do it, since there is simply no clear local, subnational, national or even global policy or legislation to show the way. As an alternative, a specialist in another Canadian province is contacted. But, now sensitized, the administration raises the same issues. The videoconference is cancelled 'due to technical difficulties'.

And the patient ... ?

Global health

Global health has been defined as those 'health problems, issues and concerns that transcend national boundaries, may be influenced by circumstances or experiences in other countries, and are best addressed by cooperative actions and solutions'.[1] Global health, similar to its predecessor, international health, maintains a strong focus on the prevention and treatment of infectious diseases such as HIV, malaria and tuberculosis. In addition, however, global health is focused on the identification and eradication of underlying conditions that contribute to the persistence of disease. These include disparities in access to care, cultural and psychosocial factors that impede the prevention and treatment of disease, and issues of extreme poverty, violence and war.[1] The use of e-health, i.e. global e-health, could influence each of these areas.

In most countries, major policy matters include the need for increased access to health care services and health reduction in inequity. Complicating factors include the ageing population, the shortage and maldistribution of health care providers, the growth of chronic disease and poor literacy. Many tools will be needed to address these health care problems, among which must be global e-health.

Global e-health

The term 'global e-health' appears to have been used from about 2000. The relationship of its components is shown in Figure 6.1. With recognition of its potential to have a profound effect on the health of the world's population, it has taken on new meaning and new significance.

A variety of definitions of telemedicine, telehealth and e-health have arisen over time, leading to some confusion and semantic debate. Common to all are the elements of the use of ICT, distance between participants, and health or medical application. Not typically included have been aspects of global application, crossing of existing boundaries and integration into current health care practice. Considering these perspectives, a definition was proffered in 2003 that was consistent with the accepted goals and terms used by the World Health Organization (WHO). Thus global e-health is:[2]

> The sustainable global integration of information and communications technologies into the practice of protecting and promoting health across geo-political, temporal, social, and cultural barriers – including research and education – to facilitate health, public and community health, health systems development and epidemiology.

Global e-health recognizes the interdependence of all nations and the mutual benefit of a flow of health information, knowledge and resources between countries.

Relevance of global e-health

MacPherson and Gushulak[3] identified the breakdown of traditional public health barriers to transmissible virulent diseases that has been caused by modern modes of

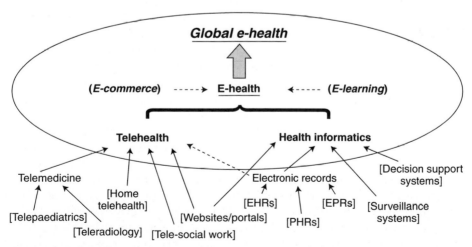

Figure 6.1 The relationship of the major components of e-health (telemedicine and health informatics) to global e-health. Also shown are subcategories of both major components, some examples of applications [square brackets], plus distinct but related elements (e-commerce and e-learning).

transportation. A potentially contagious person or product can now travel to anywhere in the world within 1–2 days. Kaul and Faust[4] noted the relevance of this in terms of political boundaries – 'In today's world, globalization has brought about interdependencies that blur the distinction between domestic and external affairs' – and noted that 'the best way to ensure one's own well-being is to be concerned about that of others'.

Given these perspectives, it is important to recognize the potential for global e-health to affect the health and health care of the world's population. There are many potential benefits:

- *System* – improved administration, communication and surveillance capabilities; better patient self-management; lower health system costs.
- *Provider* – improved distance education and remote skill development; networks for rural or isolated professionals.
- *Patient* – improved education and disease management; reduced patient costs (reduced travel, less time off work, decreased waiting time); positive influence on health outcomes.
- *Public* – improved education to maximize independent living and quality of life.

Such benefits have already been demonstrated in many industrialized countries, but usually in small-scale e-health applications. The opportunity exists to achieve benefits on a more widespread basis, but several factors will influence this, particularly in regard to developing countries. Some are health related, some are ICT related, and others touch on socio-political matters, including cultural sensitivities, governance and policy.

Global e-health and developing countries

It is reasonable to speculate that most of the world's countries have been exposed to e-health in some fashion. Developing countries perhaps have both the most to gain and the most to lose from 'e'applications, including global e-health (Figure 6.2). They have the most to gain through providing increased access to, and greater equity of, health care to their large, under-served populations. They also have the most to lose, since significant investment in time, effort and funding will be needed to raise their health and e-health infrastructure to the required levels, potentially increasing their debts and potentially diverting funding away from already stressed traditional health care delivery and support.

It will become necessary to build a sound business case for global e-health investment in developing and least developed countries, and for cogent arguments to be developed about the 'return on investment' (ROI). With more than 80% of the world's population living in developing and least developed countries, there is at least a moral argument for investment in e-health adoption and integration. However, given that exotic diseases can now more easily appear in industrialized countries, the North stands to gain from enhanced global e-health exchange with the South, which represents another tangible and valuable ROI. The WHO's recent macroeconomic study

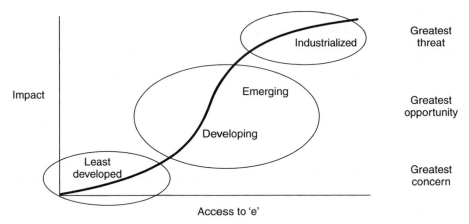

Figure 6.2 The potential impact resulting from access to 'e' applications, including global e-health. Industrialized countries must integrate e-health into existing (legacy) health and health technology systems, and this may be viewed as a threat to traditional delivery models. Developing countries, which lack legacy systems and can adopt new e-health applications relatively easily, have the greatest opportunities to gain from e-health. Of concern is the potential for the least developed countries to be excluded from the potential gains of e-health, because of the digital divide.

identifies another ROI. That study noted that investing in health in developing countries actually has a profound economic benefit for industrialized and developing countries alike.[5] The benefit for developing countries includes a fitter, healthier and more productive workforce, and decreased fecundity; the benefits for industrialized countries are – crudely – more participants (and buyers) in the global market place.

Global e-health policy perspective

Despite various international health-related collaborations, notably the WHO, health policy largely remains the sovereign domain of individual countries. But, to be effective, global e-health must become fully integrated into existing national, international and global health-related structures, in both a process and a policy sense. This will only be achieved through implementing globally accepted strategies, principles and complementary policy options. Such a goal is complicated by several matters, including existing borders and boundaries, the increasing number of stakeholders who influence health care and technology activities (particularly in developing countries), changes in governance, and the breadth and complexity of e-health-related policy matters, each discussed below. Failure to address these matters will create potentially impenetrable barriers that will deny the benefit of global e-health to much of the world's population.

Borders and boundaries

Some observers consider that national borders are becoming less meaningful.[6] Certainly, they are becoming more porous to health threats as a result of international mobility.[3] Global e-health has the ability – if developed correctly – to transcend existing geopolitical, sociocultural and temporal boundaries. By so doing, it could help to solve some of the health care problems facing the world's population. This potential also raises concerns, such as the 'jurisdictional gap' and fear of loss of control that must be addressed if e-health is to have the desired global benefits.[7-9]

Stakeholders

At one time, the WHO dominated international and global health activities. However, the world health system has grown in complexity, as well as in capacity, through an increasing number of stakeholders. These now include development banks, multilateral development agencies, development assistance agencies of industrialized countries, and non-profit private organizations such as non-governmental organizations (NGOs), big international NGOs (BINGOs), international foundations, professional bodies, health and medical assistance groups, consulting agencies, academic institutions, and finally the private sector that produces medical products, health services and ICT components. Each plays a major role in the development and dissemination of ICT and the provision of health services. Collectively, they possess much of the funding and expertise necessary for technology innovation, and are now leading global research and development.

The role of NGOs has been challenged. For many years, they have performed various service and humanitarian functions, acted as intermediaries between citizens and governments, and even tended to fill voids in governance. Now challenging their position are foundations and BINGOs, often created by private companies with access to substantial resources. For example, the Bill and Melinda Gates Foundation has assets in excess of US$36 billion. In 2007, the Foundation granted just over $2 billion for their programmes, which included the Global Health Program and the Grand Challenges in Global Health.[10] Compare this with the total WHO *biennial* budget of US$2.8 billion.[11]

Changing 'governance'

'Governance' concerns the actions and means adopted by a society to promote collective action and deliver collective solutions in pursuit of common goals – how to direct, shape or regulate use of something.[6] It is fairly straightforward to transfer this concept to the health and 'e' environments. Despite various international initiatives, 'health governance' (and associated health policy) has historically remained largely the sovereign domain of individual countries, and, with the increasing application of ICT and e-networks within countries, the concept of e-governance has arisen. E-governance deals with the whole spectrum of the relationships and networks within government that involve the use and application of ICT. The term 'e-government' is sometimes used, incorrectly, in place of e-governance. The former is a narrower concept and deals with the development of specific online services to citizens, such as e-tax, e-transportation and e-health. In a similar way, the advent of global ICT networks and globalization is challenging these recent concepts, and global e-health governance is emerging as a major issue. How does one control activities (health related and otherwise) that increasingly reside in the hands of globally distributed entities?

A notable concern is the fundamental shift in balance and growing influence of all of these entities on local, national and global health-related decisions and policy making. The dominance of the WHO, national governments and NGOs has been superseded by a dominance of private sector conglomerates and private foundations. Each stakeholder has its own priorities and interests. Despite seeking expert input to guide direction and investment, how adequately will the needs of small communities and countries be served? It will be crucial to ensure that local and national needs take precedence over corporate, donor or facilitator needs. But the reality is that global e-health policy development is no longer the sole purview of governments and the WHO. BINGOs and large multinational companies in the health and ICT sectors are extremely influential.

At a more practical level, the intensification of flows of people and goods are generating trans-border health risks that are different from those of previous eras. These new risks require novel approaches to health governance, and there is widespread belief that the current system of 'international' health governance does not sufficiently address them. E-health applications might assist. As a result, the concept of 'global e-health governance' must become a subject of greater interest, debate and development. This perhaps represents an opportunity for the WHO to remould its own policy, reclaim its confidence and influence, and take on a central role in the global e-health governance agenda.

The breadth of policy issues

E-health has been practised in some countries for several decades, and comprises health informatics and telehealth (see Figure 6.1). E-commerce and e-learning are distinct but related elements. Although originally quite localized in application, e-health solutions have became more national (crossing domestic borders) and even global (crossing national borders) – referred to as inter-jurisdictional e-health activity.[12] Such activity is often performed on the basis of 'good Samaritan', intra-professional consulting, or specific and limited inter-agency agreements. However, the need for broad policy to facilitate unfettered inter-jurisdictional activity has been recognized for many years.[13–15]

There are several commonly identified policy problems. For health informatics, they are privacy, confidentiality and security (and, more recently, patient safety) and, for telehealth, they are licensure, liability and reimbursement.[16] These have, to a large extent, usurped the limited policy debate, and the fact that they have remained unchanged for over a decade demonstrates the glacial pace of debate and action. Assuming that inter-jurisdictional e-health is a desirable goal, attention must be paid to much more than these limited matters. In earlier (unpublished) work, I identified 34 key e-health policy-related issues, and a recent paper identified almost 100 issues.[17] A three-dimensional 'global e-health policy matrix model' is being developed as a tool to assist in understanding this complex setting[18] (Figure 6.3). This tool highlights specific policy issues at the intersection of different policy levels, under specific policy themes, for specific policy stakeholders.

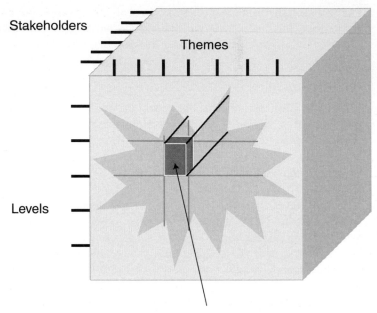

Stakeholders

Themes

Levels

Global e-health policy issues relevant to a given
policy level, theme and stakeholder

Figure 6.3 The three-dimensional e-health policy matrix model that highlights specific policy issues at the intersection of different policy levels, under specific policy themes, for specific policy stakeholders.

Definitive e-health policy is limited in scope, sparse in quantity and located primarily in a handful of industrialized countries. In other words, there is a global e-health policy void. Nascent e-health policy development can be identified in some countries, but is often indirectly related (information privacy policy) or focused on ICT rather than specifically e-health. Tools for e-health policy research[18,19] and development[20,21] have been reported. In reality, it will be too much to expect rigid global e-health policy, and a format encompassing global e-health principles and 'complementary' e-health policy[20] is much more likely. This might be structured in the form of a global e-health convention, as originally suggested by Schwarz and adopted at the Rockefeller conference on e-health policy.[22]

Earlier expectations that global e-health might revolutionize the way in which we perform health care, and maximize our well-being, have not been realized. The recent resolution by the WHO may be a turning point, drawing the attention of domestic governments of member countries to the potential of, and need for, e-health in each of their countries. The next logical step is to focus that individual effort into the larger concept of global e-health. Each jurisdiction must accept that internal e-health policy cannot be independent of the international environment. This current policy fragmentation is as much a concern as the previously described policy void. An accepted strategy is needed that attends to *glo*bal as well as lo*cal* needs within a responsive policy environment, giving rise to the idea of 'glocal' e-health policy.

'Glocal' e-health policy development: cautionary examples

In any policy development, it is possible that 'domestic' (i.e. local) policy decisions may prevent e-health from functioning on a worldwide scale (i.e. global) by putting in place – inadvertently or deliberately – administrative and policy barriers.[20] When preparing their 1998 directive on protection of personal information, the EU commented that: 'If each Member State had its own set of rules on data protection, for example on how data subjects could verify the information held on them, cross-border provision of services, notably over the information superhighways, would be virtually impossible.' This perspective exemplifies the need for 'glocal' e-health policy development.

Around the world, some policies have been developed that affect global e-health. These include:

- the policy environment in Africa, which illustrates coincidental policy development;
- the European Union's directive, and Canada's response (the Personal Information Protection and Electronic Documents Act, PIPEDA), which illustrate reactive policy development;
- the e-health policy implemented by Malaysia in the 1990s, which is an example of potentially restrictive policy development;
- the Legally eHealth initiative of the EU, which is an example of a potentially autocratic approach.

The African policy environment

Kirigia et al[23] provided an optimistic view of the e-health policy environment in Africa, and concluded that the policy environment for e-health growth internationally was very encouraging. This was based on observations of a number of international policies that encourage sustainable e-health usage, such as the World Health Assembly e-Health Resolution[24] and the health-for-all policy for the 21st century.[25]

In addition, Kirigia et al[23] pointed to 'regional development and political forums such as the New Partnership for Africa's Development (NEPAD), sub-regional economic communities, regional development banks and the United Nations Economic Commission for Africa', each of which have 'elements in their policies and/or strategies encompassing ICT development'. Finally, they noted the Blair Commission for Africa, which advocated massive investment in ICT and Internet connectivity and a 'growing realization among bilateral and multilateral donor agencies of the need for supporting investments in ICT infrastructure and Internet connectivity in developing countries as an essential strategy for economic growth'. In addition, the African Union's strategy for health in Africa lays out the planned development of health initiatives until 2015.[26]

With the exception of the WHO resolution for e-health, all of the other documents refer to 'ICT' and not specifically to e-health. While a supportive ICT environment is needed, such policy is coincidental to, and not focused on, e-health. Developing a clear, supportive, e-health-specific policy environment is necessary too.

EU directive on protection of personal information

Ironically, as the EU prepared its 1998 directive on protection of personal information, they also contributed to the creation of potentially restrictive policy. OECD guidelines for privacy protection existed, but the European Commission decided to promulgate their own directive. This directive compelled countries wanting to do business with EU countries to have a regulatory system in place to protect personal information, and required businesses to adhere to 'fair information practices'.

Lacking such legislation, Canada quickly introduced its own PIPEDA legislation in 2001 – a reactive response. But this also affected cross-border activities with Canada's largest trading partner, the USA, since they had to meet the specified requirements in order to do business with Canada and the EU. This form of reactive, snowball, and ad hoc policy development is inappropriate. Furthermore, it may well cause difficulties for developing countries, effectively setting the policy bar too high. If 'glocal' e-health policy is permitted to develop in this fashion, those countries that could benefit most may be excluded from the outset.

Malaysia's e-health policy

Malaysia was very proactive in developing both legislation (e.g. the Telemedicine Act[27]) and guidelines (e.g. for teleconsultation) for domestic telemedicine. These were intended to broaden access to health care in a borderless fashion. They achieved this for domestic purposes, but may be viewed as restrictive for global e-health activities. For example, the section 'Teleconsultation Beyond National Borders' states that 'Patients and health care professionals should be provided the opportunity to seek an expert opinion and treatment from overseas through teleconsultation'. But then two subclauses state 'Foreign experts can provide teleconsultation to health care professionals and/or patients in Malaysia *only at the invitation of the local health care personnel*' and 'All overseas experts who are invited to provide opinion or who are referred cases must be *registered with the appropriate regulatory authorities in Malaysia*'. Processes for invitation and/or registration are not provided, and penalties for transgression are severe, including fines and imprisonment.[27] Such legislation raises potential administrative barriers to borderless global e-health initiatives.

EU initiative

In support of the European eHealth Action Plan, a report called Legally eHealth[28] was intended to place e-health in a European legal and regulatory context. The report focused on how EU legislation on data protection, product and services liability, and trade and competition law applies. The report correctly noted that 'until these issues are tackled head-on in real cases, we will not begin to change the legal landscape in order to provide fertile ground for new developments'. However, if the resulting EU e-health policy is implemented then once more the EU will be forcing their requirements on the practice of global e-health. At the very least, such an approach will result in many years of retrospective policy realignment with other jurisdictions, maintaining rather than removing inter-jurisdictional barriers to global e-health practice. At the worst, it may ostracize developing countries from the global e-health community. Such approaches are not appropriate in the context of global e-health.

The way forward: a strategy

There are two basic policy options for global e-health:

1. *Continued ad hoc development followed by policy realignment.* This is the status quo. It maintains the confusion and prevents streamlined global e-health, and will require years of retrospective policy realignment to bring the many disparate approaches together. In the interim, many potential benefits of global e-health may be denied to the world's population.
2. *Progressive and collaborative complementary policy development.* A better approach, likely to permit the benefits of global e-health to be realized sooner, would be to initiate a process to guide global e-health policy development. The goal would be to identify common principles that can be agreed with relative ease, and then to use these to encourage development of domestic policy that is in line with global e-health principles, and is thereby complementary. The outcome would be removal of administrative and political barriers to global e-health.

Collaborative policy development would necessitate the creation of an inclusive and 'glocal' process whereby policy implemented at each level permits meaningful access to ICT in a country and therefore in the health sector. To guide this process, the Glocal E-health Policy Development Framework has been proposed.[21]

Conclusion

Global e-health has the ability to cross all geopolitical, socioeconomic, cultural and temporal barriers – to provide health and health care to anyone, anytime, anywhere. But how do we facilitate, yet also manage, this new paradigm? Any future activities have the potential to create functional or policy barriers. To avoid this, and to allow the benefits of global e-health to be equitably distributed, a coherent strategy is required that is based on both global and local (i.e. 'glocal') thinking.

The potential impact of global e-health is huge. However, awareness must be raised of the improvements in health care that could be achieved through global e-health. There is a need for consistency in approach to complex inter-jurisdictional issues. There is also a need for concerted development of 'glocal' e-health principles and complementary domestic policy. The current global e-health policy void is a serious concern. Inappropriate policy developed in one jurisdiction could hamper the ability of e-health to fulfil its potential.

Global e-health is no different from any other tool. To use this tool for global good requires a common vision and collective determination to achieve that vision. At present, e-health is struggling to establish itself even on a local or national basis in many countries, particularly developing countries. Policy can determine the pace and direction of change. If the potential of global e-health is to be realized, a strategy is required that will identify globally acceptable principles and thereby allow complementary domestic policy to be developed.

Further reading

Commonwealth Secretariat. *Commonwealth Health Ministers Book 2008 – E-health*. London: Henley Media Group, 2008.

eHealth ERA. *Database of European eHealth Priorities and Strategies*. Available at: www.ehealth-era.org/database/database.html.

World Health Organization. *Building Foundations for eHealth. Progress of Member States*. Geneva: WHO, 2006.

References

1. Institute of Medicine. *America's Vital Interest in Global Health*. Washington, DC: National Academy Press, 1997.
2. Scott RE, Palacios MF. E-health – challenges of going global. In: Scott CM, Thurston WE, eds. *Collaboration in Context*. Calgary: Institute for Gender Research and Health Promotion Research Group, University of Calgary, 2003.
3. MacPherson DW, Gushulak BD. Human mobility and population health: new approaches in a globalizing world. *Perspect Biol Med* 2001; **44**: 390–401.
4. Kaul I, Faust M. Global public goods and health: taking the agenda forward. *Bull World Health Organ* 2001; **79**: 869–74.
5. World Health Organization. *Macroeconomics and Health: Investing in Health for Economic Development*. Available at: whqlibdoc.who.int/publications/2001/924154550X.pdf.
6. Dodgson R, Lee K, Drager N. *Global Health Governance: A Conceptual Review*. Available at: whqlibdoc.who.int/publications/2002/a85727_eng.pdf.
7. Bettcher D, Lee K. Globalisation and public health. *J. Epidemiol Community Health* 2002; **56**; 8–17.
8. Rigby M. The management and policy challenges of the globalisation effect of informatics and telemedicine. *Health Policy* 1999; **46**: 97–103.
9. Scott RE, Lee A. E-health and the Universitas 21 organization: 3. Global policy. *J Telemed Telecare* 2005; **11**: 225–9.
10. Bill and Melinda Gates Foundation. *Foundation Fact Sheet*. Available at: www.gatesfoundation.org/MediaCenter/FactSheet/.
11. World Health Organization. *Policy and Budgets for One WHO*. Available at: ftp.who.int/gb/archive/e/e_ppb2003.html.
12. Scott RE, Jennett P, Yeo M. Access and authorisation in a glocal e-health policy context. *Int J Med Inform* 2004; **73**: 259–66.
13. Bashshur RL. Health policy and telemedicine. *Telemed J* 1995; **1**: 81–3.
14. Gobis LJ. Licensing and liability: crossing borders with telemedicine. *Caring* 1997; **16**: 18–24.
15. White AW, Wager KA, Lee FW. The impact of technology on the confidentiality of health information. *Top Health Inf Manage* 1996; **16**; 13–21.
16. Stanberry B. Legal and ethical aspects of telemedicine. *J Telemed Telecare* 2006; **12**: 166–75.
17. Khoja S, Durrani H, Fahim A. *Scope of Policy Issues for eHealth: Results from a Structured Review*. Available at: ehealth-connection.org/files/conf-materials/Scope of Policy Issues for eHealth_0.pdf
18. Scott RE. Investigating e-health policy – tools for the trade. *J Telemed Telecare* 2004; **10**: 246–8.

19. Varghese S, Scott RE. Categorising the telemedicine policy response of countries and their implications for complementarity of telemedicine policy. *Telemed J E Health* 2004; **10**: 61–9.
20. Scott RE, Chowdhury MFU, Varghese S. Telemedicine policy – looking for global complementarity. *J Telemed Telecare* 2002; **8**(Suppl 3): 55–7.
21. Scott RE. *'Glocal' e-Health – A Conceptual Policy Development Framework.* Available at: www.mrc.ac.za/conference/satelemedicine/Scott3.pdf.
22. Rockefeller Foundation. *National eHealth Policies – an Overview.* Available at: ehealth-connection.org/content/national-ehealth-policies-an-overview.
23. Kirigia JM, Seddoh A, Gatwiri D et al. E-health: determinants, opportunities, challenges and the way forward for countries in the WHO African Region. *BMC Public Health* 2005; **5**: 137.
24. World Health Organization. *WHA58.28 e-Health.* Available at: www.who.int/gb/ebwha/pdf_files/WHA58/WHA58_28-en.pdf.
25. World Health Organization. *Health-for-All Policy for the Twenty-First Century (Resolution WHA51.7).* Available at: www.paho.org/English/GOV/CSP/csp25_27.pdf.
26. African Union. *Africa Health Strategy 2007–2015.* Available at: www.africa-union.org/root/UA/Conferences/2007/avril/SA/9-13%20avr/doc/en/SA/AFRICA_HEALTH_STRATEGY_FINAL.doc.
27. Malaysian Government. *Laws of Malaysia, Act 564, Telemedicine Act, 1997.* Available at: www.parlimen.gov.my/actindexbi/pdf/ACT-564.pdf.
28. European Commission. *Legally eHealth. Putting eHealth in its European Legal Context.* Available at: ec.europa.eu/information_society/activities/health/docs/studies/legally-ehealth-report.pdf.

7 Experiences and lessons learnt from telemedicine projects supported by the IDRC

Laurent Elder and Michael Clarke

Introduction

In 1970, Lester B Pearson, then Prime Minister of Canada and a strong proponent of international development, stated the need for 'a new instrument concentrating more attention and resources on applying technology to the solution of ... economic and social problems on a global basis'.[1] In May 1970, the International Development Research Centre (IDRC) was founded by an act of the Canadian parliament. One of the Centre's priorities was Information and Communication Technologies for Development (ICT4D), since access to information and an effective means to communicate are necessary for sustainable development. IDRC's ICT4D programme now supports projects in Africa, Asia, Latin America and the Caribbean at a cost of nearly Can$20 million each year.

Exploring the means by which information and communication technology (ICT) can solve health problems was part of IDRC's early work in ICT4D. The IDRC was interested in answering questions such as the following:

- How can ICTs play a role in providing health care services to rural and remote regions of developing countries?
- Which applications afford the most potential with respect to effectiveness, adaptability and sustainability?
- What are the challenges to setting up e-health programmes in developing countries?
- How do different user groups access and use these programmes?

Early work

Much of the work supported by IDRC in the 1990s in the area of health and ICT focused on the development of health information systems. It included projects such as the Latin American Health Information Network, the National Health Information Network (Colombia) and HealthNet. The IDRC also supported the application of geographical information systems for mapping malaria risk in Africa, for endemic disease control in Botswana and Senegal, and for malaria control in the Amazon Basin. Telemedicine projects did not begin until the late 1990s, because of the generally poor telecommunications infrastructure in developing countries. It was not until the Internet started to become available in developing countries that IDRC began to investigate the potential of telemedicine.

Telemedicine in Uganda

An early project to establish telemedicine in Uganda began in 2000. The project, which received Can$452 300 in funding, focused on health problems such as cholera, malaria, HIV/AIDS and the application of telemedicine to address them. To achieve this, Makerere University School of Medicine aimed to establish telemedicine centres at Mulago and Butabika, set up the telemedicine infrastructure in the centres, conduct online consultations with the rural centres and start a continuing medical education programme.

What actually happened? As was typical of early telemedicine projects in Africa, there were difficulties in procuring appropriate telemedicine equipment and in setting up the telecommunications, which were based on VSAT. (A very small-aperture terminal, or VSAT, is a two-way satellite ground station with a dish antenna.) No online consultations actually took place between Kampala and the rural health centres, and there was no evidence of any beneficial health outcomes for the rural population.

None the less, with the support of Memorial University in Canada, the telemedicine in Uganda project helped to train staff in telemedicine activities. It also helped to focus government attention on rural health problems and it developed educational materials that are still used to this day. The project also contributed valuable lessons for future e-health projects. It set the stage for more successful e-health projects in Uganda, such as the Uganda Health Information Network and a subsequent telemedicine project in Mengo.

As far as IDRC was concerned, the project helped the organization better understand the challenges of supporting telemedicine projects in Africa and helped define some of the key questions that it would try to answer. These questions included how appropriate local capacities should be built, both technical and institutional. Second, there was a need to focus on 'e-readiness', which is the state of a country's ICT infrastructure and the ability of its consumers, businesses and governments to use ICT for their benefit. Finally, the IDRC needed to think about how it could help answer the key underlying question: is telemedicine a viable method for solving health problems in developing countries? In the Uganda project, cost–benefit analyses had not been conducted and health outcomes had not been measured, mainly because of the problems of implementing the pilot. All of these lessons helped shape IDRC's thinking about supporting the development of effective health applications (see below).

E-health applications in Asia

The IDRC programme, Pan Asia Networking (PAN), supports research into new ways of using ICT in the areas of health, education, livelihoods and governance.[2] Most of

Table 7.1 Telemedicine and e-health projects funded by the PAN Asia small grants programme

Country	Project	Organization	Grant (US$)
India	ICT-enabled life skill and sexuality education for adolescent girls	Centre for Women's Development and Research	8911
India	Using ICT to build capacities of HIV/ AIDS service providers in India	SAATHII (Solidarity and Action Against The HIV Infection in India)	29 786
India	Impact of remote telemedicine in improving rural health, India	n-Logue Communications Pvt Ltd	29 313
Indonesia	Development of ICT-based telemedicine system for primary community health care in Indonesia	Biomedical Engineering Program, Department of Electrical Engineering, Institut Teknologi Bandung (ITB)	29 479
Indonesia	Development of ICT-based mobile telemedicine system with multiple communication links for urban and rural areas in Indonesia	Biomedical Engineering Program, Department of Electrical Engineering, Institut Teknologi Bandung (ITB)	29 479
Nepal	Telemedicine in Nepal: a pilot project	HealthNet Nepal	30 000
Pakistan	ICT-assisted learning tool for the deaf in Pakistan	Sustainable Development Networking Programme, Pakistan	28 500
Philippines	A community-based child injury surveillance system: rapid data collection using SMS	Medical Informatics Unit, College of Medicine, University of the Philippines	22 642
Philippines	Mobile telemedicine and information resource system for community health workers	SynapseHealth Solutions, Inc	29 784

the activity related to health occurs in the PAN R&D Grants Program.[3] An example is the Pan Asian Collaborative for Evidence-Based eHealth Adoption and Applications (PANACeA) project, discussed in greater detail below. The health-related projects that have been funded are summarized in Table 7.1. Some recent evaluations have helped to shed light on the outcomes of some of these projects.[4] There were two activities related to telemedicine in India and Indonesia.

The first project concerned the impact of telemedicine on rural health in selected villages in India. The project aimed to field test with the help of N-Logue,[5] a low-cost medical kit, called ReMeDiTM. The equipment was developed by Neurosynaptic Communications Pvt Ltd[6] and installed in rural Internet kiosks around Tirupattur. The object was to transmit medical information to a doctor in Tirupattur.

After the service was launched, there was an increase in the number of visitors to the kiosk. However, following the initial interest, the number of visitors dropped precipitously to a few regular, repeat visitors. The drop was explained by the following factors: the kiosk operator's ability to administer the equipment properly; acceptability by the villagers; identification of the kiosk in a place where medical care is already dispensed; lack of awareness of the service; distance of the doctor from the village; and availability of competing services such as Registered Indian Medical Practitioners, Primary Health Centres and local doctors.[4] Although the project was not able to

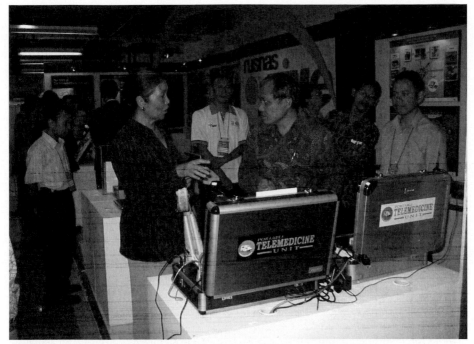

Figure 7.1 Indonesian mobile telemedicine application being demonstrated

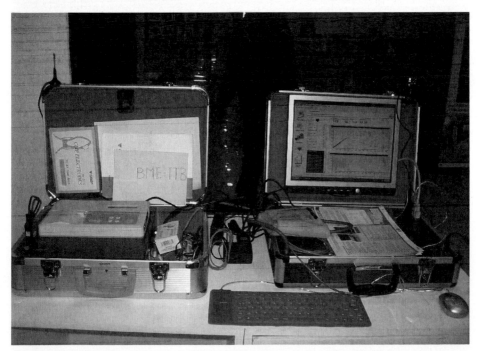

Figure 7.2 Indonesian mobile telemedicine application

document any health outcomes, it was – contrary to the Ugandan experience – able to demonstrate actual telemedicine activity.

The second project, in Indonesia, was to develop a telemedicine system for primary community health care. It was based on existing Internet technology to enhance PC-based medical stations. The pilot telemedicine network consisted of six medical stations in community health centres, and a station for the referral hospital, health office and a test laboratory. The system included teleconsultation and telediagnosis applications, medical information display software, a blood pressure and fetal heart rate interface, and an ECG interface (Figures 7.1 and 7.2).

It was found that human resource capacity building, in particular training to facilitate computer and telemedicine adoption, required substantially more time than expected. The project therefore demonstrated the significant role that human resource development plays in the implementation of telemedicine systems. However, as before, no findings were documented on the effect that the pilots had on people's health or health systems.

In a report commissioned by IDRC, the projects listed in Table 7.1 were assessed in order to evaluate their outcomes.[7] The factors examined were:

- knowledge production – any type of publication
- research targeting, capacity building and absorption – follow-on research, training of staff
- e-health solution adoption or integration – expansion or adoption of an e-health solution
- informing policy – policy documents, meetings with government officials
- broader community, institutional, or country benefit – including social and economic benefit
- health benefits to individuals or the population – more effective health care.

All projects were then ranked in terms of health outcomes and common themes were identified. The most troubling common theme was that all projects ranked 'low' with respect to demonstrated health benefits.

When Scott compared the projects, he saw that several common deficiencies had an adverse effect on nearly all of them. The deficiencies included:[7]

> Lack of planning for a sound, strategic health needs assessment, lack of planning for sustainability of (proven) solutions, lack of consideration for and mitigation of change management issues, lack of sound evaluation planning or execution, limited or no dissemination (formal or informal) of findings, and no significant or structured knowledge translation and transfer to influence decision- or policy-making around future e-health implementations. ... In addition, several general issues came to light, which also will need to be addressed. These included considerations around application software (i.e. open source versus proprietary solutions), application focus (e.g. use of traditional versus more novel technology such as GIS or m-health tools[8]), and local e-health knowledge and expertise (i.e. need for skill transfer and capacity building).

Present work

The early telemedicine projects that IDRC supported did not achieve all that was expected of them and raised more questions than it answered. Present projects include work in Africa and Asia.

Eastern and southern Africa

In 2004, the AfriAfya organization[9] undertook a study in eastern and southern Africa in conjunction with other African partners. The project was designed to study the application of ICT in the HIV/AIDS response in Uganda, Kenya, Tanzania, South Africa and Botswana. After conducting a literature review, the project staff undertook an electronic survey of individuals and organizations involved in HIV/AIDS matters. There were 990 respondents in a face-to-face survey undertaken in Tanzania and South Africa.

Unsurprisingly, the study found that South Africans and Tanzanians generally obtained their information on antiretroviral treatment (ART) from traditional media, rather than new media (Table 7.2). However, a surprisingly high proportion (30%) of South Africans obtained information from mobile phones and SMS. The assumption is that, as access to mobile telephony and the Internet rises in Africa, so will the number of people accessing health information from mobile phones.

According to the survey, illiteracy ranked highest of the factors impeding the use of ICT in both Tanzania and South Africa (although all factors scored highly in the latter). The results echo most of the research done by IDRC, which shows that illiteracy and localization matters are generally seen as among the most important factors impeding the more widespread use of ICT (Table 7.3).

Table 7.2 Sources of information on antiretroviral therapy.[10] Values shown are percentages of sample (n = 990)

ICT	South Africa (%)	Tanzania (%)
Print	75	53
Radio	88	81
TV	83	50
Video	21	20
Audiotapes	17	18
Telephones	24	4
Face-to-face meetings	77	82
Mobile phones and SMS	31	10
Computer/CDs	23	3
Email	22	2
Internet	25	2

Table 7.3 Factors impeding the use of ICTs for the fight against HIV/AIDS.[10] Values shown are percentages of sample ($n = 990$)

Factor	South Africa (%)	Tanzania (%)
Inappropriate language	81	58
Inappropriate and embarrassing messages	73	49
Lack of information, education and communication materials	80	81
Lack of feedback mechanism	82	67
Lack of enabling ICT policies	82	63
Poor infrastructure/physical access	86	80
People's attitudes	85	75
Traditional/cultural beliefs	87	80
Cost	85	68
Illiteracy	90	81

Table 7.4 Effectiveness of ICTs.[10] Values shown are percentages of sample ($n = 990$)

ICT	Don't know (%)	Harmful (%)	Extremely effective (%)
Print	7	2	46
Radio	2	8	65
TV	6	2	54
Video	30	6	14
Audiotapes	39	3	9
Telephone	43	3	8
Face-to-face meetings	6	3	61
Mobile phones/SMS	31	3	13
Computer/CDs	52	5	8
Email	59	5	9
Internet	56	9	10

The respondents perceived that radio, print media and TV, as well as face-to-face meetings, were 'extremely effective'. However, the majority of respondents did not know whether computers, email and the Internet could be effective (Table 7.4). Strangely, almost 9% saw the Internet as 'harmful', the highest percentage in that category. One can question the methodology of a perception questionnaire, as well as the terms used. For example, what does 'harmful' actually mean? What is meant by 'extremely effective'? However, one cannot deny that conventional communication methods are still perceived as the most widely used modes of information transmission.

Finally, according to the AfriAfya study, the best practices for using ICT in the fight against HIV/AIDS were:

1. Use of mobile phones and SMS
2. ICT for up-to-date HIV management information
3. ICT for mobilization
4. A combination of different forms of ICT
5. Telephone counselling.

The main lessons from this research were: that the use of 'modern' ICT is still very limited, but that there is huge potential; that institutions and health workers remain reliant on 'conventional' ICT and that there is therefore a need to integrate both 'modern' and 'conventional'to obtain the best results; and, perhaps most important, that to change perceptions and behaviours requires careful planning and patience.

Acacia project

Most mobile telecommunications infrastructure in Africa is too slow and expensive for connecting computers to the Internet. However, low-bandwidth applications have emerged that use mobile phones or personal digital assistants (PDAs) such as Palm Pilots, to connect via mobile networks. While information designed and formatted for the web is generally too bandwidth intensive to be transmitted over mobile networks, it can be formatted for small devices and low-bandwidth transmission. PDAs and smart phones are also seen as advantageous because of their robustness (no moving parts), their relative affordability, and their ability to be maintained in areas with little or no electricity infrastructure through the use of solar power rechargers. Examples of Acacia-supported mobile-enabled health applications include:

- automation of demographic surveillance activities, such as those at the core of pioneering health care initiatives, for example the Tanzanian Essential Health Interventions Project;[10]
- the use of SMS reminders in the treatment of tuberculosis in Cape Town;[11]
- delivery of continuing medical education and professional development via PDAs;[12]
- delivery of time-sensitive alerts to patients and health workers;
- maintenance of patient records for HIV-positive patients' lifelong drug treatments;
- management of specific health care initiatives such as the roll-out of ART and tuberculosis treatment initiatives.[13]

The IDRC programme Acacia has funded projects in all of these areas. The main research questions are:

- What are the most effective, relevant, affordable and scalable technologies to facilitate mobile health delivery?
- Can mobile-enabled health services and applications reduce the costs of health service management and delivery? What is the cost–benefit of using these applications?
- What kinds of health services can best be enabled through a mobile infrastructure?

- How are economies of scale being realized across the continent, and how can innovations be shared between African countries?
- What are the social effects of the introduction of these technologies in rural areas?
- What is the relationship between mobile health applications and broadband technologies, including VSAT?

Pan Asia Networking

In the Pan Asia Networking programme, more pervasive technologies, such as mobile phones and PDAs, are expected to be important for health applications.[14] Since mobile phone use is more widespread in Asia than in Africa, it is clear that there is great potential in Asia. The PAN programme emphasizes that more research is needed to gauge which applications and projects in the area of health have made a difference, to understand why they have or have not been successful, and, when warranted, to scale them up. However, the fast pace of innovation in both ICT and health research means that there is also a need for developing, implementing and evaluating new applications, particularly in the area of demographic surveillance of disease incidence and medical compliance, using new technologies such as mobile devices.

Another important matter in Asia is pandemics. Severe acute respiratory syndrome (SARS) and Avian influenza are serious threats to the health of Asians, as well as the rest of the world. A key to reducing the spread of these infectious diseases is to ensure that appropriate information on outbreaks is captured and communicated to the relevant experts as quickly as possible. ICT can therefore play an important role in helping to prevent or control pandemics, although more research and experimentation are needed to identify the best means of communication in rural and remote areas, where many of these outbreaks begin.

The questions that PAN would like to answer are:

- Which ICT health applications have had the most beneficial outcomes on people's health and health systems? What are the best ways of ensuring that beneficial outcomes can reach the segment of the population that does not have adequate access to health services?
- What is the potential of using new pervasive technologies, such as mobile phones, to make the delivery of health services or information more effective?
- What types of applications are best suited to help prepare for, or mitigate the effects of, pandemics such as SARS and Avian influenza?

PANACeA project

The PANACeA project (Pan Asian Collaborative for Evidence-Based eHealth Adoption and Application) will support research on e-health solutions in Asia. The research programme includes:

- a portable system for telemedicine and health information in rural and remote areas;

- a pilot programme in Mongolia and the Philippines of remote consultation to improve health services for rural mothers;
- a disaster/emergency telemedicine system;
- a cost–benefit analysis of hospital information management system data mining and data warehousing;
- an evidence-based approach to mainstreaming e-health initiatives in primary care;
- basic intervention research on e-health for persons with disabilities;
- online tuberculosis diagnostic committees for clinically suspect, sputum-negative patients in the TB-DOTS programme;
- use of mobile phones for referral of pregnant women.

The research programme also includes research activities such as reviews of telemedicine and health informatics in Asia.

Future work

IDRC will continue to support research and development projects in telemedicine and e-health in its next five-year planning cycle beyond 2010. Sufficient evidence has been generated from work carried out by IDRC partners and others to show that implementing telemedicine and e-health applications can have many benefits, including direct benefits to patients. The benefits include reductions in medical errors, cost savings, real-time monitoring of public health incidents, and provision of validated data and information for health systems decision and policy making. However, there is a continuing need to support research that demonstrates these benefits within the framework of a cost–benefit analysis in order to justify the often substantial initial investments associated with telemedicine. This, of course, is particularly significant in the context of developing countries with limited financial resources and telecommunications infrastructure.

Telemedicine and e-health applications that are shown to be appropriate, affordable and effective in one region can be adopted in other regions, provided that they are localized and contextualized. This should be within the capacity of the networks of ICT workers and researchers that IDRC now supports around the world.

IDRC's work on telemedicine and e-health research in developing countries depends on innovation. Unfortunately, in several projects, satisfactory results were not achieved, for the reasons indicated above. However, it should be noted that the average failure rate for ICT projects is about 50%[15] and is no different in the health care sector specifically.[16] Such high failure rates are not acceptable in most countries. The research that IDRC supports in this area should improve the likelihood of success.

Our research programmes will also continue to respond to emerging technologies and markets. As pointed out above, we have developed a number of research collaborations focusing on the use of mobile telephony as a device for the monitoring, management and delivery of health care. The needs of people living in developing countries are evident, but, ultimately, depend on a healthy society with full access to effective health care. IDRC is committed to helping them achieve just that.

Further reading

AED-Satellife. *Uganda Health Information Network*. Available at: pda.healthnet. org/.

Dansky KH, Thompson D, Sanner T. A framework for evaluating eHealth research. *Evaluation and Program Planning* 2006; **29:** 397–404.

E-health. *Interview with Michael Clarke*. Available at: www.ehealthonline.org/inter-view/interview-details.asp?interviewid=161.

IDRC. *Acacia Initiative*. Available at: www.idrc.ca/en/ev-5895-201-1-DO_TOPIC. html.

IDRC. *Telemedicine/Health*. Available at: www.idrc.ca/en/ev-22782-201-1-DO_ TOPIC.html.

References

1. IDRC. *History of IDRC*. Available at: www.idrc.ca/en/ev-26547-201-1-DO_TOPIC.html.
2. IDRC. *Pan Asia Networking*. Available at: www.idrc.ca/pan.
3. IDRC. *ICT R&D Grants Programme*. Available at: www.idrc.ca/panasia_grants/.
4. Dougherty M. *Exploring New Modalities. Experiences with Information and Communications Technology Interventions in the Asia–Pacific Region*. Bangkok: UNDP Asia–Pacific Development Information Programme, 2006. Available at: www.idrc.ca/uploads/user-S/11685405431ExploringNewModalities.pdf.
5. N-Logue Communications Pvt Ltd. *N-logue*. Available at: www.digitaldividend.org/case/case_nlogue.htm.
6. Neurosynaptic Communications Pvt Ltd. *ReMeDi*. Available at: www.neurosynaptic.com.
7. Scott R. IDRC Internal Report, 2006 (available from the authors).
8. MoHCA. *Mobile Healthcare Alliance*. Available at: www.mobilehealthcarealliance.org/index.shtml.
9. IDRC. *The Impact of ICTs in HIV/AIDS Programs in Eastern and Southern Africa*. Available at: www.idrc.ca/en/ev-87732-201-1-DO_TOPIC.html.
10. IDRC. *Tanzania Essential Health Interventions Project (Archive)*. Available at: www.idrc.ca/en/ev-3170-201-1-DO_TOPIC.html.
11. Bridges.org. *Testing the Use of SMS Reminders in the Treatment of Tuberculosis in Cape Town, South Africa*. Available at: www.bridges.org/publications/11.
12. IDRC. *Uganda Health Information Network (UHIN)*. Available at: www.idrc.ca/en/ev-86353-201-1-DO_TOPIC.html.
13. IDRC. *Free State HIV Therapy Database (ART-HIV)*. Available at: www.idrc.ca/en/ev-86361-201-1-DO_TOPIC.html.
14. IDRC. *PAN Prospectus 2006–2011*. Available at: www.idrc.ca/en/ev-9622-201-1-DO_TOPIC.html.
15. IT Cortex. *Failure Rate: Statistics over IT Projects Failure Rate*. Available at: www.it-cortex.com/Stat_Failure_Rate.htm.
16. Gauld R. Public sector information system project failures: lessons from a New Zealand hospital organization. *Government Information Quarterly* 2007; **24**: 102–14.

8 Strategies to promote e-health and telemedicine activities in developing countries

Sisira Edirippulige, Rohana B Marasinghe, Vajira H W Dissanayake, Palitha Abeykoon and Richard Wootton

Introduction

Logic suggests that employing information and communication technology (ICT) to deliver health care at distance (i.e. telehealth or e-health) would be useful to address at least some of the problems in developing countries. There is a growing body of literature to attest to this argument.[1-3] In the early 1990s, there was a general expectation that e-health would solve the main problems in health care in developing countries. However, the progress actually made with e-health in developing countries has been rather limited to date. It is also true that the use of e-health in industrialized countries is limited.[4]

What are the factors that have prevented developing countries from using e-health? What strategies might promote the use of e-health?

Role of national governments in promoting e-health

Governments as policy-making organizations play a pivotal role in formulating regulations in the health sector. The contribution of the government is particularly important in developing countries, where the public health system is usually the major provider of services. Government policies often have a significant impact on governing, financing and regulating the health sector in developing countries.[5]

Most developing countries in recent years have recognized the importance of ICT in their economic development and social progress.[6-8] A number of countries in the developing world have initiated national policies towards integrating ICT into their economic plans.[9-12] However, it is surprising that, in most cases, these national ICT initiatives have not considered the health sector as an important sector.

We believe that the exclusion of the health sector in national ICT initiatives is a major cause of the slow progress of e-health in developing countries. The factors contributing to this situation are described below.

Reasons for non-adoption of e-health

The reasons for the non-adoption of e-health include:

- lack of awareness of the benefits among policy makers
- lack of evidence for the benefits
- limited finance
- prejudice
- lack of expertise
- health system inertia.

First, we assume that one powerful reason for this situation is a lack of awareness of policy makers about the benefits of e-health.[13] Although policy makers in developing countries commonly believe that ICT can be used in the development of industry, agriculture and other economic and social activities, they are not aware of the benefits that the health sector can derive through the use of ICT. There can be many reasons for this. The health/medical sector is a very sensitive area where traditional ways of working have evolved over centuries and, as a result, there is resistance to change. Health is also closely linked with privacy and security concerns. Therefore, the introduction of ICT into health care institutions may not be as straightforward as in other sectors, such as commerce and education.

Lack of evidence about the benefits of e-health may be another reason for policy makers being unaware of e-health. Even in industrialized countries, there is a dearth of hard evidence with regard to the successful use of e-health. Similar evidence from developing countries is even scarcer. The lack of a sustainable business case to demonstrate cost-effectiveness is the root cause.

Although policy makers in developing countries are aware of the benefits of e-health, for a range of reasons they are reluctant to include this tool in their ICT initiatives. First, this may be due to limited financial capability. Policy makers are more likely to spend their limited resources on interventions that are known to produce health gain, such as sanitation, clean drinking water and vaccination, rather than funding e-health projects. The critical state of the health sector and its financial limitations may not allow policy makers to change their traditional patterns of spending health funding, even when they are aware of the benefits of e-health. In some of the wealthier developing countries that have good health care services, there seems to be a lack of people within the health sector who can champion the cause of e-health with policy makers.

Reluctance to use e-health may also stem from certain prejudices. Policy makers in developing countries may regard e-health as a family of methods imported from the industrialized world that have little relevance in their own countries. E-health may even be seen as the imposition of new methods from the Western world or former colonial authorities, i.e. as a form of neocolonialism.

Even when they have an understanding of the benefits of e-health, policy makers in developing countries may be hesitant to use it owing to a lack of expertise, infrastructure, technical knowledge and skills.[14,15] Starting an e-health project requires the presence of people with a certain level of technical expertise, and this may not be available in many developing countries.[16] In addition, the telecommunication infrastructure in developing countries is still limited.[17] These factors make it difficult for developing countries to launch e-health projects on their own.

Aspects such as inertia, reluctance to change and a lack of political will are also important factors that prevent policy makers from considering e-health as an alternative for addressing health problems in developing countries. Reluctance to change traditional methods of practice has been a serious obstacle to integrating e-health in the industrialized world too.[18] The introduction of a new practice is always demanding, and in that respect the role of champions or enthusiasts is extremely important. The lack of such champions in policy-making circles may be a strong reason for the current situation.

Another important factor, perhaps due to a combination of the factors mentioned above, is the need for long-term investment in telehealth and e-health, in order to build an infrastructure and the human resources required to demonstrate success. This is impeded by the relatively short political cycle, which requires short-term political rewards for investments.

Strategies at national level

Strategies to promote e-health at national level include:

- raising awareness of policy makers
- expanding e-health education
- changing the attitude of policy makers
- using expatriate communities.

One way of addressing the problems outlined above is to alert policy makers to the benefits of e-health. There needs to be a systematic way of making them aware of the current state of e-health practice and successful applications. It is important to make them aware of aspects of e-health that are applicable in developing countries. To do so, improving access to the evidence base in e-health is extremely important. Making updated information about successful e-health projects available to policy makers is one way of achieving this goal. Enthusiasts within the health sector, both IT and health professionals, may also play a pivotal role in making policy makers aware of the benefits of e-health.

The importance of e-health education has so far been overlooked. Evidence shows that access to systematic education in e-health is limited in both industrialized and developing countries.[16,19] Systematic education in e-health for health personnel must be at the heart of any strategy designed to facilitate e-health. An understanding of the benefits of e-health, current applications, technical requirements and the ethical/legal aspects would enable health professionals to adopt this new technique. In this task, local academics and researchers can play an important role. It is important to encourage academics to publish the outcomes of any e-health projects internationally. By doing so, local academics and health scientists can influence policy makers to facilitate the wider use of e-health.

On the other hand, policy makers must adopt an open-minded approach to these new changes. Political will and commitment, which have often been lacking in developing countries, are important elements in bringing about changes in these societies. The willingness of policy makers to use ICT in health is important in integrating this tool into the health sector.

While the continuing brain drain is a serious problem in developing countries, little attempt has so far been made to use expatriate communities to the benefit of the development of these countries. This is certainly not a problem specific to e-health. However, in promoting e-health, expatriate experts (particularly experts in the areas of health and ICT) can make a significant contribution by bringing their knowledge, skills and expertise. Mobilization of experts from expatriate communities must be promoted, as these people have knowledge and skills not only in the subject area, but also about specific needs and cultural issues. From the policy makers' side there must be an attitudinal change to accept and facilitate these experts.

In any environment, however, change is driven by individuals who have the motivation and desire to do so. In countries such as Sri Lanka, where national level e-health initiatives have lagged behind, there are numerous anecdotal examples of successful institutional level initiatives driven by such champions of e-health. Thus, it is clear that what is lacking in some countries is not resources or finances but leadership. Identifying such individuals within the heath care system of the country and providing the necessary support to them to bring about the desired change are very important.

Role of international agencies

International agencies such as the World Health Organization (WHO), the United Nations (UN), the World Bank and certain regional organizations (e.g. the African Union and SAARC) have recognized the value of ICT in development.[20–22] In fact the WHO has been instrumental in promoting e-health in a number of ways.[23] Some of these organizations have been involved in e-health projects in different parts of the world.[24]

Regardless of the enthusiasm of these organizations for e-health, their activities have so far been piecemeal and fragmented. In most cases, the primary responsibility of these organizations has been limited to providing funds. Often, the outcome of these initiatives has been unhappy: once the initial funding dried up, the e-health projects stopped functioning.[24] Another feature of these projects has been their disconnectedness. That is, most of them have functioned in isolation, and have not had links to other health work within the region concerned. There may be a number of factors contributing to this situation. International organization(s) initiating e-health projects in developing countries often have very limited understanding of the local situation. They may also have limited authority and recognition.

Another feature of e-health projects undertaken in developing countries is that they are commonly nothing more than a replication of projects carried out in industrialized countries. There is often no attempt to understand the specific needs of the locality and to find appropriate solutions to address those needs.

Thus, one of the main problems with international involvement in developing countries undertaking e-health projects has been a lack of coordinated management. This certainly invites another important question: 'Who should drive e-health globally?' There is no conclusive answer to this question. There is no authoritative organization to oversee e-health activities around the world – or in developing countries in particular. The question as to whether the UN, the WHO, the World Bank or any other

---

Box 8.1 Summary of the report of the WHO Global Observatory for eHealth[26]

Key findings
1. Active involvement of the WHO in the development of generic e-health tools, and guidance in creating and implementing e-health services would be welcomed by Member States.
2. The need for guidance in a broad range of e-health areas was expressed in particular by countries that do not belong to the Organization for Economic Co-operation and Development (OECD).
3. OECD countries did not express consistent views of their needs in e-health areas.
4. There is a need to raise awareness as to what e-health tools and services already exist at global and national levels.

Proposed action
The WHO, in collaboration with public and private sector partners, should take action in the following key areas:
1. *Provision of generic tools.* The WHO should facilitate the development of those generic e-health tools most sought after by its Member States, including tools for monitoring and evaluation of e-health services; drug registries; institutional patient-centred information systems that could be extended to include electronic health record systems; and directories of health care professionals and institutions.
2. *Access to existing tools.* As a parallel and complementary action, electronic directories of existing e-health tools and services should be created, with an emphasis on open-source solutions.
3. *Facilitating knowledge exchange.* An international knowledge exchange network to share practical experiences on the application and impact of e-health initiatives should be built. This would be Internet based and could be complemented by international e-health conferences to facilitate networking.
4. *Providing e-health information.* The WHO should create a digital resource of e-health information to support the needs of Member States in key areas such as e-health policy, strategy, security and legal matters.
5. *Education.* The use of e-learning programmes for professional education should be promoted in the health sciences, as well as in ongoing professional development. Collaborations should be developed to generate databases of existing e-learning courses. The WHO should advocate the inclusion of e-health courses within university curricula.

organization should take the responsibility for e-health activities in developing countries remains unanswered. What makes responding to this question even harder is that it implies a number of other questions: whether this organization has the capacity to fulfil the expectations; whether it is willing to take this role; whether the role would be acceptable to the members of the international community. These are hard questions to answer. Without answers to these questions, it is difficult to formulate a global strategy for e-health.

The role of the WHO in promoting e-health globally has to be acknowledged. The WHO has recognized the need for e-health to address health issues in developing countries.[25] It has also been instrumental in forming strategies, policies and standards for the utility of e-health. For example, the WHO Global Observatory for eHealth (GOe) was established to provide Member States with strategic information and guidance on effective practices, policies and standards in e-health.[26] The GOe produced the first WHO Global Survey on e-health, *eHealth Tools & Services: Needs of the Member States*, in 2005 (Box 8.1).[27]

The WHO has formed an e-health standardization coordination group as a platform to promote stronger coordination among the key players in all technical areas of e-health standardization.[28] The WHO has also initiated and assisted a number of e-health projects in different parts of the world. For example:

- The Telemedicine Alliance was implemented with the collaboration of the European Union and the International Telecommunication Union.[29]
- The WHO Regional Office for the Eastern Mediterranean (EMRO), in collaboration with the Islamic Republic of Iran Ministry of Health and Medical Education, organized the Fourth Regional e-Health Conference, which aimed to promote e-health.[30]
- The WHO has initiated several e-health projects in African countries to address health issues, advance health and medical education, and raise awareness of policy makers in the use of ICT in health.[31]
- A number of e-health projects have been undertaken in Sri Lanka (Table 8.1).

However, there is little evidence to show the success of any of these activities. One of the most critical problems has been the WHO's role in funding e-health.

Strategies at international level

Strategies to promote e-health at international level include appointing an e-health governing body and linking international aid to e-health.

As already mentioned, there is a critical need for a global governing body to oversee e-health activities. Setting up such an organization with appropriate legal and regulatory rights should be a priority. While this body would have authority relating to e-health activities across the world, it should also have the necessary financial capability to fund its activities. An organization with no financial capability will be doomed to failure. A global authority in e-health would be instrumental in defining matters such as standards of practice, regulations and funding. Among other things, the agenda

Table 8.1 E-health projects in Sri Lanka

Date	Project	Description
2001	Three-day course on basic and specialist skills in general surgery	The course was conducted by the Royal College of Surgeons of England and was delivered by distance education[11]
2001	Feasibility study in partnership between the WHO and the Norwegian Centre for Telemedicine	This aimed to examine the potential for telemedicine in addressing problems of the health care sector in Sri Lanka[12]
2003	Pilot e-health project funded by the WHO in collaboration with the Ministry of Health of Sri Lanka	This low-cost, store-and-forward telemedicine system was designed to connect doctors in remote hospitals with specialists for consultation[13]
2003	WHO-initiated pilot programme	This was designed to create a national telemedicine system, paying attention to wireless communication technologies in telehealth[14]
2005	'E-health Emergency Hospital' project	The objectives of the project were to improve recording and reporting, improve communication via the Internet and email, and improve access to specialist advice in cases of emergency[14]

of such an organization should include education and training as a priority. Accreditation by this global e-health body would provide much-needed recognition for e-health education to flourish. The existence of a global body would also assist the private sector to explore business opportunities in this new field.

It is important that international development assistance schemes should be linked to the promotion of e-health. Currently, there are various overseas development funds that assist health and ICT projects. Yet, development assistance funds are not designed to help e-health. International donors must acknowledge that promotion of e-health is an integral part of the development of health in developing countries. Similarly, international aid for infrastructure development should be tied to the promotion of e-health.

Conclusion

Although e-health has been generally accepted as a useful technique for improving access to health services in developing countries, for various reasons it has made very little progress. Policies at national and international level have not yet been able to facilitate e-health. At the national level, efforts must be made to raise awareness of policy makers, health personnel and business communities about the benefits of e-health. Policy makers must also have a more open-minded attitude towards e-health. At the international level, there is a pressing need for a global authority to oversee e-health. This organization must have the financial and legal capacity to promote e-health. Overseas development assistance schemes must include e-health as an integral part of the development and promotion of health generally.

Further reading

Eysenbach G. Poverty, human development, and the role of e-health. *J Med Internet Res* 2007; **9**: e34.

Khoja S, Scott RE, Casebeer AL et al. E-health readiness assessment tools for health-care institutions in developing countries. *Telemed J E Health* 2007; **13**: 425–31.

Latifi R. The do's and don't's when you establish telemedicine and e-health (not only) in developing countries. *Stud Health Technol Inform* 2008; **131**: 39–43.

Wootton R, Youngberry K, Swinfen P, Swinfen R. Prospective case review of a global e-health system for doctors in developing countries. *J Telemed Telecare* 2004; **10**(Suppl 1): 94–6.

References

1. Al-Shorbaji N. WHO EMRO's approach for supporting e-health in the Eastern Mediterranean. *East Mediterr Health J* 2006; **12** (Suppl 2): S238–52.
2. International Telecommunication Union. *Telemedicine & eHealth Directory, 2004.* Available at: www.itu.int/ITU-D/cyb/publications/2004/180ANN1E.pdf.
3. E-Health Innovation Professionals Group. *The Impact of e-Health and Assistive Technologies on Healthcare.* 2005. Available at: www.health-informatics.org/tehip/tehipstudy.PDF.
4. Ray P, Androuchko L, Androuchko V. A comparative overview of e-health development in developing and developed countries. 2006. Available at: www.medetel.lu/download/2006/parallel_sessions/abstract/0406/Ray1.doc.
5. Kumaranayake L, Mujinja P, Hongoro C, Mpembeni R. How do countries regulate health sector? Evidence from Tanzania and Zimbabwe. *Health Policy Plan* 2000; **15**: 357–67.
6. Islamic Development Bank. *Importance of ICT to Economic Development.* Available at: www.msctc.com.my/idb/2-3.htm.
7. Wang EH. ICT and economic development in Taiwan: analysis of the evidence. *Telecommunications Policy* 1999; **23**: 235–43.
8. International Telecommunication Union. *World Telecommunication/ICT Development Report 2006: Measuring ICT for Social and Economic Development.* Available at: www.itu.int/dms_pub/itu-d/opb/ind/D-IND-WTDR-2006-SUM-PDF-E.pdf .
9. Islam KMB. *National ICT Policies and Plans towards Poverty Reduction: Emerging Trends and Issues.* Available at: www.uneca.org/disd/events/accra/Poverty/ICT%20for%20Poverty%20Reduction-%20Paper%20by%20Baharul%20Islam.pdf.
10. World Summit on the Information Society. *Plan of Action: Civil Society's Priorities.* Available at: www.genderit.org/wsis/WSIS-CS-ActionPlan.doc.
11. United Nations Economic and Social Council. Economic and Social Commission for Asia and the Pacific. *Report on the Current Economic Situation in the Region and Related Policy Issues.* Available at: www.unescap.org/EDC/English/Commissions/E63/E63_3E.pdf.
12. Kearns P. *An International Overview of Trends in Policy for Information and Communication Technology in Education.* Available at: www.dest.gov.au/sectors/higher_education/publications_resources/summaries_brochures/towards_the_connected_learning_society.htm.
13. World Health Organization Regional Office for the Eastern Mediterranean. Intercountry Meeting on Telemedicine (Riyadh, Saudi Arabia, 7–9 February 1999). *Conclusions and Recommendations.* Available at: www.emro.who.int/HIS/ehealth/Meetings-TelemedicineSAA1999.htm.
14. Drury P. The eHealth agenda for developing countries. *World Hosp Health Serv*, 2005; **41**: 38–40.
15. Metaxiotis K, Ptochos D, Psarras J. E-health in the new millennium: a research and practice agenda *Int J Electron Healthc* 2004; **1**: 165–75.
16. Edirippulige S, Marasinghe RB, Smith AC et al. Medical students' knowledge and perceptions of e-health: results of a study in Sri Lanka. In: *MEDINFO 2007.* Amsterdam: IOS Press, 2007: 1406–9.
17. Parliamentary Office of Science and Technology. *ICT in Developing Countries.* Available at: www.parliament.uk/documents/upload/postpn261.pdf.

18. World Bank. *2006 Information & Communications for Development (IC4D) – Global Trends and Policies.* Available at: www.worldbank.org/ic4d.
19. Edirippulige S, Smith AC, Young J, Wootton R. Knowledge, perceptions and expectations of nurses in e-health: results of a survey in a children's hospital. *J Telemed Telecare* 2006; **12**(Suppl 3): 35–8.
20. UNESCO Secretariat. *Information and Communication Technologies in Development: A UNESCO Perspective.* Available at: www.unesco.org/webworld/telematics/uncstd.htm.
21. Boucher P. *Guidelines Public/Private Collaboration for ICT Development in Health Department of Knowledge Management and Sharing.* Available at: www.who.int/kms/initiatives/Guidelines.pdf.
22. United Nations. *Fourth Annual Report of the Information and Communication Technologies Task Force.* New York: United Nations, 2006.
23. Merchant JA, Cook TM, Missen CC. *The Role of Information and Communications Technology.* Available at: www.who.int/bulletin/volumes/85/12/07-048975/en/print.html.
24. Marasinghe RB, Edirippulige S, Smith AC et al. A snapshot of e-health activities in Sri Lanka. *J Telemed Telecare* 2007; **13**(Suppl 3): 53–6.
25. World Health Organization. *World Health Assembly Resolution on E-health* (WHA58.28, May 2005). Available at: www.euro.who.int/telemed/20060713_1.
26. World Health Organization. *Global Observatory for eHealth (GOe).* Available at: www.who.int/kms/initiatives/ehealth/en/.
27. World Health Organization. *eHealth Tools & Services: Needs of the Member States.* Available at: www.who.int/kms/initiatives/tools_and_services_final.pdf.
28. World Health Organization. *eHealth Standardization Coordination Group.* Available at: www.who.int/ehscg/en/.
29. World Health Organization Regional Office for Europe. *Reports and Guidelines from the Telemedicine Alliance and Telemedicine Bridge Projects.* Available at: www.euro.who.int/telemed/Publications/20060718_2.
30. World Health Organization Regional Office for the Eastern Mediterranean. *Fourth Regional e-Health Conference: Building the Electronic Health Record* (Teheran, Islamic Republic of Iran, 7–9 September 2004). *Conclusions and recommendations.* Available at: www.emro.who.int/his/ehealth/meetings-iran2004-recommendations.htm.
31. World Health Organization Regional Office for Africa. *Knowledge Management in the WHO African Region: Strategic Directions.* Available at: afrolib.afro.who.int/RC/RC%205⁶/Doc_En/AFR-RC56-16%20Knowledge%20Management%20-%20Final.pdf.

SECTION 3

EDUCATIONAL

9 Telemedicine in low-resource settings: Experience with a telemedicine service for HIV/AIDS care

Maria Zolfo, Verena Renggli, Olivier Koole and Lut Lynen

Introduction

In December 2003, the World Health Organization (WHO) and the Joint United Nations Programme on HIV/AIDS launched the '3 by 5' initiative to help low- and middle-income countries provide treatment to three million people living with HIV/ AIDS. Although the target date of December 2005 was not met, the global efforts to scale up access to antiretroviral therapy (ART) have brought positive changes world-wide. At the end of 2006, more than two million people living with HIV were being treated with ART in low- and middle-income countries.[1]

It has been an enormous challenge to introduce ART in a safe and effective way in resource-limited settings. The lack of human resources and clinical expertise has required approaches such as task shifting and continuum-of-care models where non-HIV specialists, nurses and lay providers all play a role in HIV/AIDS care. The public health approach that was proposed by the WHO in 2003 has provided the tools necessary to deliver decentralized HIV care, including ART with limited resources.[2]

It is clear that supportive supervision and clinical mentoring is the cornerstone of this public health approach in most of the resource-constrained clinical settings, where the health system is already weak and overwhelmed. Telemedicine (using the telephone, email, Internet or videoconferencing) is one possible way of offering clinical mentoring. We have established a telemedicine service for physicians working in HIV/AIDS services in low-resource settings.

The HIV/AIDS TELEmedicine service

The Institute of Tropical Medicine in Antwerp (ITMA) has run a short course on ART (SCART) every summer since 2003. The course provides three weeks of training on ART and clinical management of HIV infection for more than 40 physicians from resource-poor countries. After completing the course, a hybrid web/email forum is offered to the participants to support their decision-making and assist in the management of difficult HIV/AIDS cases in their daily clinical practice (Figure 9.1).[3]

The patient's history, physical examination, laboratory findings and questions to be answered are sent to a network of HIV/AIDS specialists using a discussion forum accessed through the TELEmedicine website (Figure 9.2). All postings submitted to this discussion forum are stored in a database and available for consultation. An internal email account is also available for direct contact between members, facilitating the exchange of recent literature, policy documents and interaction between sites. In addition, a system of email warning messages can be used to give early notice when a new posting is available on the discussion forum.

The TELEmedicine website contains interesting clinical cases and answers to common questions. This information can be consulted through a search function for continuing medical education (CME). Policy documents, guidelines and supporting material on HIV/AIDS care in low-resource settings and links to other important websites are also accessible.[4,5] The website conforms with the Health On the Net Foundation Code of Conduct.[6] This code is designed to improve the reliability of health information on the web. It defines a set of rules for website developers to ensure that readers always know the source and the purpose of the information that they are reading.

Service usage

Between April 2003 and March 2007, the TELEmedicine service received 642 second-opinion requests, from more than 35 resource-constrained countries. Three-quarters of the teleconsultations concerned management of complex medical problems in a specific patient and one-quarter were questions in the field of organization of health services for HIV prevention, treatment and care, vaccination programmes and guidelines.

In the first three years of activity (April 2003–March 2006), there were 491 queries. Of these, 47% ($n = 230$) were related to the general use of antiretrovirals, side effects, second-line regimens, prevention of mother-to-child transmission (PMTCT), immune reconstitution syndrome, TB/HIV and management of other co-infections during ART; 40% ($n = 197$) were related to the diagnosis and treatment of specific opportunistic infections and 13% ($n = 64$) to general topics such as the organization of health services for AIDS care, directly observed TB therapy, vaccination programmes and guidelines (Figure 9.3).

During the first three years of TELEmedicine activity, we noticed a significant increase in the proportion of questions related to organizational issues of HIV programmes: from 8% during the first year to 27% during the third year ($P < 0.001$). The opposite occurred for questions on general use of antiretrovirals (from 14% to 5%), management of side effects (from 12% to 5%) and management of specific opportunistic infections (from 44% to 30%); these differences were significant ($P < 0.05$).

There was a clear reduction in the numbers of questions on general use and side effects of antiretrovirals and a significant increase in questions concerning the

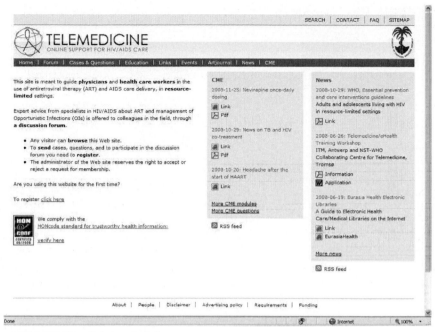

Figure 9.1 TELEmedicine website[3]

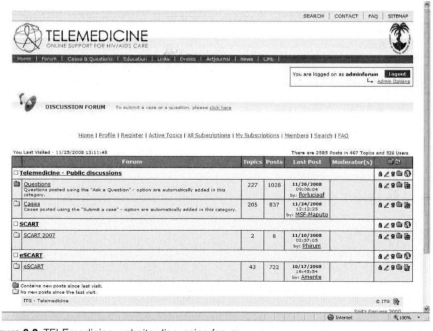

Figure 9.2 TELEmedicine website discussion forum

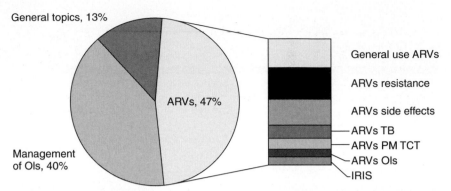

General topics, 13%

ARVs, 47%

Management
of OIs, 40%

General use ARVs

ARVs resistance

ARVs side effects

ARVs TB

ARVs PM TCT

ARVs OIs

IRIS

Figure 9.3 Telemedicine referrals (first three years of service). ARVs, antiretrovirals; IRIS, immune reconstitution inflammatory syndrome; OIs, opportunistic infections; TB, tuberculosis; PMTCT. prevention of mother-to-child transmission

organizational issues of ART programmes. This is related to the maturing of the HIV/ AIDS programmes. Thus, in the last two years, we have received many questions about ART roll-out: how to increase access to treatment and care, how to implement PMTCT services in ART clinics, and how to extend care to paediatric HIV cases. These questions do not arise in the early stages, when the burden of first-line access to HIV care is the main problem. It is also clear that management of opportunistic infections remains a challenge, and training programmes should not neglect this aspect of HIV care.[7]

User satisfaction

A survey was conducted in 2006 to evaluate clinicians' perception of the TELEmedicine service. The members were divided into 'active users' (i.e. clinicians who participated in the discussion forum) and 'passive users' (i.e. clinicians who consulted the TELEmedicine forum but did not post clinical cases and/or questions there).

There was a response rate of 53% among active users (18/34). Among these respondents, the service was judged to have been useful in influencing the management of the patients in 100% of cases, and 67% of the users perceived that the advice was useful in more than 75% of cases. The service was beneficial for the establishment of the diagnosis (78%), for the referring clinician's education (55%) and for reassurance (39%).[8]

Computer skills

Lack of access to information remains one of the major barriers to the practice of evidence-based medicine in low-resource settings. The problems include limited access to computer facilities, to literature databases and to CME programmes.

At the end of the short courses in 2004 and 2005, we assessed physicians' access to the web and their abilities to use computers while working in the field. Out of the total of 84 trained physicians, who were mainly African and Asian nationals working for international organizations or for the ministry of health, 75 completed the questionnaires. While 11% of the physicians stated that they did not have access to the web, almost all of them (74/75) said that they had their own email account. Of the respondents, 69% preferred to access the Internet in the evening (17:00–midnight). A connection speed of at least 28.8 kbit/s was available to 40% of them. For 83%, the operating system they used was Windows 2000/XP, 93% had a CD reader and 63% had a sound card on their computers. Two-thirds of the users reported that they were able to download files and to use software such as Acrobat, Excel, PowerPoint, WinZip and Word.

Online course

Although web access and information and communication technology (ICT) ability and use remain limited in low-resource settings, our selected group of physicians who attended the short course showed a good level of basic informatics knowledge, ability to use computers and access to the Internet.[9] This type of information helped us to plan the delivery of online modules through the website for CME purposes and to start the conversion of the face-to-face course to an online training modality (eSCART).

The eSCART content is structured into 13 different modules and uses a problem-based learning approach with clinical cases, tutorials, additional readings and self-assessments. At a workload of 4–5 study hours per week, the 3-week face-to-face course requires a minimum of 3 months' online training. To expand the availability of the eSCART course, we intend to work with appropriate international organizations and offer adaptations for HIV/AIDS programmes in low-resource settings.

Other telemedicine approaches

Consultations

Some HIV/AIDS programmes in low-resource settings have developed a consultation system that allows newly trained providers to ask questions of an expert through direct telephone calls, email and call centres. Telephone contact is usually set up so that health care workers and patients can make a toll-free or low-cost phone call to a central location.

Call centre in Uganda

The AIDS Treatment Information Centre at the Infectious Disease Institute (IDI) of Makerere University in Kampala hosts a call centre that responds to providers' treatment questions. The centre operates during normal office hours.[10] It is staffed by clinical pharmacists, who are supported by the IDI faculty. The call centre automatically records the caller's telephone number, and the staff return the call at no cost to the caller. The centre automatically develops a database of the most frequently asked questions.[11]

Satellife (HealthNet)

This is an international not-for-profit organization that uses the Internet for health information purposes in the developing world.[12] The organization aims to improve the communication and exchange of information in the fields of public health, medicine and the environment. There are global discussion groups (e.g. in nutrition, essential drugs, paediatric management and nursing). Using a low-Earth-orbit satellite and telephone lines for telecommunication, the organization provides email access in 140 countries, to a total of about 10 000 health care workers. Special emphasis is placed on areas of the world where access is limited by poor communications, economic conditions or disasters. Where adequate telecommunication links exist, Satellife and other organizations provide higher-capacity email and Internet connections. These allow the transmission of email attachments such as image files. The patient's findings can be described in an email message, and digital photographs of the patient and their investigations, such as electrocardiograms and X-ray films, can then be attached. This 'store-and-forward' telemedicine does not allow real-time interaction, but it permits specialist support in the management of difficult cases (see Chapter 19).

Case conferences

Another way to mentor health care workers is through case conferences, i.e. regular meetings to discuss complex problems in HIV care and to provide updates on practices or guidelines. For example, telephone conferences are used by the Heineken Company for mentoring its health care workers. In the period October 2001 to December 2003, the company had 10 health care workers operating in 5 different African countries. A total of 268 problems were raised during 45 telephone conferences. There were 79 questions (29%) about ART, 53 (20%) about the diagnosis and treatment of opportunistic infection, 43 (16%) about antiretroviral toxicity, 40 (15%) about care organization and policy, 32 (12%) about laboratory or drug supply, and 21 (8%) about biological parameters. The level of satisfaction among local company physicians was 65% for logistics, 89% for scientific relevance, 84% for applicability of advice and 85% overall. The most common complaints concerned the poor quality of the telephone connection and language problems for francophone participants. This showed that database-supported telephone conferencing could be useful for mentoring company health care workers in their routine care of HIV-infected workers and family members.[13]

Twinning

An established relationship between two institutions to share expertise is referred to as twinning. Ideally, these are long-term partnerships (at least three years), with clear, common objectives that serve as a basis for exchanging expertise and experience for the benefit of both institutions. A twinning broker, such as the Twinning Center,[14] develops and supports twinning partnerships. The Twinning Center is also exploring mechanisms to support collaboration between institutions in resource-constrained settings.[11]

Another example of this approach is the collaboration between the Moi University Faculty of Health Sciences in Kenya and both the Indiana University School of Medicine and the Brown University School of Medicine in the USA.

Twinning increases resources for individual institutions by facilitating a flow of funds and an exchange of information and expertise from one institution to the other.

There is, however, a limit to the number of available twinning programmes, and trainers from foreign institutions are not always knowledgeable about local conditions, language or policy.[15]

Other web-based collaboration and telemedicine systems

There are a number of other web-based collaboration and telemedicine systems, not restricted to the field of HIV.

AIDSPortal

This is an Internet portal that provides tools to support global collaboration and knowledge sharing among new and existing networks of people responding to the AIDS epidemic.[16] AIDSPortal offers: networking (members can access a directory of people and organizations to locate others interested in similar problems or working in a particular place); policy dialogue (the most up-to-date information on policy initiatives and international processes is easily accessible through AIDSPortal, and people can share information about their engagement); country-led management (supporting constructive dialogue between national responses and experiences and international processes); and access to information (AIDSPortal facilitates access to information given the time and resource constraints facing organizations responding to HIV and AIDS).

Community-based HIV treatment programme in Haiti

Partners In Health and Zanmi Lasante launched a community-based HIV treatment programme in Haiti's impoverished central plateau. It is a web-based medical record system linking remote areas in rural Haiti. It is used to track clinical outcomes, laboratory tests, drug supplies, communications, data analysis and drug supply management. Decision support is particularly useful for interpreting laboratory results. Technicians at two clinical sites enter patients' CD4 cell counts. Each night, a program checks for patients with low CD4 counts who are not receiving the appropriate drug regimen. A warning email message is sent to all 20 Zanmi Lasante clinicians and contains a link to the electronic medical records of patients who require additional treatment. Reminders can also be generated for patients who require extra drugs or investigations.[17]

Cell-Life

This is a platform for communication, information and logistical support to manage HIV/AIDS patients, enabling close monitoring of ART adherence and providing support to health care workers visiting AIDS patients in remote areas. The system supports communications technology, such as mobile phones and the Internet.[18,19]

RAFT (Réseau en Afrique Francophone pour la Télémedecine)

The RAFT project permits remote collaboration, case discussion and data sharing over low-bandwidth networks between the Geneva University Hospitals and 10 French-speaking African countries.[20,21] The core activity of the RAFT is the webcasting of interactive courses. Other activities include videoconferences, teleconsultations based on the iPath system, collaborative knowledge base development, support for medical laboratory quality control, and the evaluation of the use of telemedicine in rural areas (via satellite connections) in the context of multisectorial development. The project uses Linux and other open source software.

iPath

This is Internet-based software for the exchange of medical knowledge, distance consultations, group discussions and distance teaching in medicine and allows image sharing in pathology, radiology and dermatology.[22,23] It is being used in Africa, Asia and the Pacific. It is built with open source software, which is available free at www. sourceforge.net. More than 200 discussion groups use the iPath system.

Conclusions

More than two million people infected with HIV are now receiving ART in middle- and low-income countries. However, this has created extraordinary demands on health care workers in areas where health systems were already weak and overwhelmed. Thus, there are several problems in scaling up treatment programmes. A number of approaches are being tried, including mobilization of national and private partners, decentralization of HIV/AIDS services, and training and mentoring of health care workers.

It is evident that training and supervision are critical factors. Over the past few years, private donors and large organizations, such as the President's Emergency Plan for AIDS Relief and the Global Fund, have begun to be involved in pre-service training and mentoring of health care workers dealing with HIV/AIDS care in low-resource settings. Some developing countries have established collaborations with external partners to access training curricula or shape existing didactic material into a new model of teaching (training of trainers, onsite refresher courses, CME and distance learning), and some of the programmes have even expanded the range of support, offering attachments or onsite mentoring.

Telemedicine is one of the approaches to mentoring health care workers in low-resource settings, even though exhaustive data about its effectiveness are not yet available. In many settings, connectivity and computer literacy are still major limitations. In our experience, the opportunity for continued dialogue with physicians in the field has been valuable. It has allowed the identification of HIV/AIDS knowledge gaps and provided answers to some critical questions. Decisions on how to best support programmes on HIV/AIDS care in low-resource settings should really be made after taking into account the questions raised in the field.

The Institute of Tropical Medicine in Antwerp offers both face-to-face training courses and online training in ART. The TELEmedicine website also supports the management of difficult HIV/AIDS clinical cases via a discussion forum, where a network of international specialists is available to give second opinion advice. This is just one example of mentoring health care workers and providing direct support in the management of HIV/AIDS clinical cases. We believe that by giving clinicians the opportunity to access support and clinical mentoring, it is possible to lower the threshold for launching ART programmes. In addition, updating staff through CME helps to maintain quality in ART programmes, even in resource-limited settings.

Acknowledgements

This work was supported by the Belgian Directory General of Development Cooperation. We thank Vera Van Boxel and Joris Menten for the data analysis and Carlos Kiyan for offering advice.

Further reading

Latifi R. *Establishing Telemedicine in Developing Countries: From Inception to Implementation*. Amsterdam: IOS Press, 2004.

Norris AC. *Essentials of Telemedicine and Telecare*. Chichester: Wiley, 2002.

Sørensen T. *Guidelines for a country feasibility study on telemedicine*. Norwegian Centre for Telemedicine, 2003. Available at: www.telemed.no/guidelines-for-a-country-feasibility-study-on-telemedicine.64916-7398.html.

Swinfen Charitable Trust Website. Available at: www.swinfencharitabletrust.org.

Wootton R, Craig J, Patterson V. *Introduction to Telemedicine*, 2nd edn. London: Royal Society of Medicine Press, 2006.

References

1. World Health Organization. *Towards Universal Access: Scaling up Priority HIV/AIDS Interventions in the Health Sector*. Geneva: WHO, 2007. Available at: www.who.int/hiv/mediacentre/univeral_access_progress_report_en.pdf.
2. World Health Organization. *Antiretroviral Therapy for HIV Infection in Adults and Adolescents: Recommendations for a Public Health Approach*. Geneva: WHO, 2006. Available at: www.who.int/hiv/pub/guidelines/artadultguidelines.pdf.
3. TELEmedicine website. Available at: telemedicine.itg.be.
4. Zolfo M, Lynen L, Dierckx J, Colebunders R. Remote consultations and HIV/AIDS continuing education in low-resource settings. *Int J Med Inform* 2006; **75**: 633–7.
5. Zolfo M, Lynen L, Huyst V, Lynen L. Telemedicine for HIV/AIDS care in low resource settings. *Stud Health Technol Inform* 2005; **114**: 18–22.
6. Health On the Net Foundation. *Quality and Trustworthiness of the Medical and Health Web*. Available at: www.hon.ch/visitor.html.
7. Zolfo M, Koole O, Renggli V et al. Online consultations for HIV/AIDS care in resource-limited settings. In: *Proceedings of the 11th Congress of the International Society for Telemedicine*, 26–29 November 2006, Cape Town, South Africa.
8. Zolfo M, Renggli V, Koole O et al. Telemedicine survey on users' satisfaction. In: *Proceedings of the 11th Congress of the International Society for Telemedicine*, 26–29 November 2006, Cape Town, South Africa.
9. Zolfo M, Lynen L, Renggli V et al. Computer skills and digital divide for HIV/AIDS doctors in low resource settings. In: Proceedings of Med-e-Tel, 5–7 April 2006, Luxexpo, Luxembourg.
10. AIDS Treatment Information Centre Website. Available at: www.idi.ac.ug/index.php?m=menu&i=170.

11. World Health Organization. *WHO Recommendations for Clinical Mentoring to Support Scale-up of HIV Care, Antiretroviral Therapy and Prevention in Resource Constrained Settings*. Geneva: WHO, 2006. Available at: www.who.int/hiv/pub/guidelines/clinicalmentoring.pdf.
12. AED-SATELLIFE website. Available at: www.healthnet.org.
13. Clevenbergh P, Van der Borght SF, van Cranenburgh K et al. Database-supported teleconferencing: an additional clinical mentoring tool to assist a multinational company HIV/AIDS treatment program in Africa. *HIV Clin Trials* 2006; **7**: 255–62.
14. HIV/AIDS Twinning Center website. Available at: www.twinningagainstaids.org.
15. McCarthy EA, O'Brien ME, Rodriguez WR. Training and HIV-treatment scale-up: establishing an implementation research agenda. *PLoS Med* 2006; **3**: e304.
16. AIDSPortal website. Available at: www.aidsportal.org.
17. Jazayeri D, Farmer P, Nevil P et al. An Electronic Medical Record system to support HIV treatment in rural Haiti. *AMIA Annu Symp Proc* 2003: 878.
18. Cell-Life website. Available at: www.cell-life.org.
19. Skinner D, Rivette U, Bloomberg C. Evaluation of use of cellphones to aid compliance with drug therapy for HIV patients. *AIDS Care* 2007; **19**: 605–7.
20. AFT website. Available at: raft.hcuge.ch.
21. Geissbuhler A, Bagayoko CO, Ly O. The RAFT network: 5 years of distance continuing medical education and tele-consultations over the Internet in French-speaking Africa. *Int J Med Inform* 2007; **76**: 351–6.
22. iPath website. Available at: telemed.ipath.ch/ipath.
23. Brauchli K, Oberholzer M. The iPath telemedicine platform. *J Telemed Telecare* 2005; **11**(Suppl 2): 3–7.

10 Medical Missions for Children: A global telemedicine and teaching network

Philip O Ozuah and Marina Reznik

Introduction

Advances in information and communication technology (ICT) have provided new ways of delivering health care.[1] The World Health Organization (WHO) has recognized the role of 'health telematics' in improving access to medical and health care, health education, global health promotion, training of health personnel and the management of emergency situations.[2] This is particularly relevant in developing countries, where there are often growing health disparities, and where children are particularly affected by inequalities of access.

Telemedicine has become increasingly popular in both industrialized and developing countries.[1] In developing nations, telemedicine has important effects on many aspects of health systems.[3] It has the potential to improve health care by removing time and distance barriers, providing medical education and medical care, and optimizing the use of the limited health services available in these under-served communities.[4]

There have been many reports suggesting the potential advantages and benefits of telemedicine as a useful technique for delivering health care in the developing world.[5-8] However, few authors have described the actual clinical experience of using telemedicine there.[9-13] The reported use of telemedicine for children in developing countries is even more limited.[14-17] Medical Missions for Children (MMC) is a US not-for-profit organization that operates a global videoconferencing network. It delivers expertise from medical specialists and technicians based in hospitals in the USA to children needing care in developing countries by using telemedicine.[18]

Medical Missions for Children

The goal of MMC is to improve health care for children in medically under-served communities by using telemedicine. It has the following aims:[18]

1. To provide medical diagnoses and treatment via telemedicine to children and mothers in under-served communities around the world.

2. To facilitate medical knowledge transfer from those who have it to those who need it using the latest in communication technology.
3. To support applied medical research utilizing state-of-the-art communications infrastructure.

MMC works with a network of 27 American hospitals, who mentor participating hospitals in under-served countries.[18] It provides videoconferencing equipment for the hospitals in the developing world, as well as satellite time for the communication. Videoconferencing equipment (donated by Polycom) includes ViewStation HXD 9000, ViewStation VSX 7000 and HDX equipment, which communicates at bandwidths from 384 kbit/s to 4 Mbit/s. Physicians from the mentoring hospitals volunteer their time and expertise to participate via videoconference in remote examinations of patients, consultations about diagnosis and treatment, and education about new procedures, drugs and medical equipment.

History

MMC was founded in March 1999 by Peg and Frank Brady at St Joseph's Children's Hospital in Paterson, New Jersey, as a way of screening ill children from developing countries prior to doctors travelling to treat them. After eight years of operation, MMC serves children in over 100 countries throughout Latin America, the Caribbean, Europe, Africa, Asia, the Pacific and the Middle East. At least three patient consultations or diagnostic sessions are held by videoconference each day, with 1000–1200 direct consultations conducted every year. Since its inception, MMC has provided diagnostic consultations to almost 25 000 children, using the expertise of more than 600 physicians from 27 mentoring hospitals via telemedical support.

Programmes

MMC's work is accomplished through five programmes.

1. Telemedicine Outreach Programme

MMC operates a distance medicine network in more than 100 countries, called the Telemedicine Outreach Programme. This programme, a partnership with the World Bank, allows physicians to be electronically linked to patients in remote locations. MMC maintains a network of 27 mentoring hospitals in the USA and Europe that participate in the programme.[18]

2. Medical Broadcasting Channel

The Medical Broadcasting Channel (MBC) was launched in November 2005. It was developed as a means of helping physicians and other health care professionals to stay abreast of the latest developments in the medical field. High-quality, up-to-date medical education is delivered to physicians and allied health care workers around the world by satellite broadcasting and Internet streaming. The Intelsat 903 satellite is used to broadcast medical content to an area that encompasses 9 million physicians, 14 million nurses, 5 million health care workers, 89 000 hospitals, and 16 000 universities and medical schools.[18]

MBC is also available via the Internet2, the high-speed research version of the Internet. This network can support the transmission of TV-quality video and is available in 88 countries around the world.[19] The network is available to more than 300 000 institutions, including universities, government agencies, hospitals, medical schools, corporations and research facilities.

Eight daily seminars on different medical topics ranging from paediatrics to geriatrics are transmitted three times a day via satellite and the Internet. By providing and disseminating this latest medical information, MMC helps to increase the level of expertise in each participating hospital, as well as alleviating the disparity of care between industrialized nations and the developing world.

3. Global Video Library of Medicine
The Global Video Library of Medicine (GVLM) provides health care workers around the world with free access to an archive of more 25 000 hours of medical video. GVLM is the digital repository of thousands of video-based medical lectures, news programmes, symposia and training sessions, all of which are available to health care providers throughout the world. It provides a reliable source of clinical and medical research content via the public Internet.[18] It is available to health care professionals as well as the general public. Its Video-on-Demand capability allows researchers to search for and retrieve medical content. GVLM also serves as the content source for MBC.

4. Giggles Children's Theatre
The Giggles Children's Theatre performs three times each week to bring the healing powers of laughter and entertainment to hospitalized children in the city of Paterson, New Jersey (Figure 10.1). From the comfort of the Giggles Theatre, children are able to travel the globe on interactive virtual field trips that include swimming with sharks, visiting zoos and museums, and exploring rainforests.

The theatre provides a short escape from the fear and monotony that often accompany a hospital stay. Giggles presentations are also delivered via closed circuit television to the bedside of children too ill to come to the theatre and are broadcast via satellite and Internet2 to other children's hospitals around the world.[18]

5. MMC-produced television shows
The belief in creating knowledgeable patients who can work as a team with the physician to manage their illnesses led MMC to produce three television programmes for the Public Broadcasting System and MBC. The programmes educate individuals about health problems that could affect them and their families. The programmes are:[18]

- *Plain Talk about Health*, which was designed to take the medical jargon out of important conversations about health.
- *Tomorrow's Medicine Today*, which includes interviews with the directors of the 27 institutes of the US National Institutes of Health (NIH) and researchers from around the world.

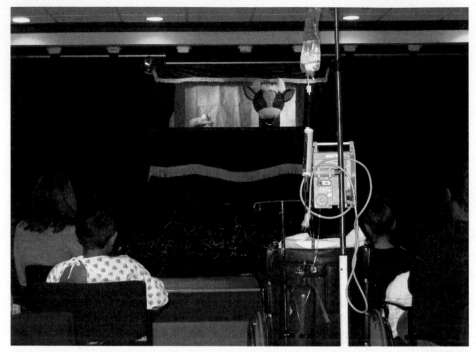

Figure 10.1 A Giggles Children's Theatre presentation of Aesop's Fables

- *Take Care*, which presents a patient describing his symptoms and the subsequent review and diagnosis by specialists.

Case report

The first child helped by MMC, Yordano, was an 11-year-old boy from rural Panama who was born with a cranial deformity resulting in the absence of one eye, difficulty in swallowing and learning difficulties. Yordano comes from a family of six. His father is a painter and his mother is a seamstress. He has an 18-year-old brother, a 5-year-old brother and a healthy twin brother. Yordano was the first child to use the MMC telemedicine network. He was examined by the physicians at St Joseph's Children's Hospital in New Jersey, and it was decided that he could be helped. A computer model of his head was created with the help of interactive telemedicine to collect the measurements. Then, using a computer, physicians designed titanium implants to correct his deformity. A physical model was made to confirm that all the parts fitted properly. Yordano's doctors in Panama were involved with the preparation. However, it was decided that his surgery should be performed at St Joseph's. Yordano and his mother arrived in the USA in November 2001 for the initial surgery. Subsequently, Yordano had 11 surgical procedures performed at St Joseph's to reconstruct his skull and jaw, to create an eye socket for a prosthetic eye and to receive a new titanium jaw (Figures 10.2–10.4). After this surgery was completed, educational sessions were held by the surgeons from the USA, who used the MMC network to review the procedure with 50 physicians from Panama. The plan is for Yordano to have one more operation in Panama to align his jaw. He is now 17 years old and doing well.

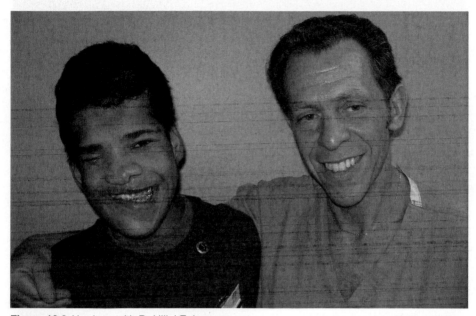

Figure 10.2 Yordano with Dr Hillel Ephros

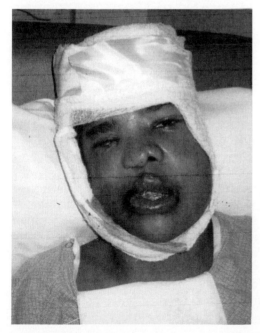

Figure 10.3 Yordano, post surgery

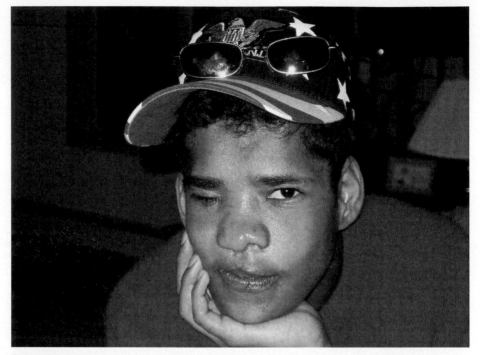

Figure 10.4 Yordano, seven years after the first operation

MMC and the Children's Hospital at Montefiore

The Children's Hospital at Montefiore in the Bronx, New York, acts as a mentoring hospital for the University College Hospital in Ibadan, Nigeria. The object is to provide health education and better access to medical care for children in Nigeria. The International Center for Child Health at the Children's Hospital at Montefiore (CHAM) houses telemedicine equipment to facilitate encounters between CHAM staff and Nigerian medical professionals, providing a forum for medical information exchange in the form of training sessions, seminars, symposiums and consultations via videoconferencing.

Working in partnership with the MMC, CHAM is sponsoring the College of Medicine at University College Hospital in Ibadan. MMC has provided the telemedicine equipment for the hospital in Nigeria. A curriculum of the hospital's educational needs and interests is being developed by medical staff in Nigeria in collaboration with CHAM faculty members. An agreement between MMC and the World Bank allows CHAM to connect with the Medical Missions site (via three ISDN lines) and access the World Bank satellite to reach the College of Medicine via Ibadan's satellite dish. The World Bank pays for the satellite time.

Our Nigerian partner has responsibility only for providing space for the telemedicine equipment and administrative support to ensure the quality and sustainability of

the programme. They also provide an appropriate mechanism for assessing and discussing the medical and educational needs of Nigeria, to ensure that the programme
contributes to the enhancement of paediatric health care.

Conclusion

There are many potential benefits of using telemedicine to deliver health care in the
developing world.[7–9] However, there are few reports that describe the use of telemedicine for children in developing countries. MMC, a non-profit-making organization,
has a well-established telemedicine network between mentoring hospitals in the USA
and hospitals in developing nations. Since its inception, the programme has provided
direct medical consultation and services to some 25 000 children in developing
countries.

Further reading

Reznik M, Marcin JP, Ozuah PO. Telemedicine and under-served communities in
developing nations. In: Wootton R, Batch J, eds. *Telepediatrics: Telemedicine and
Child Health*. London: Royal Society of Medicine Press, 2005: 193–8.
Swinfen Charitable Trust Website. Available at: www.swinfencharitabletrust.org.

References

1. Wootton R, Craig J, Patterson V, eds. *Introduction to Telemedicine*, 2nd edn. London: Royal Society of Medicine Press, 2006.
2. World Health Organization. *Health-for-all Policy for the Twenty-First Century* (Document EB101/INF. DOC./9). Geneva: WHO, 1998.
3. Edworthy SM. Telemedicine in developing countries. *BMJ* 2001; **323**: 524–5.
4. Zhao Y, Nakajima I, Juzoji H. On-site investigation of the early phase of Bhutan Health Telematics Project. *J Med Syst* 2002; **26**: 67–77.
5. Einterz EM. Telemedicine in Africa: potential, problems, priorities. *CMAJ* 2001; **165**: 780–1.
6. Fraser HS, McGrath SJ. Information technology and telemedicine in sub-Saharan Africa. *BMJ* 2000; **321**: 465–6.
7. Groves T. SatelLife: getting relevant information to the developing world. *BMJ* 1996; **313**: 1606–9.
8. Kastania AN. Telemedicine models for primary care. *Stud Health Technol Inform* 2004; **104**: 89–98.
9. Wootton R. The possible use of telemedicine in developing countries. *J Telemed Telecare* 1997; **3**: 23–6.
10. Wootton R. Telemedicine and developing countries – successful implementation will require a shared approach. *J Telemed Telecare* 2001; **7**(Suppl 1): 1–6.
11. Vassallo DJ, Swinfen P, Swinfen R, Wootton R. Experience with a low-cost telemedicine system in three developing countries. *J Telemed Telecare* 2001; **7**(Suppl 1): 56–8.
12. Patterson V, Hoque F, Vassallo D et al. Store-and-forward teleneurology in developing countries. *J Telemed Telecare* 2001; **7**(Suppl 1): 52–3.
13. Latifi R, Muja S, Bekteshi F, Merrell RC. The role of telemedicine and information technology in the redevelopment of medical systems: the case of Kosova. *Telemed J E Health* 2006; **12**: 332–40.
14. Lee S, Broderick TJ, Haynes J et al. The role of low-bandwidth telemedicine in surgical prescreening. *J Pediatr Surg* 2003; **38**: 1281–3.

15. Person DA, Hedson JS, Gunawardane KJ. Telemedicine success in the United States Associated Pacific Islands (USAPI): two illustrative cases. *Telemed J E Health* 2003; **9**: 95–101.
16. Graham LE, Zimmerman M, Vassallo DJ et al. Telemedicine – the way ahead for medicine in the developing world. *Trop Doct* 2003; **33**: 36–8.
17. Qaddoumi I, Mansour A, Musharbash A et al. Impact of telemedicine on pediatric neuro-oncology in a developing country: the Jordanian–Canadian experience. *Pediatr Blood Cancer* 2007; **48**: 39–43.
18. Medical Missions for Children. *Global Telemedicine and Teaching Network.* Available at: www.mmissions.org/index.html.
19. Medical Missions for Children. List of Countries Aided by MMC's Telemedicine Outreach Program. Available at: www.mmissions.org/top/countries.html.

11 Telementoring in India: Experience with endocrine surgery

Saroj K Mishra, Puthen V Pradeep and Anjali Mishra

Introduction

Telementoring – mentoring through the use of telecommunication – provides access to more experienced staff. This is an application of tele-education in general. In surgery, telementoring allows a remotely located surgeon to obtain the help of centrally located, more experienced surgeons in performing complicated procedures. This may occur before, or even during, surgery, when expert advice can improve intraoperative decision making.

Intraoperative assistance has been described by several authors.[1,2] At the Sanjay Gandhi Postgraduate Institute of Medical Sciences (SGPGIMS) in Lucknow, we have developed telementoring further, so that a mentor's input is continuously provided for the overall clinical care of the patient, to assist in diagnosis, preoperative treatment planning and postoperative care.[3] Telementoring has been incorporated into the training and teaching programme of the Department of Endocrine Surgery at the SGPGIMS. This department is one of only two in India that provide curriculum-based training in this relatively new subspecialty. Hence, the short-course training given in house to general surgeons is further consolidated with telementoring. This model may be relevant to other developing countries where there is a shortage of staff in certain subspecialties.[4,5]

Telemedicine in India

Public health care in India is primarily a responsibility of the state or province. The health system has a three-tiered structure: the primary health care centres cover a group of villages, secondary level health centres are at district level and medical colleges, located in big cities, provide tertiary care. Private sector hospitals account for almost 60% of health care.

Both government and private agencies have begun telemedicine projects. Government agencies that support these activities are the Indian Space Research Organization (ISRO), the Department of Information Technology, the Ministry of

Communications and IT, the Department of Science and Technology, and the Ministry of Defence. In addition, self-funded activities are being carried out by various corporate hospitals. A few mobile telemedicine units using satellite connectivity provided by ISRO have been introduced for community ophthalmology care. At present, ISRO's telemedicine network consists of about 200 nodes spread across the country.

The Department of Information Technology has produced guidelines and standards for the practice of telemedicine in India, which are aimed at enhancing interoperability among the various telemedicine systems being set up in the country.[6] This document aims to streamline the establishment of telemedicine centres and to standardize services available from different telemedicine centres. In addition to suggesting standards for various equipments needed for setting up telemedicine centre, it also provides guidelines for conducting telemedicine interactions.

The Ministry of Health and Family Welfare has recently launched two national projects. The first is oncoNET India, which will connect 25 regional cancer centres with four peripheral medical colleges/hospitals each, creating a network of about 100 telemedicine nodes exclusively for cancer care. The second is the Integrated Disease Surveillance Project, in which all the district hospitals in India will be networked with regional medical colleges. The object is to improve surveillance of diseases of public health importance and to deliver continuous professional education of peripheral health care staff. A national task force on telemedicine has been working under this ministry for over two years in formulating policies to facilitate the growth and integration of telemedicine into health care.[7] During the government's next five-year plan, it is expected that new telemedicine projects will be introduced based on an evaluation of existing telemedicine projects.

SGPGIMS infrastructure

In 1999, the Department of Endocrine Surgery at the SGPGIMS started experimenting with the use of videoconferencing to deliver education to a remote medical college. This followed a successful trial of multisite videoconferencing of a four-day postgraduate course in endocrine surgery and a workshop on minimally invasive endocrine surgery. Endocrine surgery, as a subspecialty of surgery, is not well developed in India. To facilitate knowledge exchange across the country, the department carried out a technical trial. Gradually, the educational interest expanded to include remote health care delivery. More projects began, and the telemedicine infrastructure grew. Currently, the infrastructure at the SGPGIMS telemedicine centre consists of several telemedicine workstations, equipped with teleradiology, pathology and videoconferencing units with large display devices. It can carry out medical data transfer and videoconferencing with six remote locations simultaneously.

The equipment used for telemedicine includes multimedia PCs with 43 cm monitors, as well as studio-type videoconference systems with flat-panel 74 cm television screens. Peripherals include an X-ray digitizer and a trinocular microscope with digital camera attachment. Initially, the connectivity was through a 128 kbit/s ISDN line. Subsequently, satellite-based connectivity with a 384 kbit/s bandwidth was obtained from ISRO. There is one K_u-band demand assigned multiple access (DAMA) and an extended C-band very small aperture terminal (VSAT).

The telemedicine centre at the SGPGIMS uses various modules in telemedicine care (teleconsultation, tele-follow-up, pre-referral screening, treatment planning and telementoring), distant medical education and remote assistance in skill development of health care professionals, as well as research and development in the field of telemedicine.[8] All telemedicine sessions are real-time.

Partners

The SGPGIMS telemedicine network partners are both national and international. National partners are listed in Table 11.1.

The international partners are Ranguil University, Toulouse, France and the Holy Family Hospital, Rawalpindi, Pakistan. Both of the overseas centres are connected with 384 kbit/s ISDN.

The technical partners are ISRO, the Centre for Development of Advanced Computing (CDAC), Pune and Mohali, and the Online Telemedicine Research Institute (OTRI), Ahmedabad.

Currently, the Orissa Telemedicine Network project is operational and the Uttaranchal network is in the implementation phase. A network involving eight medical colleges in Uttar Pradesh is being designed.

Telementoring and tele-education at the SGPGIMS

The first successful telementoring session was conducted in 2004, when a parathyroid tumour removal was performed at the Amrita Institute of Medical Sciences under expert guidance from the SGPGIMS. There had been two previous unsuccessful attempts at tumour removal by the same surgeon in 2001. This experiment was the

Table 11.1 National telemedicine partners of the SGPGIMS

Institution	Location	Distance from Lucknow (km)
All three medical colleges of the state of Orissa	Cuttack, Berhampur and Burla	1500
Two district hospitals of Uttaranchal State	Almora and Srinagar	500
All India Institute of Medical Sciences	New Delhi	700
Postgraduate Institute of Medical Sciences and Research	Chandigarh	500
Amrita Institute of Medical Sciences	Kochi, Kerala	2500
Christian Medical College	Vellore, Tamil Nadu	2000
Rohtak Medical College	Rohtak, Haryana	550

first of its kind reported from India.[5,9] The patient benefited, since he had the operation performed locally, without having to travel to a distant specialist centre. In fact, the general condition of this patient was so poor that he could not have travelled to the specialist endocrine surgical unit. For the telementoring session, both institutions were provided with dedicated 512 kbit/s VSAT connectivity. Video and audio quality was good enough for the expert at the SGPGIMS to guide the remote team satisfactorily.

We have also used telementoring as a tool in subspecialty growth in general[4] and in reinforcing endocrine surgical training.[5] This has been done to meet local require-ments, since there is a lack of specialist endocrine surgical centres in India. As far as structured endocrine surgical training is concerned, only two centres in India provide the MCh (Master of Surgery) degree. They have an annual intake of three candidates. In addition to the MCh training, short-course training (1–3 months) is also provided by the department at the SGPGIMS. The short-course training is reinforced by the use of telemedicine. During a short training post of three months, the trainees rotate through clinical and laboratory services and attend all the academic sessions con-ducted by the department. Following their return to their parent institute, telementor-ing is used to monitor their endocrine surgical practice and to guide them in solving diagnostic problems, in treatment planning and postoperative care.[5] The trainees also receive mentoring from experts in associated specialties such as nuclear medicine, endocrine pathology and interventional radiology.[5]

The tele-CME (continuing medical education) programmes conducted by the Department of Endocrine Surgery at the SGPGIMS are regularly transmitted to these trainee locations so that they receive updates on recent developments.[10] Table 11.2 shows the details of the tele-CME transmitted to the medical college in Cuttack, where two of the short-term trainees are currently located.

The trainees also consult their mentors at the SGPGIMS in discussing complex endocrine surgical problems, treatment planning, intraoperative and postoperative consultation, and follow-up plan. Figure 11.1 shows the numbers of such sessions held from 2001 to 2007. Figure 11.2 shows a tele-CME and a tele-education session in progress.

The benefit of telementoring and tele-education is that the trainees are able to manage many of the common endocrine surgical diseases without referring them to the SGPGIMS.[5] The added confidence due to the continuous presence of the mentor

Table 11.2 Conferences, CME and workshops held

	Year	No. of hours of transmission
5th Postgraduate Course in Endocrine Surgery (5 days)	2001	37
6th Postgraduate Course in Endocrine Surgery (5 days)	2003	40
Indian Thyroid Society Conference	2004	9
7th Postgraduate Course in Endocrine Surgery (5 days)	2005	36
8th Postgraduate Course in Endocrine Surgery (5 days)	2007	34

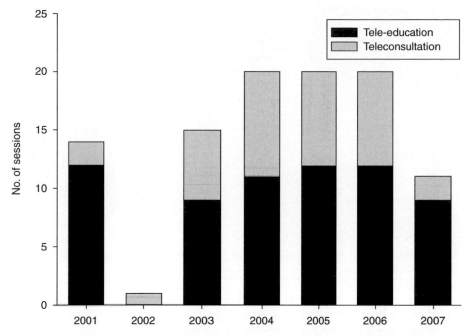

Figure 11.1 Number of telemedicine sessions held per year for reinforcement of training

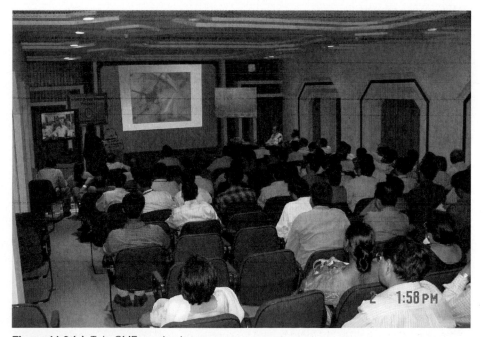

Figure 11.2 (a) Tele-CME session in progress

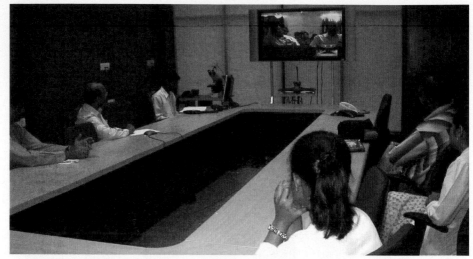

Figure 11.2 (b) Tele-education session in progress

increases their output in terms of the range of endocrine surgical procedures performed and reduces the complication rates.[5]

Although our initial experience has been successful, there is a need to develop standards and an accreditation system to facilitate general adoption of the techniques. The government has now set up a national task force for telemedicine that is going to address these matters.

Other telementoring and tele-education in India

There are few reports of telementoring in medicine from other centres in India. However, some institutions, such as the All India Institute of Medical Sciences and the Apollo Telemedicine Centre, are involved in telementoring experiments (personal communications). The 50-bed hospital at Aragonda, Andhra Pradesh (in the southern part of India) receives guidance for managing its patients from the specialists at the Apollo hospitals in Chennai or Hyderabad. Under expert guidance from specialists at Chennai, the Apollo Telemedicine Centre at Aragonda has also helped primary care physicians in making decisions about complex neurosurgical cases and treating certain minor problems locally without referring them to the tertiary centre at Chennai.[11]

Telementoring and tele-education in other developing countries

Telemedicine has increasingly been used to solve certain health care problems faced by the developing world, but there is a paucity of published reports. This is especially true regarding telementoring. Until the number of publications increases, it will be difficult to judge the true extent of telemedicine applications being carried out in the developing world.[12]

Publications in the field of telementoring in endocrine surgery from the developing world are very few in number. Even though there is paucity of telementoring applications in the field of endocrine surgery in developing countries, there are reports in other specialties. Lee et al[13] reported telementored laparoscopic varicocelectomy and nephrectomy in Bangkok, Thailand, which was 17 500 km from the mentoring location at the Johns Hopkins Hospital in Baltimore, USA. This experiment was conducted using ISDN lines at a bandwidth of 384 kbit/s. The authors concluded that transfer of knowledge and teaching–learning were achieved and that the video pictures transmitted had acceptable resolution and clarity. Similarly, transcontinental telementored procedures (laparoscopic bilateral varicocelectomy and a percutaneous renal access for a percutaneous nephrolithotomy) were carried out in collaboration between surgeons in Baltimore and Sao Paulo and Recife in Brazil.[14]

Telementoring has been conducted using low-bandwidth mobile telemedicine applications to support a mobile surgery programme in rural Ecuador.[15] This involved a mobile operating room, which was taken to a remote region of Ecuador (see Chapter 18). Using a laptop computer equipped with telemedicine software, a videoconferencing system and a digital camera, surgical patients were evaluated and operative decisions were made via ordinary telephone lines. The surgeons in the mobile unit in Ecuador were telementored by an experienced surgeon located at Yale University in the USA. Apart from five preoperative evaluations, a laparoscopic cholecystectomy was successfully telementored from the Department of Surgery at Yale University School of Medicine to the mobile surgery unit in Ecuador. The use of real-time surgical telementoring to teach complex ophthalmological procedures was successfully performed in real time via an ISDN line at a bandwidth of 128 kbit/s from the Saint Francis Medical Centre in Honolulu, Hawaii, to ophthalmologists at the Makati Medical Center in Manila, Philippines, more than 8000 km away.[16]

Telemedicine has also been used asynchronously (store-and-forward) for consultations and patient management by practitioners at remote location. Vassallo et al[17] reported the establishment of a telemedicine link by the Swinfen Charitable Trust in July 1999, to support a lone orthopaedic surgeon practising in Savar, near Dhaka, Bangladesh. Evaluation of the telemedicine-based advice for 27 referrals revealed it to be useful and cost-effective (see Chapter 19).

A trial telemedicine system to facilitate consultation between medical students pursuing elective study at a remote location in the developing world and specialists at a central location was established between Gizo Hospital in the Solomon Islands and Emory University Hospital in Atlanta, USA. A visiting medical student used this facility to relay images and investigation reports to specialists in Atlanta. This was used for telemedicine-aided learning, thus providing expert support to medical students in remote locations.[18] A pilot study at the Patan Hospital, Kathmandu, Nepal by the Swinfen Charitable Trust has shown that a low-cost telemedicine link is technically feasible and can be of significant benefit for diagnosis, management and telemedicine based education in a developing world setting.[19] Remote monitoring of paediatric patients at the Children's Field Hospital in Gudermes, Chechnya, not only allowed significant number of patients to be treated locally but also enabled the doctors at the peripheral location to receive advice about operative techniques[20] (see Chapter 25).

Problems concerning telementoring and tele-education in developing countries

Common health care delivery problems faced by developing countries are infrastructural and organizational in nature. Infrastructural problems include unreliable electricity supplies, poor telephone services, lack of transport and lack of medical supplies. Organizational problems include a lack of CME for health staff, poor training and supervision of health care workers, shortage of doctors and health care workers, and too many patients. Telemedicine may be useful in assisting with many of these difficulties. The major challenges with telemedicine in developing countries are unrealistic expectations, unsustainable funding models, lack of trials and evaluation data, and lack of published results and sharing of expertise.

During the audit of the telemedicine programmes at the SGPGIMS (2001–2005), it was found that only 61% of the scheduled sessions were held successfully, i.e. 39% of sessions could not be conducted owing to technical or human resource problems. Technical problems (23%) included power failure at the remote end, disconnection of the VSAT link and shifting of the VSAT service (Indian National Satellite System) to a new transponder. Human resource problems (77%) included non-availability of doctors at the expert end (36%) or at the remote end (35%), non-availability of technical staff at the remote end (7%) and others.[21]

The legal and ethical barriers that are commonly cited in telemedicine generally are also relevant in developing countries. These include questions about medicolegal liability and recommendations for good clinical practice, for which guidelines and protocols are still evolving. This is especially true for cross-border practice.[22] Other concerns include standards, interoperability, product liability, intellectual property rights and sharing of health information. Ethical and political matters need to be addressed.[23]

At present, professional boundaries are definitely barriers to the practice of telementoring both within and between countries. This may be assisted by national health care regulatory bodies or by international agencies such as the World Health Organization, which in consultation with its member countries has the potential to develop a global regulatory framework. In the meantime, accreditation of telementoring-based programmes needs to be carried out by appropriate agencies in each country or at a global level. Standardization of equipment, networks, technique, professional competence and process needs to be worked out. Legal questions regarding the sharing of responsibility as a result of the consequences of actions taken during telementoring must be addressed. There are as yet no guidelines on these matters. The health care regulatory body within each country needs to develop legislation for safe practice via telemedicine.

Conclusion

Telemedicine has the potential to improve the utilization of available resources for health care in developing countries. Our experience in the specialty of endocrine surgery in India has demonstrated the effectiveness of telemedicine applications in training, education and skills development. We have successfully used telementoring for continuous reinforcement of endocrine surgical training and also in the operating theatre for guided tumour removal. Even though telemedicine-enabled applications are being explored in India and other developing countries, few published reports have yet appeared. Deploying and sustaining telemedicine and telementoring requires the commitment and support of all those involved if success is to be achieved.

Further reading

Anvari M, Durst L. Development of a new telementoring program. *Healthcare Q* 2000; **3**(3): 26–30. Available at: www.longwoods.com/product.php?productid= 16718.

NASA. *NEEMO 9 Mission Journal.* Available at: www.nasa.gov/mission_pages/ NEEMO/NEEMO9/mission_journal_4.html.SGPGIMS. *Telemedindia.*

References

1. Rosser JC, Wood M, Payne JH et al. Telementoring. A practical option in surgical training. *Surg Endosc* 1997; **11**: 852–5.
2. Bruschi M, Micali S, Porpiglia F et al. Laparoscopic telementored adrenalectomy: the Italian experience. *Surg Endosc* 2005; **19**: 836–40.
3. Mishra SK, Mishra A, Pradeep PV. Telementoring in endocrine surgery. In: Kumar S, Marescaux J,eds. *Telesurgery.* Heidelberg: Springer-Verlag, 2008.
4. Pradeep PV, Mishra A, Kapoor L et al. Surgical sub-specialty growth in developing country: impact of telemedicine technology; a case study with endocrine surgery. In: *Proceedings of the 8th International Conference on E-Health Networking, Application and Services (Healthcom 2006)*, New Delhi: 34–9.
5. Pradeep PV, Mishra A, Mohanty BN et al. Reinforcement of endocrine surgery training: impact of telemedicine technology in a developing country context. *World J Surg* 2007; **31**: 1665–71.
6. Ministry of Communications and Information Technology. *Recommended Guidelines & Standards for Practice of Telemedicine in India.* Available at: www.mit.gov.in/telemedicine/Report%20of%20TWG%20 on%20Telemed%20Standardisation.pdf.
7. Mishra SK, Gupta SD, Kaur J. Telemedicine in India: initiatives and vision. In: *Proceedings of the 9th International Conference on E-Health Networking, Application and Services (Healthcom 2007)*, 19–22 June, Taipei, Taiwan: 81–3.
8. SGPGI. Telemedicine. Available at: www.sgpgi-telemedicine.org.
9. Pradeep PV, Mishra SK, Vaidyanathan S et al. Telementoring in endocrine surgery: preliminary Indian experience. *Telemed J E Health* 2006; **12**: 73–7.
10. Pradeep PV, Mishra A, Kapoor L et al. Applications of tele-health technology in endocrine surgery: Indian experience. In: *Proceedings of the Telemedicine 2007 Conference*, 31 May–1 June 2007, Montreal, Canada.
11. Ganapathy K. Telemedicine and neurosciences in developing countries. *Surg Neurol* 2002; **58**: 388–94.
12. Wootton R. Telemedicine and developing countries – successful implementation will require a shared approach. *J Telemed Telecare* 2001; **7**(Suppl 1): 1–6.

13. Lee BR, Bishoff J T, Janetschek G et al. A novel method of surgical instruction: international telementoring. *World J Urol* 1998; **16**: 367–70.
14. Rodrigues Netto N Jr, Mitre AI, Lima SV et al. Telementoring between Brazil and the United States: initial experience. *J Endourol* 2003; **17**: 217–20.
15. Rosser JC Jr, Bell RL, Harnett B et al. Use of mobile low-bandwith telemedical techniques for extreme telemedicine applications. *J Am Coll Surg* 1999; **189**: 397–404.
16. Camara JG, Rodriguez RE. Real-time telementoring in ophthalmology. *Telemed J* 1998; **4**: 375–7.
17. Vassallo DJ, Swinfen P, Swinfen R, Wootton R. Experience with a low-cost telemedicine system in three developing countries. *J Telemed Telecare* 2001; **7**(Suppl 1): 56–8.
18. Mukundan S Jr, Vydareny K, Vassallo DJ et al. Trial telemedicine system for supporting medical students on elective in the developing world. *Acad Radiol* 2003; **10**: 794–7.
19. Graham LE, Zimmerman M, Vassallo DJ et al. Telemedicine – the way ahead for medicine in the developing world. *Trop Doct* 2003; **33**: 36–8.
20. Ehrlich AI, Kobrinsky BA, Petlakh VI et al. Telemedicine for a children's field hospital in Chechnya. *J Telemed Telecare* 2007; **13**: 4–6.
21. Kapoor L, Basnet R, Chand RD et al. An audit of problems in implementation of telemedicine programme. In: *Proceedings of the 9th International Conference on E-health Networking, Application and Services*, 19–22 June 2007, Taipei, Taiwan: 87–9.
22. Stanberry B. Legal and ethical aspects of telemedicine. *J Telemed Telecare* 2006; **12**: 166–75.
23. Kapoor L, Basnet R, Pradeep PV et al. Integrating telemedicine in surgical applications. *Comput Soc India Commun* 2007; **30**: 17–20.

SECTION 4

CLINICAL

12 Teledermatology in developing countries

Steven Kaddu, Carrie Kovarik, Gerald Gabler and H Peter Soyer

Introduction

The inherent visual nature of dermatology makes it suitable for telemedicine. Several teledermatology projects have recently been initiated in developing countries, and the number is gradually increasing.[1–7] Preliminary results underline a number of potential benefits to patients, remote health care workers and health care systems of host countries. These benefits (Box 12.1) include easy extension of specialized dermatological services to geographically remote areas with few dermatologists, reduction of patients' waiting time for appointments, faster screening for skin diseases, promotion and coordination of scientific health projects, and education of health workers and lay people.[1–6,8] Local physicians benefit from the mentoring and educational aspects of the consultations, as well as the access to improved research facilities and professional

---

Box 12.1 Potential benefits of teledermatology

Benefits to patients

- Enhanced access to a trained dermatologist
- Prompt specialist opinion, leading to more accurate diagnosis and treatment outcomes
- Reduction of patient's waiting time
- Reduction of travel expenses

Benefits to local health care workers

- Improved and efficient access to specialized dermatology care
- Improved management of patients with skin problems
- New opportunities for continued medical education
- Enhanced professional collaboration
- Enhanced collaboration in research
- Access to online atlases and databases
- More efficient screening of patients with skin problems
- Better follow-up of patients with selected skin problems

Benefits to local health care system

- Reduction in health care costs
- Reduction in patient's and physician's travel costs
- Reduction in total number of hospital admissions, as well as faster discharges
- Increase efficiency in the use of human resources
- Increased and effective support for local health professionals
- Compilation of online databases

---

interactions. Consulting experts also get special opportunities to review rare or unusual dermatological cases.

As in other telemedicine systems, teledermatology employs both store-and-forward methods (asynchronous) and real-time approaches (synchronous).[9] Both modalities have previously been shown to be quite reliable and accurate when compared with traditional face-to-face consultation.[9-13] Store-and-forward systems are more widely used, owing to their lesser technological requirements and affordability. Images are submitted by email or presented on a web-based system. Although the real-time approach represents a reasonable substitute for in-person consultation and has the advantage of enhancing patient–doctor interaction, it is more time-consuming and expensive.

Teledermatology may involve providing assistance, follow-up or teaching. Tele-assistance models aim at teleconsultation, telescreening and/or second opinion.[7,14] The majority of teledermatology projects in developing countries deal with dermatology consultations. Telescreening projects have been used to manage waiting lists for treatment of dermatoses with different healing times or to support prevention programmes such as those surveying skin tumours.[15] Telefollow-up systems deal with transmission of medical information regarding follow-up and treatment progression of patients from remote centres (e.g. to follow up patients treated for certain chronic skin conditions such as leg ulcers and leprosy) and for postoperative evaluation.[5,16] Tele-education is proving to be a versatile model, helpful in staff development such as by tutoring and assessing medical and paramedical workers.[7] Most teledermatology collaborative projects also involve some degree of tele-education in addition to tele-assistance. Thus, in addition to long-distance consultation, they also provide continuing medical education (CME) for physicians who submit cases. Applications for tele-education mainly integrate text and images (static or dynamic) and/or virtual reality models to achieve health education.

The use of web applications for discussion forums represents another application of teledermatology. The main objective of such applications is to create a quick and easy method for teleconsultation from a pool of expert consultants. The philosophy behind these 'DermOnline' communities is open access teleconsultation in dermatology, which means that these platforms are free to all users and that the users themselves generate the content by sending and answering the teleconsultations. These communities have moderators who check both the subscribers and the content of the requests in order to guarantee friendly and orderly virtual interaction.

Teledermatology in developing countries

There are several teledermatology networks and projects in developing countries.

The telederm.org application and networks

The telederm.org application was initiated by the Department of Dermatology of the Medical University of Graz, Austria, in 2002. The primary goal was to develop a software application that would facilitate worldwide exchange of knowledge and expertise in dermatology and dermatopathology. The application is now used by several teledermatology networks, some of which are active in developing countries, including the telederm.org project and the Africa Teledermatology Project.[7,17–19] Versions of the application are available in German, Italian, Chinese, Turkish languages, Serbian and Hebrew.

The program provides the functionality to store and forward medical cases with attached images. Within a particular network, users are categorized as either clients or experts. Clients can only submit cases to selected experts, whereas experts have the right to review cases, write comments and suggest a diagnosis, or further forward cases to other selected experts within the system (Figure 12.1). All users can subscribe for notifications so that they get an automatic email if, for example, a new comment is added to one of their cases or if a new case is entered on the site. Every network has at least one administrator who is able to register users and/or reassign consultations to preferred experts.

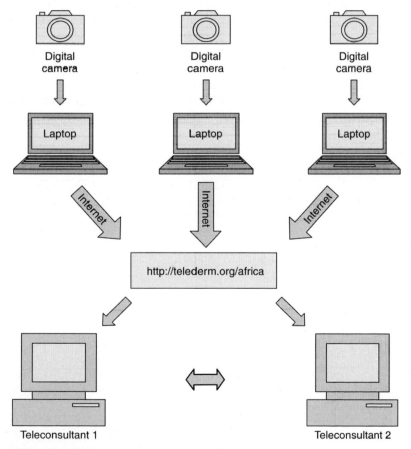

Figure 12.1 Africa Teledermatology project data flow

All requests are archived in a database with a personal archive for each user. A client can choose to send a request for consultation only to a selected expert, or he or she can submit a request to an open forum as a 'discussion case'. In the former situation, the user receives a personal answer and interactions remain private. Cases submitted as 'discussion cases' are visible to all users, who can review the cases and submit on-line opinions.

The telederm.org project

This teledermatology network was initiated in April 2002 with the aim of creating an easy-to-use platform for teleconsultation services where physicians could seek diagnostic advice in dermatology from a pool of expert consultants and discuss challenging cases.[18] An online discussion forum was included in October 2003. At present, more than 1300 physicians are subscribed to the telederm.org project from over 90 countries worldwide. Through this application, participants from different medical specialties are matched with dermatologists with a range of experience in diagnosis and management of various skin diseases. By providing a platform for interactive discussion between physicians at the point of care and experts from different countries, the telederm.org project seeks to raise the level of competence of physicians and dermatologists at the point of care on a worldwide level.

The telederm.org project is a non-profit venture under the auspices of the International Society of Teledermatology. The main academic institutions involved are the Department of Dermatology, Medical University of Graz, Graz (Austria) and the Dermatology Group, School of Medicine, University of Queensland, Brisbane (Australia). Moderators of the telederm.org community come from a range of different countries, including Turkey, Croatia, Romania, China, Pakistan, USA and India. The telederm.org project has 1024 users, with an average of 38 new users per month. It handles about 27 new cases per month.

The Africa Teledermatology project

The Africa Teledermatology project[20] was initially conceived as the 'Uganda Tele-Dermatology- and E-Learning-Project' in February 2007, with sponsorship from the Kommission für Entwicklungsfragen (KEF) der Österreichischen Akademie der Wissenschaften. Its main objective was to facilitate improvement of the treatment of skin diseases in Uganda by establishing an Internet channel for long-distance dermatological consultation between the medical Universities of Makerere and Mbarara in Uganda and the Department of Dermatology, University of Graz. In collaboration with the Department of Dermatology at the University of Pennsylvania, USA, the scope of the project was expanded, with the eventual inclusion of a number of other medical centres in eastern, central and southern Africa, which led to the formation of the Africa Teledermatology project. The main purpose of this work is to support African health workers in the diagnosis and management of patients with skin diseases, especially those having skin conditions related to HIV/AIDS.

The Africa Teledermatology project uses the telederm.org application (Figure 12.2). There are links on the application homepage to educational resources and a dermatology curriculum. An online archive of tropical skin conditions should emerge

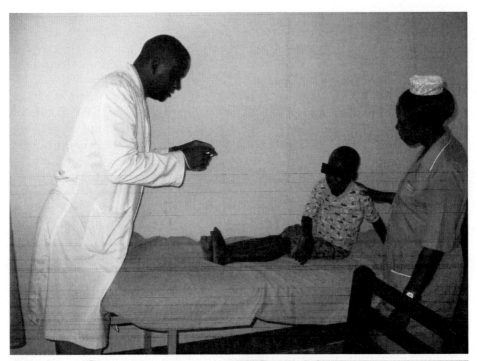

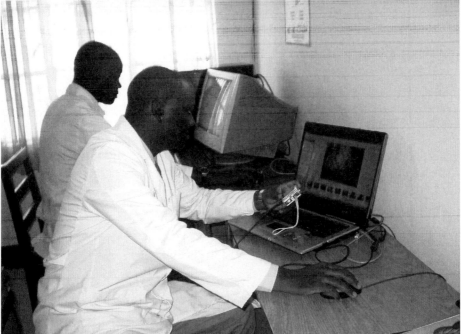

Figure 12.2 Dematologists and medical staff at Mbarara university hospital, Uganda selecting and processing difficult cases of skin diseases for teleconsultation

that will serve as an Internet source of educational material for training and updating of medical specialists and health personnel. A secondary goal of the project is to establish a platform for dermatology research collaboration. The ultimate objective is the integration of the various aspects of teledermatology and teledermatopathology into health care systems of developing countries.

In the first 12 months, 160 teledermatology-supported patient encounters have been processed. Of these, 35% of cases were children and 25% represented HIV-associated skin conditions. A number of Internet learning facilities for medical personnel have been set up on the project website, including an online case presentation with discussion, dermatology lectures and an international forum of physicians with an interest in tropical dermatology. Through this initiative, scientific cooperation has been established with a number of specialists from well-known medical/dermatology centres worldwide, who have contributed their experience in management of difficult skin conditions submitted by colleagues in Africa.

iPath application and networks

The iPath software was developed by the Department of Pathology of the University Hospital Basel as an open source framework for building web- and email-based telemedicine applications.[21–23] iPath provides the functionality to store medical cases with attached images and other documents in closed user groups. Within these groups, users can review cases, suggest diagnoses and submit comments. In addition, users can subscribe for notifications so that they receive an automatic email message if, for example, a new comment is added to one of their cases or if a new case is entered in a group. All users are organized into one or more discussion groups. Every discussion group has at least one moderator who can assign other users to the group and who can delete erroneous data.

At present, iPath hosts several telemedicine networks active in developing countries, several of which involve teledermatology. These include the following.

Solomon Islands National Telemedicine Network
This is a joint project of the National Referral Hospital in Honiara, South Pacific Medical Projects and the University of Basel.[24] It aims to use telemedicine to improve health care delivery in provincial hospitals in the Solomon Islands. There is special emphasis on the fields of dermatology, radiology, orthopaedics and paediatrics.

LT Telepatologija
This is regional network of pathologists and other medical specialists in the Baltics, based on the iPath platform.[25] Its purpose is to support clinicopathological case discussions, consultations and CME.

RAFT-Forum (telemedicine platform of the Réseau de Télé-enseignement et de Télémédecine en Afrique Francophone)
The main activity of this forum is the webcasting of interactive courses for physicians and other health care workers in French-speaking countries of Africa, including Mali, Mauritania, Senegal, Morocco, Tunisia and Madagascar.[26] The main goal is to

encourage knowledge sharing across medical institutions in the various participating countries. Topics for discussion are proposed by the partners of the network. The technology used for the webcasting works with an Internet connection, a Java-enabled web browser (e.g. Internet Explorer or Mozilla) and the free software RealPlayer.

Telemedicine Sur
This is a telemedicine platform for medical discussions, CME and consultations for medical specialists and health practitioners in Latin America.[27] Specialties involved include mainly pathology, dermatology and venereology, as well as paediatrics.

West Africa Doctors and Healthcare Professionals Network
This is a West African telemedicine network, again based on the iPath software.[28] Its goal is to enhance the communication capabilities of doctors, particularly in the areas of information access, distance learning (CME), telemedicine- and knowledge-based support of diagnosis, and management of patients in various specialties.

HealthNet Nepal
This is a health information and communication network in Nepal that provides low-cost email, Internet access and a wide range of medical and public health resources to the Nepalese health community.[29] The network began in 1994, and is subscribed to by over 230 health institutions and organizations, including hospitals, clinics, university departments, research sites and non-governmental organizations (NGOs) in both urban and rural areas. The network enables health professionals throughout Nepal to communicate and exchange knowledge.

Teledermatology project in Port St Johns, South Africa
This project was initiated in 1999 at Port St Johns, a small and poor provincial town on the east coast of South Africa, with the aim of improving access to dermatological care for patients and family practitioner clinical skills.[30,31] The scope of the project was to connect general practitioners from Port St Johns to a network with dermatology specialists. The project started with email-based store-and-forward teledermatology, but, since 2002, it has been using the iPath software. In the first year, the server in Basel was used, but, since 2003, the project has been connected to a telemedicine network run by the Telemedicine Unit of the University of Transkei (UNITRA) in Umtata.

ITG telemedicine – the Institute of Tropical Medicine website

The project was begun in 2003 by the Department of Clinical Sciences at the Institute of Tropical Medicine, Antwerp, Belgium.[32] Its aim was to facilitate the introduction of antiretroviral therapy (ART) for patients affected by HIV/AIDS in developing countries by providing training, distance support and education to health care providers working in these settings. Advice is given through email messages from a server list, and afterwards through a discussion forum on a telemedicine website. Details of the patient's history, physical examination, images, laboratory findings and questions to be answered have been received from a number of different countries.

Swinfen Charitable Trust

The Swinfen Charitable Trust was set up in 1998 by Lord and Lady Swinfen to 'assist poor, sick and disabled people in the developing world' by providing access to expert medical advice from consultants all around the world.[33] It offers provincial hospitals in developing countries the opportunity to submit cases to specialists worldwide. Communication is via a simple email telemedicine system using an automatic email messaging service developed by the Centre for Online Health at the University of Queensland, Brisbane, Australia. The core of the network is an automatic email routing system that directs the messages about each case to the parties concerned (i.e. the referring doctor and the specialists being consulted). The Swinfen Charitable Trust has been able to establish telemedicine links between remote hospitals in the developing world with international medical consultants in order to receive advice free of charge. The remote hospitals and clinics are supplied with high-resolution digital cameras and tripods, and medical staff are taught how to use the equipment. The Swinfen Charitable Trust operates in over 30 countries, including Afghanistan, Cambodia, East Timor, Iraq, Nepal, Papua New Guinea and Sri Lanka, and offers specialist advice in a wide range of fields including dermatology, dentistry, paediatrics, obstetrics and gynaecology, oncology, orthopaedics, ophthalmology, neurology, plastic surgery and trauma (see Chapter 19).

Teledermatology outcomes

There have been few previous studies focusing on teledermatology outcomes, and these have mainly involved projects in industrialized countries.[34–36] Generally, diagnostic accuracy and clinical effectiveness represent the most popular clinical outcome measures. The possible explanation for their repetitive evaluation is the rapidly changing technology, especially that of the digital cameras used in teledermatology.

As far as developing countries are concerned, there have not yet been any large studies focusing on the clinical outcomes of teledermatology, despite general consensus supporting the increased diagnostic accuracy and clinical effectiveness possible using the technique. Problems in assessment of clinical outcomes in projects in developing countries include mainly patient loss to follow up and inadequate medical record systems, although similar problems may also apply to traditional face-to-face consultations in this setting.

The economic value, clinical benefits and sustainability of teledermatology in developing countries remain to be formally proved. This is primarily because evaluations of these economic outcomes require complex analysis of the direct and indirect costs to national health providers and patients, as well as assessment of the impact of teledermatology services on earlier diagnosis and expert management.

Quality

A number of factors may lower diagnostic accuracy in teledermatology. These include poor-quality images, insufficient clinical information supplied, intrinsic difficulties of cases submitted, interference of technology in the perception of three-dimensional images, lack of ability to palpate or physically examine the patient, and lack of proper training of physicians who submit cases or who give opinions, among others. Poor-quality images may be of low resolution or may have a high level of compression. Clinical information may be confusing owing to image files from similar patients being separately sent or inconsistently coded. It is necessary that medical workers be adequately trained to take good images and instructed how to properly send cases before being involved in teledermatology projects. It is also advisable to include a link to working instructions on the homepage of teledermatology web applications; for example, see the Africa Teledermatology project website.[20]

Legal problems

The increasing availability of health information about individuals in electronic data-bases and through online networks has offered tremendous benefits to physicians, health care workers and patients. However, it has also created new legal challenges. There are presently extensive discussions concerning the potential risks and complex legal problems associated with telemedicine health care services provided to patients from remote locations using telecommunication. Legal problems relate generally to problems concerning the privacy of identifiable health information, and the reliability and quality of health data, as well as medical liability. Since telemedicine in developing countries is mainly practised across state borders, providers must be aware of the potential risks concerning medical liability in the respective countries where the patients are located. There is a need for developing countries to adopt rules and regulations to address legal aspects involved in the use of telemedicine in order to safeguard the rights of patients. Matters that need to be considered include mainly safeguards about data forwarding, security of the patient's data (including images), confidentiality and the responsibilities of health workers involved in telemedicine.

Generally speaking, local physicians are directly responsible for treatments deriving from teleconsultations in dermatology. The medico-legal position of remote expert dermatologists is similar to that when the telephone, fax, email or letter is used for consultation, since all these methods amount to the provision of advice from a distance, and normal standards of care and skill should therefore apply. In teledermatology, there is an obligation to practise to a reasonable level of skill. The referring doctor must give accurate clinical information and submit representative images of reasonable quality. Complicated treatment procedures recommended by remote experts need the patient's permission before being carried out.

Integration and intercultural context

Preliminary studies have confirmed the feasibility and benefits of integrating teledermatology into the medical care systems of developing countries. However, there are major challenges to sustainability, including political, economic, technical as well as cultural barriers. Many governments in developing countries are gradually recognizing the potential of telemedicine to improve health care delivery and reduce national health care budgets. Obviously, dermatology is not a main focus of government and NGO health policies in developing countries, since available resources are normally allocated to medical conditions with more serious consequences, such as malaria, tuberculosis and HIV/AIDS rather than to non-lethal skin disorders.

As a basis for introducing and sustaining teledermatology services in developing countries, it is crucial that the relevant national governments modernize internal communication in hospitals and remote medical centres. Internet services need to be widely accessible, even in rural parts of the developing world. The availability of email services in remote areas has potential benefits for poor countries. It is cheap, requires relatively simple hardware and software, and can easily deliver stored information. The deployment of fixed or mobile telecentres promises to be valuable in bringing telemedicine services to remote areas.

Cultural barriers may play a negative role in the sustainability of teledermatology programmes, and may be based on individual, institutional or societal attitudes. Individual patients may feel uncomfortable or refuse to be involved in teledermatology owing to a lack of trust in the ability of the technology to improve their health. This attitude may be based on inadequate information as a result of political and economic differences, cultural attitudes, language barriers and differences in perceptions of 'health and wellness'. Studies have shown that patients who are well acquainted with computers and the Internet tend to be more open to the use of telemedicine.[37] There is a need for proper explanation in advance, together with information for patients about teledermatology, such as what it is and what its benefits are, before patients are offered teledermatology.

Local physicians and health workers may also adopt a negative attitude to the use of teledermatology services for a number of reasons. They may be uncomfortable about sending consultations in English, feel that teledermatology cannot improve the health of their patients, distrust the safety and privacy of the systems used, prefer the option of transferring patients, or feel that teledermatology services cannot lower their health care costs. Moreover, because of the limited number of doctors in developing countries, local physicians and health workers may be concerned that teledermatology systems will be time-consuming and generate unnecessary extra work. It is therefore crucial that leaders at local hospitals and medical centres be engaged early enough in the process of introducing teledermatology services and be made aware of the potential and relative advantages of the technique. Participating local physicians and health workers should also receive comprehensive education and training packages, as well as support to improve their technical and media skills, prior to their involvement in teledermatology projects. It is an advantage to add formal guidelines and protocols of instructions on the homepages of web applications. In order to facilitate faster adoption, local health workers selected to participate in teledermatology projects should preferably have prior experience in the use of the Internet.

In summary, consideration of a range of economic, political and technical factors in the host country or institution during the planning and early stages of implementation of teledermatology projects should help to ensure the viability and sustainability, as well as the integration, of teledermatology programmes (Box 12.2).

Box 12.2 Practical steps in setting up a teledermatology project

1 Review prior telemedicine and teledermatology activities in the region of interest.

2 Assess current technologies and telecommunications, as well as human resources available.

3 Assess clinical, educational and administrative needs and priorities.

4 Assess the ability of teledermatology to meet the needs and willingness of health professionals to use the technology.

5 Review the current policies (or lack of policies) that may affect the practice of teledermatology in both the remote sites and the referral centres.

6 Plan and distribute information and educational packages to all individuals potentially involved.

7 Find out about available technology and telecommunications links at all potential sites, and make sure that the technology is available at remote sites.

8 Identify teledermatology technology that best meets the needs of the communities, technical requirements and security, and is compatible with the referral centres.

9 Establish contacts with potential remote centres.

10 Establish a team of individual to help in strategic planning, implementation and evaluation of the initial phases of the project.

11 Contract and choose a vendor to install the required IT infrastructure at each of the remote sites.

12 Identify the telecommunications options and work with the vendor(s) to test and implement the preferred option.

13 Educate and train potential users about the teledermatology system and how to use it.

14 Educate and train potential technicians how to repair the technology

15 Educate the administrators/managers at the teledermatology sites about how it may affect current workflow.

16 Initiate and conduct a preliminary evaluation of design, implementation and technical performance, as well as clinical staff and patient satisfaction

17 Develop an ongoing education and training programme focused on individuals who are not part of the original rollout.

Financial aspects

Most teledermatology activity in developing countries represents pilot projects receiving subsidized funding from external governments and NGOs, or from foreign universities and hospitals. There is very little available information concerning the cost-effectiveness and sustainability of these services. Economic analyses of the viability of teledermatology projects are also complicated owing to the rapidly declining cost of hardware and telecommunications, and the presence of a number of hidden costs and benefits, such as the opportunity cost of a patient's time and the intangible benefit of an earlier correct diagnosis, which are hard to quantify. Nevertheless, for the adoption of teledermatology services in countries with low resources, it is necessary to obtain reasonable estimates of the financial consequences, including the costs of implementation and subsequent operation. Proper prior financial planning will help to ensure success and sustainability.

Implementation expenses in teledermatology projects mainly comprise the costs for equipment (in a store-and-forward system, these include digital camera and accessories, computers, image editing programs, a back-up system and a printer), equipment maintenance, telecommunication and staff training. Sustainability expenses tend not to depend on the number of users/patients served. They include costs related to the operation and running of the project, acquiring the physical space, supplies and travel.

Future developments

The number of medical centres using teledermatology in developing countries is increasing, and the technique could soon become an integral part of the health care system in some countries. Future technical developments may improve the delivery of teledermatology consultations in developing countries. For instance, the use of mobile phones with built-in cameras represents a potential alternative to bulky digital cameras and computers in more remote areas.[16,38,39] Teledermatopathology, a related field to teledermatology, could refine dermatology teleconsultation by providing a channel for confirming diagnoses as well as for training and supervision and collaborative research. Until now, establishing teledermatopathology services has been mainly hampered by the high implementation costs.

There is an urgent need for physicians and health policy makers in the developing world to establish standards and regulations concerning the practice of telemedicine and teledermatology. Future studies should define the ethical, legal, economic and technical standards required of telemedical referrals in individual countries that would ensure acceptance, economic viability and effectiveness, as well as security, privacy and confidentiality of patients. Studies focusing on teledermatology outcomes should be conducted to confirm its clinical benefits and cost-effectiveness.

Finally, the global increase in the number of teledermatology networks implies a need to establish a common international teledermatology forum. Such a forum could serve to educate and assist users and policy makers in different parts of the developing and industrialized world on how to optimize teledermatology services, especially through identification of proven low-cost technology approaches.

Further reading

FreeMedicalJournals.com. Available at: www.freemedicaljournals.com.

I Do Imaging: Free Medical Imaging Software. Available at: www.idoimaging.com/index.shtml.

Krupinski E, BurdickA, Pak H et al. *American Telemedicine Association's Practice Guidelines for Teledermatology*. Available at: www.liebertonline.com/doi/abs/10.1089/tmj.2007.0129.

Pak H, Burg G. Store-and-forward teledermatology. *eMedicine*. Available at: www.emedicine.com/derm/topic560.htm.

Wootton R, Oakley A, eds. *Teledermatology*. London: Royal Society of Medicine Press, 2002.

References

1. Schmid-Grendelmeier P, Masenga EJ, Haeffner A, Burg G. Teledermatology as a new tool in sub-saharan Africa: an experience from Tanzania. *J Am Acad Dermatol* 2000; **42**: 833–5.
2. Schmid-Grendelmeier P, Doe P, Pakenham-Walsh N. Teledermatology in sub-Saharan Africa. *Curr Probl Dermatol* 2003; **32**: 233–46.
3. Caumes E, Le Bris V, Couzigou C et al. Dermatoses associated with travel to Burkina Faso and diagnosed by means of teledermatology. *Br J Dermatol* 2004; **150**: 312–16.
4. Fraser HSF, McGrath St JD. Information technology and telemedicine in subSaharan Africa. *BMJ* 2000; **321**; 465–6.
5. Miot HA, Paixão MP, Wen CL. Teledermatology – past, present and future. *An Bras Dermatol* 2005; **80**: 523–32
6. House M, Keough E, Hillman D et al. Into Africa: the telemedicine links between Canada, Kenya and Uganda. *CMAJ* 1987 15; **136**: 398–400.
7. First World Congress of Teledermatology and Annual Meeting of the Austrian Scientific Society of Telemedicine, 9–11 November 2006, Graz, Austria. Available at: www.teledermatology-society.org/worldcongress.
8. Kristiansen IS, Poulsen PB, Jensen KU. Economic aspects – saving billions with telemedicine: fact or fiction? *Curr Probl Dermatol* 2003; **32**: 62–70.
9. Eedy DJ, Wootton R. Teledermatology: a review. *Br J Dermatol* 2001; **144**: 696–707.
10. Du Moulin MF, Bullens-Goessens YI, Henquet CJ et al. The reliability of diagnosis using store-and-forward teledermatology. *J Telemed Telecare* 2003; **9**: 249–52.
11. Pak HS, Harden D, Cruess D et al. Teledermatology: an intraobserver diagnostic correlation study, Part II. *Cutis* 2003; **71**: 476–80.
12. Piccolo D, Smolle J, Wolf IH et al. Face-to-face diagnosis versus telediagnosis of pigmented skin tumors: a teledermoscopic study. *Arch Dermatol* 1999; **135**: 1467–71.
13. Granlund H. Aspects of quality: face-to-face versus teleconsulting. *Curr Probl Dermatol* 2003; **32**: 158–66.
14. Taylor P, Goldsmith P, Murray K et al. Evaluating a telemedicine system to assist in the management of dermatology referrals. *Br J Dermatol* 2001; **144**: 328–33.
15. Oliveira MR, Wen CL, Neto CF et al. Web site for training nonmedical health-care workers to identify potentially malignant skin lesions and for teledermatology. *Telemed J E Health* 2002; **8**: 323–32.
16. Braun RP, Vecchietti JL, Thomas L et al. Telemedical wound care using a new generation of mobile telephones: a feasibility study. *Arch Dermatol* 2005; **141**: 254–8.
17. Soyer HP, Hofmann-Wellenhof R, Massone C et al. Telederm.org: freely available online consultations in dermatology. *PLoS Med* 2005; **2**: e87.
18. Massone C, Hofmann-Wellenhof R, Gabler G et al. Global teledermatology: a specific web application for dermatological consultation. *Internet Health* 2004; **3**: e3. Available at: www.Internet-health.org/ih200431e03.html.
19. Massone C, Soyer HP, Hofmann-Wellenhof R et al. Two years experience with Web-based teleconsulting in dermatology. *J Telemed Telecare* 2006; **12**: 83–7.
20. Africa Teledermatology Project. Available at: telederm.org/africa.
21. iPath. Available at: ipath.ch.
22. Brauchli K, O'Mahony D, Banach L, Oberholzer M. iPath – a telemedicine platform to support health providers in low resource settings. *Stud Health Technol Inform* 2005; **114**: 11–17.
23. Brauchli K, Christen H, Haroske G et al. Telemicroscopy by the Internet revisited. *J Pathol* 2002; **196**: 238–43.
24. Solomon Islands Telemedicine Network. Available at: telemed.ipath.ch/solomons.
25. LT Telepatologija – Lithuania. Available at: ipath.ch/site/node/441. Also, in Lithuanian, at: telemed.ipath.ch/lithuania.
26. RAFT. Available at: raft.hcuge.ch.
27. Telemedecina Sur. Available at: telemed.ipath.ch/tmsur.
28. West Africa Doctors and Healthcare Professionals Network. Available at: www.wadn.org.
29. HealthNet Nepal. Available at: www.healthnet.org.np.
30. Teledermatology in Port St Johns, South Africa. Available at: ipath.ch/site/node/22.
31. O'Mahony D, Banach L, Mahapa DH et al. Teledermatology in a rural family practice. *SA Fam Pract* 2002; **25**: 4–8.
32. Telemedicine: Online Support for HIV/AIDS Care. Available at: telemedicine.itg.be/telemedicine/site/Default.asp.

33. Swinfen Charitable Trust Website. www.swinfencharitabletrust.org.
34. Wootton R, Bloomer SE, Corbett R et al. Multicentre randomised control trial comparing real time tele-dermatology with conventional outpatient dermatological care: societal cost-benefit analysis. *BMJ* 2000; **320**: 1252–6.
35. Heinzelmann PJ, Williams CM, Lugn NE, Kvedar JC. Clinical outcomes associated with telemedicine/ telehealth. *Telemed J E Health* 2005; **11**: 329–47.
36. Aoki N, Dunn K, Johnson-Throop KA, Turley JP. Outcomes and methods in telemedicine evaluation. *Telemed J E Health* 2003; **9**: 393–401.
37. Qureshi AA, Kvedar JC. Patient knowledge and attitude toward information technology and teledermatology: some tentative findings. *Telemed J E Health* 2003; **9**: 259–64.
38. Massone C, Lozzi GP, Wurm E et al. Cellular phones in clinical teledermatology. *Arch Dermatol* 2006; **141**: 1319–20.
39. Massone C, Lozzi GP, Wurm E et al. Personal digital assistants in teledermatology. *Br J Dermatol* 2006; **154**: 801–2.

13 Cross-cultural telemedicine via email: Experience in Cambodia and the USA

Paul Heinzelmann, Rithy Chau, Daniel Liu and Joseph Kvedar

Introduction

The Khmer empire was once the largest and most powerful in South-East Asia. The descendant country of Cambodia is now home to over 14 million people. The Vietnam War and the violent reign of the Khmer Rouge in the 1970s left millions dead or traumatized. The collapsed health system was left with an enormous burden of infectious diseases, malnutrition and psychological trauma. In 1979, there were thought to be fewer than 50 doctors left in the entire country.[1]

The average annual rate of 0.3 medical contacts per person remains the lowest in the region. This may be primarily due to a lack of access, as Cambodia has the lowest ratio of physicians to population in the region.[2] Despite the fact that 85% of Cambodians live in rural areas, only 13% of government health workers work there.[2] The problems associated with the lack of access are compounded by frequent misuse of prescription drugs and indigenous health practices that are at times dangerous.[3] For example, animist healers may sometimes treat open fractures with a splint and a topical application called 'ma'lou'. This compound is made from chewed betel nut and lime paste, and has been known to result in serious infection or even death.

Poor health system performance has led to poor health outcomes. One out of 12 children never lives to reach the age of five years,[4] and among antenatal clinic attendees, HIV is estimated at 2.2%, the highest reported for any country in Asia.[5] The tuberculosis case rate (508 per 100 000 persons) is approximately 100 times that of the USA and is the highest rate in Asia.[6] Malaria remains endemic, and has a prevalence of 5 per 1000 persons.[7] Meanwhile, there is a growing prevalence of chronic non-communicable disease, and traumatic injuries and deaths from landmines and road traffic accidents continue steadily.

Cambodia ranks among the lowest countries on the United Nations Human Development Index (it was ranked 129 of 177 countries in 2006)[8] and among the highest in poverty. Forty percent of Cambodians live on less than US$10 per month, and some 45% of the population has to borrow money to pay for health care services, which in turn has become the main cause of indebtedness and loss of land ownership.[9] Table 13.1 compares Cambodia's health indicators and resources with those of the USA.

Table 13.1 Health indicators and resources: the USA versus Cambodia[19]

	USA	Cambodia	Year
Health indicators			
Life expectancy at birth (years) males	75	51	2005
Life expectancy at birth (years) females	80	57	2005
Under-5 mortality rate (per 1000 live births)	8	143	2005
Infant mortality rate (per 1000 live births)	7	98	2005
Deaths due to HIV/AIDS (per 100 000 population per year)	5	114	2005
Mortality rate for non-communicable diseases (per 100 000 population per year)	460	853	2002
Mortality rate for cardiovascular diseases (per 100 000 population per year)	188	392	2002
Health care resources			
Physicians (density per 1000 inhabitants)	2.6	0.2	2000
Nurses (density per 1000 inhabitants)	9.4	0.6	2000
Pharmacists (density per 1000 inhabitants)	0.9	0.04	2000
Total expenditure on health (% of GDP)	15.4	6.7	2004
General government expenditure on health (% of total expenditure on health)	44.7	25.8	2004
Private expenditure on health (% of total expenditure on health)	55.3	74.2	2004
Out-of-pocket expenditure (% of total private expenditure on health)	23.8	85.4	2004
Per capita total expenditure on health (US$)	6096	23.6	2004
Gross national income per capita (purchasing power parity[a]) (US$)	41 950	2490	2005

[a]Purchasing power parity is a currency conversion rate that both converts a common currency and equalizes the purchasing power of different currencies. It eliminates the differences in price levels between countries in the process of conversion.

Telecommunications

During the 1990s, the advent of the Internet and the growth of mobile phone technology dramatically changed the way that people communicate and share information on a global scale. Disparities in access to these networks inadvertently left Cambodia and many other regions isolated by a 'digital divide'. None the less, broad public access to the Internet within Cambodia was boosted by foreign investment in the late 1990s from countries such as Canada and Australia via a link through Singapore.[10] Like many developing countries, diffusion has been slow, with only 2 of every 1000 citizens becoming Internet users by 2002.[11]

Early investment in mobile phone networks gave Cambodia the distinction of being the first country in the world where mobile phone subscribers outnumbered fixed line subscribers. By 2000, four out of five telephone subscribers were using a mobile

Table 13.2 Information and communication technology (ICT) indicators[20]

	USA	Cambodia	Year
ICT diffusion[a]	0.81	0.21	2004
ICT connectivity[a]	0.75	0.01	2004
ICT access[a]	0.87	0.41	2004
ICT policy[a]	1.0	0.38	2004
Mobile phone subscribers per 1000 inhabitants	49	3	2002
Personal computers per 1000 inhabitants	659	2	2002
Internet users per 1000 inhabitants	551	2	2002

[a]*Diffusion* is the average of three factors: *connectivity*, which is based on the number of Internet hosts, PCs, telephone main lines, mobile subscribers per capita; *access*, which is based on the estimated number of Internet subscribers, adult literacy rate, cost of a local call and GDP; and *policy*, which is based on the presence of Internet exchanges, level of competition in telecommunications, level of competition in the Internet service provider market.

phone – the highest ratio in the world.[10] Various information and communication technology (ICT) indicators in Cambodia and the USA are compared in Table 13.2.

Humanitarian non-profit organizations and social entrepreneurs have begun to recognize the opportunity to use these growing communications networks for social change. The non-profit organization American Assistance for Cambodia (AAfC) and its founder provide one example. Bernard Krisher formed the AAfC in 1993 with the aim of rehabilitating Cambodia. Since that time, the AAfC has built over 300 elementary schools throughout rural Cambodia and has provided approximately one-third of them with access to the Internet.[12] This growing Internet infrastructure established by AAfC has become the backbone for a cross-cultural, multi-organizational telemedicine project that allows physicians at the Harvard Medical School in Boston and clinicians at the Sihanouk Hospital Centre of HOPE in Phnom Penh to support patient care in under-served regions of Cambodia.

Telemedicine programme

The telemedicine programme is a collaboration between the AAfC, Operation Village Health (a project of the Center for Connected Health of the Partners HealthCare system in Boston) and the Sihanouk Hospital Centre of HOPE in Phnom Penh. The aim is to provide remote consultation and supporting tools to build capacity and improve local care for those living in rural Cambodia.

The local health care providers (Cambodian nurses and doctors) play a central role in the work. After assessing the patient (i.e. history and physical and diagnostic tests), they transcribe a document of their findings into English and transmit this, together with attached images, via email to the consulting clinicians in Boston and Phnom Penh for review. Coordinators at each facility direct the cases to the appropriate medical specialist. After reviewing the medical cases, the offsite clinicians return their recommendations. The supportive guidance delivered in this way not only enhances the quality of care, but also provides a unique educational opportunity.

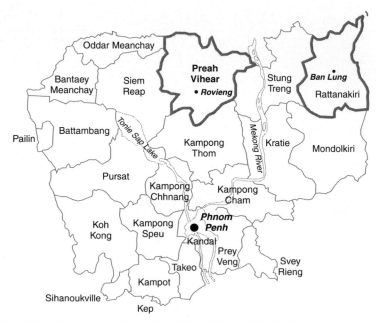

Figure 13.1 Sites of operation of the telemedicine clinics in Cambodia

The programme currently operates at two sites in northern Cambodia (Figure 13.1). In the first seven years, approximately 1000 telemedicine-supported patient encounters were completed at the two sites.

Site 1: Rovieng Health Centre

The Rovieng district is located in the Preah Vihear province, and is home to 6493 families (approximately 32 000 people). The region is served by two health centres, which are located 15 km apart. The region is primarily an agricultural community, and the estimated average annual income is less than US$50. Indigenous medical practices are still commonly used, and include techniques that involve direct skin contact (i.e. cupping, pinching and coining), animistic healing practices and the use of various herbal remedies.[13] Most visitors to the health centre have never met a Western-trained physician in person.

The pilot telemedicine programme began in February 2001 at one of the health centres in Rovieng. Each month, 25–40 people gather there to have their medical conditions assessed and, if appropriate, triaged for telemedicine consultation. Typically, 15–20 of these cases are documented in English and sent via email to Western-trained clinicians located in Phnom Penh and Boston. To date, telemedicine patients have come from 35 of the 57 villages in the district. On many occasions, those living near the health centre provide accommodation for people who have travelled longer distances by allowing them to stay for several days in their homes.

This site is 235 km and about 6 hours by road from the major hospitals in the capital city of Phnom Penh. It is also about 4 hours from the nearest referral hospital. Despite the existence of these more sophisticated facilities, cost, uncertainty and time constraints prevent most village inhabitants from seeking care outside the village.

To facilitate improved local care, a nurse from Sihanouk Hospital Centre of HOPE travels by road from Phnom Penh to Rovieng each month. Those patients who cannot be easily diagnosed and treated by the nurse have their cases sent by email to consulting physicians using the satellite Internet connection at the adjacent elementary school. The local nurse must assess each patient and transcribe the details of the encounter before these recommendations are provided. Once received by the relevant consultant, recommendations for patient management are generally returned to the nurse within 12 hours.

The telemedicine clinic operates as follows:

Day 1: Nurse and driver travel from Phnom Penh to Rovieng.
Day 2: Nurse assesses patients, performs local laboratory tests, photographs patients and sends transcribed cases in English to consultants for review via email. Consulting clinicians in the USA and Phnom Penh review cases and return their recommendations within 12 hours.
Day 3: Same activities as Day 2.
Day 4: Nurse reviews and implements consultant recommendations.
Day 5: Blood samples for any off-site testing are collected; nurse and driver return to Phnom Penh with blood samples in a cooler.

To enhance local diagnostic capacity, five point-of-care laboratory tests were introduced in October 2004. The availability of these tests has decreased the need for more expensive off-site laboratory testing, allowing quicker and more accurate diagnosis. The five tests were:

(1) blood glucose
(2) haemoglobin
(3) urine analysis (glucose, ketones, pH, specific gravity, protein, leucocyte esterase, nitrites)
(4) urine chorionic gonadotrophin (pregnancy test)
(5) faecal occult blood.

The choice of these tests was based on several factors, including the prevalence of local disease, ease of use, storage requirements, low cost, and the ability to use them without reliance on running water or electricity. Simple algorithms for using these tests were also created so that the nurse could use them independently. Several manufacturers kindly donated test kits to launch the service.

Site 2: Rattanakiri Referral Hospital

Based on the success of telemedicine in Rovieng, a second site opened in April 2003 at the Rattanakiri Referral Hospital (RRH) in Banlung, the capital of the Rattanakiri province. This province is home to a mixture of 13 ethnic and tribal groups, and is generally considered to be the poorest of the provinces. Non-Western indigenous health practices are widely practised. Unlike the cases from Rovieng, these referrals are initiated by Cambodian physicians working at the RRH, who have greater access to local resources, including ECG measurement, laboratory tests and basic X-ray imaging. Accordingly, the cases tend to be more complex, although there is usually more information for consulting physicians to consider in formulating their recommendations. As with the Rovieng site, the cases are sent each month as email messages using a satellite connection to the Internet. Turnaround time for receipt of consultant recommendations is also less than 12 hours. The telemedicine clinic operates as follows:

Day 1:   Patients in need of teleconsultation are selected by local physicians.
Day 2:   Cases are transcribed into English; relevant images (e.g. skin, ECG, X-ray or ultrasound) are attached and sent via email to consulting clinicians; consulting clinicians in USA and Phnom Penh review cases and return their recommendations within 12 hours.
Day 3:   Local physicians review and implement the recommendations
Day 4:   Any remaining arrangements for off-site testing or referral are made.

This site received its initial financial support from the Markle Foundation and is now largely supported by private individual donations, most notably from Edward and Laurie Bacharach.

Effects on local care

Retrospective reviews of the telemedicine work have been completed by staff at the Center for Connected Health and the Harvard Medical School. These studies have examined the types of patients participating in the telemedicine programme, the clinical impact on the community, and the utility and cost savings associated with the portable point-of-care laboratory. To date, the majority of these formal evaluations and reviews have focused on operations at the Rovieng site. The results are summarized below.

Demographics and case mix

A retrospective review evaluated all cases completed at the Rovieng site from January 2005 to May 2006.[13] There were 196 teleconsultations for 106 patients. The majority of patients were female, and two-thirds of all patients sought telemedicine care on more than one occasion (Table 13.3). Most visits for new patients were for non-communicable chronic diseases (Table 13.4). The most frequent diagnosis among all patients was dyspepsia (Table13.5).

Clinical impact

In a previous study, the first 214 cases of the programme were reviewed.[14] The mean duration of the chief complaint among first-time clinic visitors was 37 months for the first 6 months of the study period. By the last six months of the study period, this had dropped to 8 months (Figure 13.2). The proportion of patients referred for care at offsite facilities decreased by 51% per year of clinic operation (95% confidence interval 27–75%; $p < 0.001$) (Figure 13.3). These data suggest that longstanding chronic conditions among villagers are now being addressed and that appropriate care can be delivered locally.

Table 13.3 Patient utilization and demographics: Rovieng, January 2005–May 2006

	Number	%
Total number of visits	196	100
Follow-up visits	132	67
New patient visits	64	33
Total patients	86	100
Female	64	74
Male	22	26
Age (years): 0–14	7	8
15–64	65	76
≥65	14	16

Table 13.4 Most frequent complaints among new patients: Rovieng, January 2005–May 2006 ($n = 64$)

	Number	%
Epigastric pain	9	14
Cough	6	9
Neck mass	5	8
Joint pain	5	8
Shortness of breath	5	8
Palpitations	5	8
Dizziness	5	8
Polydipsia / polyuria	4	6
Oedema	4	6

Table 13.5 Most frequent diagnoses: Rovieng, January 2005–May 2006. There were 196 consultations for 106 patients, some of whom had multiple diagnoses.

Diagnosis	Visits, including this diagnosis	Patients
Dyspepsia	45	30
Hypertension	73	27
Anaemia	40	22
Diabetes (type 2)	48	15
Thyroid disease	23	12
Total	229	106

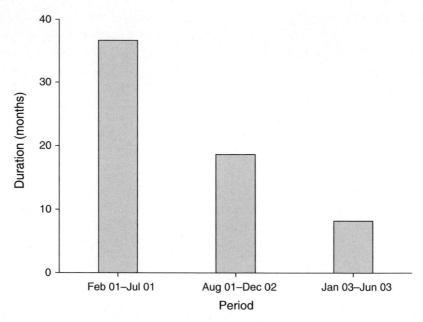

Figure 13.2 Duration of patients' primary chief complaint at initial visit, during three phases of the study period. (Reproduced with permission from *Telemed J E Health* 2005; **11**(1), published by Mary Ann Liebert, Inc.)

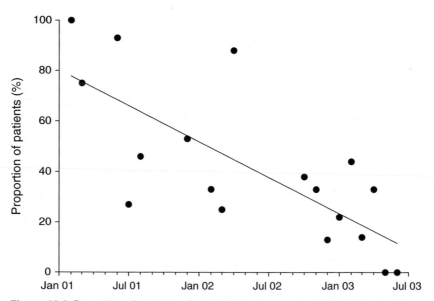

Figure 13.3 Proportion of patients referred off-site for care during the study period. (Reproduced with permission from *Telemed J E Health* 2005; **11**(1), published by Mary Ann Liebert, Inc.)

Point-of-care testing

Comparisons were made between the 57 patient encounters occurring after the introduction of the laboratory tests and 119 encounters occurring in the year before, which served as historical controls. Overall, the proportion of patient cases receiving laboratory testing did not increase (Fisher's exact test, $p = 0.71$). Meanwhile, the proportion of cases requiring off-site referral for the completion of laboratory testing decreased significantly from an average of 69% to 35% ($p < 0.001$). The costs associated with laboratory testing also decreased, from an estimated average of US$41 to US$17 per month.[15]

Lessons learned

Several valuable lessons have been learned during seven years of operation. The project has demonstrated the feasibility of using store-and-forward telemedicine across time zones, socioeconomic strata and cultures. More specific observations have also been made, and can be categorized as human, economic or technology factors (Table 13.6).

Human factors

Human factors are arguably the most important for success. This requires not only commitment at the organization level, but also adoption by the users: the patients, local care providers and consulting physicians.

Patients

Demand by patients for telemedicine services at the Rovieng Health Centre has remained high, particularly among women aged 15–64 years. The sustained patient volume and rate of return visits suggest that cross-cultural telemedicine can compete successfully with conventional and local indigenous practices. This is probably due to several factors.

The willingness of families to accommodate one another during the monthly telemedicine clinics signals a high degree of 'social capital' within this community. The monthly schedule of the clinics encourages adherence among patients through frequent opportunities to educate, inform and reinforce the benefits of the prescribed medication. The social nature of these monthly gatherings brings community members together, and may also play a role in adherence – much like that of a support group or

Table 13.6 Proposed characteristics of programme success

Factor	Characteristics
Human	Willingness to participate/collaborate, adoption, satisfaction, cultural competence, supportive political environment
Economic	Sustainability, affordability, marketability, profitability
Technological	Usability, interoperability, scalability, transferability

'group visit' (a model of chronic care management gaining popularity among US primary care physicians). The significance of this is most evident in instances where patients are asked to begin long-term medication regimens that may have little effect on their sense of wellbeing – or even produce undesirable side effects. For example, antihypertensive medications are now frequently prescribed to treat the surprisingly high prevalence of high blood pressure in this community. The high return rate among villagers and the apparent adherence to modern drug regimens suggests that the concept of chronic disease management is being incorporated into the local culture.

It is important to note that, at present, there is no direct cost to patients for telemedicine visits or for the prescribed medications recommended in the consultations, which undoubtedly encourages a high return rate. To better understand patient expectations, their satisfaction and willingness-to-pay were assessed in 2003 using a verbally administered survey.[7] All patients surveyed ($n = 63$) were either 'satisfied' or 'very satisfied' with the use of telemedicine as an alternative to the seeking of care within the traditional Cambodian health system. Of those surveyed, 78% were willing to pay for these services. Of those willing to pay, the mean amount was US$0.63 per visit.

Local providers

Initially the dialogue between local and consulting clinicians was a fairly unstructured exchange, akin to an instant messaging Internet 'chat'. However, as the telemedicine programme has matured, this has evolved into a structured format using a standardized template for history and physical examination (Box 13.1).

The visiting telemedicine nurse in Rovieng is part of the SHCH staff, and participation is mandated in the job description. In contrast, telemedicine at the RRH depends on the interest and willingness of the local physicians to participate. Patients that are managed using telemedicine require more local physician time, although there is no additional physician remuneration. It could be argued that the inherent opportunity cost to physicians who participate under this arrangement might ultimately become a barrier to sustainability. Possible methods of maintaining the participation of local Cambodian physicians include reducing lengthy translation/transcription times and improving cultural competence among US consultants to ensure that their recommendations are relevant to the local context and available resources.

Consulting physicians

Informal inquiries of consulting clinicians in the USA and Phnom Penh have revealed several potential areas for quality improvement. To maximize the value of the consulting physician's recommendations and avoid a 'garbage-in–garbage-out' situation, measures should be taken to ensure the completeness of the initial clinical data collected and documented by the local provider. Convenient and reliable web access to patient medical records could enhance continuity of care for those with recurring or chronic conditions.

Overall, a high degree of cultural competence among consulting and local clinicians has been important to the successful introduction of Western-based medical concepts such as chronic disease (i.e. diabetes and hypertension) and prevention.

Box 13.1 Standardized template for history and physical examination

Patient:

Chief complaint:

History of present illness:

Past medical/surgical history:

Social history:

Allergies:

Family history:

Review of systems:

Physical examination:

Vital signs: (blood pressure, pulse, respiration, temperature, weight)

General:

Head, eyes, ears, nose, throat:

Chest:

Abdomen:

Musculoskeletal:

Neurological:

Genitourinary:

Rectal:

Previous laboratory studies:

Laboratory studies requested:

Assessment:

Plan:

Comments/notes:

Examined by: Date:

Economic factors

Grants, foundations and private donations from organizations such as the Asia Development Bank and Japanese corporate sponsors have funded the efforts of AAfC. Satellite services (estimated cost US$285 per site per month) have been secured as corporate gift-in-kind donations from a Thai telecommunications company. By 'piggy-backing' the telemedicine programme onto this existing Internet infrastructure, large capital investments have been avoided.

None the less, certain problems remain, such as the cost implications of telemedicine. As mentioned above, the local physician time required per patient is greater than for traditional care in cases originating at the RRH. Furthermore, strict adherence by local clinicians to the recommendations of US consulting physicians who are uninformed about local resource constraints could result in increased utilization and, therefore, cost.

At present, the programme continues to rely on volunteers and donations from charitable organizations. As a result, alternative economic schemes (i.e. fee-for-service or a pooled payment model) may eventually need to be introduced if this model of care is to be transferred to other regions or implemented on a broader scale. Some revenue has been generated via the online sales of locally produced products such as coffee, scarves and other handicrafts, but, to date, this has contributed little to the overall operating budget.

Technological factors

Reliable electrical power and Internet connectivity are central to the operation of the programme. The use of solar panels supplemented by portable generators has proven to be feasible for the operation of computers and satellite communications equipment. Telecommunication employs a low-to-moderate range of bandwidth and uses a store-and-forward, asynchronous email mode of communication. These characteristics contribute to the potential for scalability, especially as the use of email and familiarity with computers among Cambodians grow. Expansion of Internet connectivity, however, has been restricted by poverty, the lack of a rigorous academic community to nurture networking, the complexity of using the Khmer language with computing and application development, a shortage of dial-up telephone lines and restrictive government regulations.[10]

In terms of laboratory technologies to support remote consultations, the point-of-care laboratory tests appear to be feasible, clinically useful and likely to reduce the need for slower, more expensive offsite testing.

Future directions

The data from the retrospective reviews and lessons learned have helped to plan a strategy for the future.

Human factors

As there is a high level of demand for management of chronic illnesses such as diabetes and hypertension, an increased emphasis on continuity of care is planned for patients at the Rovieng site.

Recently, the non-governmental organization HealthNet International has been contracted by the Cambodia Ministry of Health to reform health care delivery in several provinces, including Rattanakiri. As a result, the telemedicine component at the RRH is also being restructured. Expected benefits include greater local ownership and accountability of the programme through stronger administrative oversight and physician participation. This change is expected to integrate telemedicine more formally into the hospital's service and enable a greater measure of evaluation and quality control. In addition, it is hoped that this new arrangement will facilitate a stronger relationship with the Ministry of Health and potentially enable broader use of telemedicine to support government-sponsored public health initiatives.

To build local capacity, an increased emphasis on clinician education is anticipated. Linking educational content directly to patient care recommendations is being considered as one way to enhance the experiential learning that already occurs. Skills training in the use of computers, project management and administration would also enable greater local ownership of the programme.

Economic factors

To date, the programme has successfully enlisted the voluntary participation of highly skilled medical specialists and clinicians whose time would otherwise not be affordable. This approach will continue to be crucial for the future sustainability of the programme, as will philanthropic and gift-in-kind contributions from socially minded individuals and corporations.

Technology factors

A more sophisticated clinical information management system is required. This would facilitate continuity of care through web access to patient records and enable more robust data analysis for population tracking and research. Several web-based platforms or electronic medical records are being explored. Examples include the system created by the Swinfen Charitable Trust (see Chapter 19) and open-source formats (i.e. OpenMRS and OpenVista).

To improve the efficiency and completeness of local clinician assessment and transcription, digital pen technology combined with standardized clinical forms is being explored. This may be an improvement over keyboard data entry.

Conclusion

Cambodia's health system faces a significant disease burden, as well as provider shortages and limited resources. The low-bandwidth, store-and-forward telemedicine programme that began in 2001 has expanded to a second site. Experience suggests that this model of care is not only feasible, but also acceptable to patients and care providers, and has positive clinical effects. Continued challenges to its operational efficiency and effectiveness remain, as do methods of data collection to assess the clinical effects. With stakeholders in the USA and Cambodia, this collaborative project seeks to become a sustainable, scalable and transferable model of cross-cultural telemedicine for low-resource settings.

From a broad perspective, the process of globalization will undoubtedly have an impact on the health of populations in both the industrialized and the developing world.[16] Telemedicine and telehealth applications are likely to emerge as future tools to transform the way care is delivered across cultures, geography and time zones. It is clear that utilizing communication technologies to decrease health disparities is possible in places such as rural Cambodia, but large-scale deployment of telehealth in the developing world will depend on the positive convergence of human, economic and technological factors.[17]

Acknowledgements

We thank Kathy Fiamma, Dr Kavitha Reddy, Dr Sherene Idriss, Heather Bello, Nedialka Douptcheva and Marco Senelly.

Further reading

King H, Keuky L, Seng S et al. Diabetes and associated disorders in Cambodia: two epidemiological surveys. *Lancet* 2005; **366**: 1633–9.
Telemedicine in Low Resource Settings (Discussion Group). Available at: www. dgroups.org/groups/telemedicine/index.cfm.

References

1. Ricciardi L. *A Model for Remote Health Care in the Developing World: The Markle Foundation Telemedicine Clinic in Cambodia.* Available at: www.markle.org/markle_programs/healthcare/projects/cambodia_telemedicine.php#report1.
2. Kvedar J, Heinzelmann PJ, Jacques G. Cancer diagnosis and telemedicine: a case study from Cambodia. *Ann Oncol* 2006; **17**(Suppl 8): 37–42.
3. Kemp C. Cambodian refugee health beliefs and practices. *J Community Health Nurs* 1985; **2**: 41-52
4. World Health Organization. *The World Health Report 2000 – Health Systems: Improving Performance.* Geneva: WHO, 2000. Available at: www.who.int/whr/2000/en/index.html.
5. Centers for Disease Control. Screening HIV-infected persons for tuberculosis – Cambodia, January 2004–February 2005. *MMWR Morb Mortal Wkly Rep* 2005; **54**(46): 1177–1180.
6. World Health Organization. *Global Tuberculosis Control – Surveillance,` Planning, Financing.* Geneva: WHO, 2005. Available at: www.who.int/tb/publications/global_report/en.
7. World Health Organization Regional Office for the Western Pacific. *Malaria Annual Data.* Available at: www.wpro.who.int/sites/mvp/data/malaria.
8. United Nations Development Programme. *Human Development Report 2006.* Available at: hdr.undp.org/hdr2006/statistics.
9. World Health Organization. *Country Cooperation Strategy: Cambodia.* Available at: who.int/countries/en/cooperation_strategy_khm_en.pdf.
10. Wright D. The International Telecommunication Union's report on Telemedicine and Developing Countries. *J Telemed Telecare* 1998; **4**(Suppl 1): 75–9.
11. World Health Organization. *Core Health Indicators.* Available at: www.who.int/whosis/database/core/core_select.cfm.
12. American Assistance for Cambodia. Available at: www.cambodiaschools.com.
13. Reddy KK, Idriss SZ, Chau R et al. Cross-cultural telemedicine approach to epidemic diabetes: model for developing nations. *Telemed J E Health* 2007, **13**: 198 (Abst T5C1).
14. Brandling-Bennett HA, Kedar I, Pallin DJ et al. Delivering health care in rural Cambodia via store-and-forward telemedicine: a pilot study. *Telemed J E Health* 2005; **11**: 56–62.
15. Heinzelmann PJ, Jacques G, Kvedar J. Telemedicine by email in remote Cambodia. *J Telemed Telecare* 2005; **11**(Suppl 2): 44–7.
16. Huynen MM, Martens P, Hilderink HB. The health impacts of globalization: a conceptual framework. *Global Health* 2005; **1**: 14.
17. Graham LE, Zimmerman M, Vassallo DJ et al. Telemedicine – the way ahead for medicine in the developing world. *Trop Doct* 2003; **33**: 36–8.
18. Heinzelmann PJ, Lugn NE, Kvedar JC. Telemedicine in the future. *J Telemed Telecare* 2005; **11**: 384–90.
19. World Health Organization. *WHO Statistical Information System (WHOSIS).* Available at: www.who.int/whosis.
20. World Health Organization. *The Digital Divide: ICT Development Indices 2004.* New York and Geneva: United Nations, 2005.

14 Telepathology and telecytology in developing countries

Sangeeta Desai

Introduction

The field of surgical pathology and cytology involves a cascade of operator-dependent technical, scientific and medical processes. The preparation and interpretation of surgical pathology and cytology material requires trained technical personnel, excellent technical support, skill, experience and some basic infrastructure. Developing nations such as India are typically flawed by vast socioeconomic differences. In India, there is a truly heterogeneous and uneven development of health care facilities, which results in major disparities: some medically privileged areas have expertise on par with the industrialized world, while other remotely located, rural, under-served populations are almost totally deprived of any medical facilities. Telemedicine provides a method of bridging this gap.[1–5]

Telepathology for the developing world

Telepathology is the practice of pathology at a distance using telecommunications. It involves viewing images on a video monitor rather than directly through a microscope. The minimum requirements for telepathology are:

- a light microscope (motorized for dynamic telepathology);
- a high-resolution camera (either a digital camera or a video camera with a frame grabber card);
- a workstation for the telepathologist;
- access to a telecommunications network.

Telepathology can be performed using a static, or 'store-and-forward', approach; it can also be conducted using a dynamic, or real-time, approach; or it may employ a hybrid of the two.[1,2] There are obvious disadvantages associated with static telepathology, the major one being sampling error, which reflects the passive nature of this exercise. In contrast, dynamic telepathology overcomes the basic drawback of static telepathology, although techniques such as ultra-rapid virtual slide processing[6] are prohibitively expensive in a developing country setting. Sampling error in static telepathology consultation could be reduced by the referring pathologist sending a set of images covering both ambiguous and unambiguous areas. There is general agreement that a reasonably accurate histopathological diagnosis is possible on the basis of the examination of judiciously selected digital images. It has been our observation that mutual trust, rapport and close interaction between referring pathologist and telepathologist, and adequate training of the referring pathologist, are very important to achieve successful teleconsultations.[2]

The quality of the images is largely dependent on the quality of the basic starting material, which is the stained slide. The mode of transmission and the image compression will not compromise the quality of images if chosen carefully. It has been suggested that successful telepathology diagnoses can be achieved using adaptive colour reduction algorithms to reduce image file size, thus facilitating transmission without sacrificing quality.[7]

The single most important factor that influences selection of the system in the developing world is the cost. The potential customer, in addition, also faces the problem of commercial pressure by the vendors. Dealing with single-vendor proprietary systems, i.e. buying the camera, software and microscope in a package, implies an inability to negotiate costs. However, it is heartening to note that the costs of most of the components of telepathology system are declining.

Constraints

There are a number of constraints that limit the introduction of telepathology in the developing world. These include the following.

Inadequate infrastructure

The essential components of any telepathology system, i.e. the microscope, a camera with software and a computer, may not available in rural areas of developing countries. Procurement of these items may be difficult. Telecommunication facilities may not be developed at all, or they may be so poorly developed that it may be difficult or impossible to transmit cases. Moreover, the development and availability of telecommunication facilities may be non-uniform.[3,4,8,9]

Non-uniform processing of pathology material

The limiting step in telepathology is availability of a well-processed histology or cytology glass slide. In the developing world, the lack of infrastructure, equipment and uniform standards makes for poor pathology material or suboptimal technical material.

Lack of accreditation

Telepathology is a combination of surgical pathology, information technology and imaging. All three processes lack defined standards. A few centres conduct accreditation for histopathology, but there are no standards laid down for telepathology in particular.

Low level of training

A well-processed stained slide is the most important factor for success in telepathology. Lack of trained manpower for histopathology processing has a very negative effect on the subsequent quality of a telepathology consultation. As training is required for surgical pathology and cytology specimen processing, it is also required for information technology and handling of camera and computer. The natural tendency of the staff to initially resist any new technology may also need to be managed carefully.

Lack of dedicated personnel

It is often difficult to find dedicated personnel to carry out telepathology or to staff a telemedicine department. The staff are expected to perform multitasking, especially in a low-volume centre.

Applications of telepathology

Intraoperative consultation between pathologist and surgeon requires rapid and accurate diagnosis, which is rendered on a frozen section and provides the necessary guidance to the operating surgeon. For interpretation of intraoperative frozen sections, transmission of live images is required using dynamic telepathology. The same also holds true for primary diagnosis of routine surgical pathology. Although this technique is well developed in certain parts of Europe and the USA,[5,10] in developing countries, the constraints of cost mean that intraoperative consultation is rare.

However, telepathology has proven its merit in developing countries where dynamic teleconsultation is not required, for example to obtain second opinions,[3,4,8,9] expert-to-expert consultations, quality assurance, distance education, consensus diagnosis for pathology review in clinical trials and proficiency testing. In the USA, ultra-rapid turnaround time in surgical pathology has recently been demonstrated in breast cancer clinics. These combine digital mammography imaging and interpretations, the latest advances in rapid specimen processing (microwave and automated immunostaining), and biopsy diagnosis by telepathology, producing a 'one-stop shop' for patients being investigated.[6] Although this is attractive, promising and useful for the industrialized world, it is not practical in the developing world because of the high costs.

Another potential use of telepathology is for consultations generated in the industrialized world to be outsourced to experts in developing countries. This is currently practised in the field of radiology at some centres. However, credentialing requirements, issues related to licensure and malpractice coverage need to be resolved for this approach.[11] If these factors are dealt with appropriately then this model of telepathology may have potential.

Telepathology is not yet validated in the field of exfoliative cytology, which involves microscopic examination of cells that are shed from the lesion. Most cytologists would agree that telecytology is not a preferred mode for reporting exfoliative cytology. However, it is worth noting that there have been a few studies of telecytology involving fine-needle aspiration cytology (FNAC).[9]

Tele-surgical pathology and telecytology

The distinction between tele-surgical pathology and telecytology is based on the inherent differences between the cytology and surgical pathology material. Surgical pathology material consists of cells and tissue architecture. Hence, the telepathologist and referring pathologist can make use of the tissue architecture as a reference point to discuss the case and/or obtain additional images from any suspicious areas. Cytology smears mainly consist of cells with a few stromal fragments and are spread over a large area. The whole smear needs to be scanned. Hence, telecytology requires more comprehensive and optimized initial sampling of the smears, which increases the number of images produced. Telecytology largely depends on the images chosen by the referring pathologist. Hence, it is desirable to have the problematic areas adequately represented in the initial images in telecytology.[9]

Experience of telepathology in Mumbai

The Tata Memorial Hospital in Mumbai, India is a tertiary cancer referral centre, delivering comprehensive care to cancer patients in the Indian subcontinent. The hospital has a static telepathology link with two rural cancer centres located 500 km from Mumbai (Figure 14.1). The process to establish a static telepathology link with one of

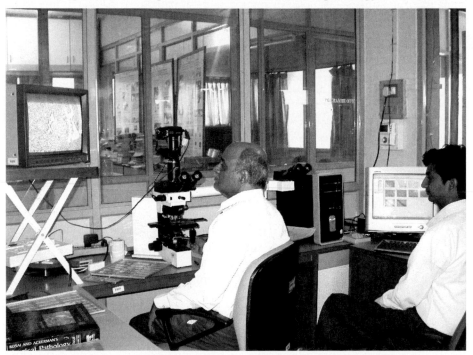

Figure 14.1 Static telepathology workstation at the referring pathologist's end in Barshi, Solapur, India

the rural cancer centres, the Nargis Dutt Memorial Cancer Hospital, began in October 2000 and came to fruition in January 2002. The delays were mainly due to hurdles related to the communication link. However, once it became fully operational, tele-pathology was able to sustain itself.[3,5,8,9] The communication medium employed is the ordinary telephone system, with the 56 kbit/s dial-up modem providing access to the Internet. A set of compressed images in conjunction with clinical data are sent as email attachments.

The performance of static telepathology was assessed by comparing the diagnoses rendered on telepathology and glass slides, respectively. The comparison was cate-gorized as follows:

(1) complete concordance
(2) minor discrepancy (clinically unimportant)
(3) major discrepancy (clinically important)
(4) qualified diagnosis
(5) deferred diagnosis.

Analysis of tele-surgical pathology consultations

In a study of 299 static telepathology consultations accrued over a period of 3 years to December 2004, there were 251 surgical pathology, 2 international consultations and 46 cytology cases.[3,4,8,12] Concordance (absolute concordance, qualified diagnosis or minor, clinically unimportant discrepancies) for tele-surgical pathology was 96% (199 of 207 cases). The diagnosis was deferred in 30 cases.

Our experience of deferred diagnoses on telepathology indicates that the 'probable' diagnosis rendered in complex cases such as lymphoid neoplasia, sarcoma and round cell tumours matched the final glass slide diagnosis in 47% of cases. The 'probable' telepathology diagnosis rendered on potentially difficult cases does give the referring pathologist a direction or impart a different thought process during decision making.[12]

We believe that static telepathology consultation helps the referring pathologist to unravel the diagnosis while dealing with potentially complex cases, even in the event of deferral. Static telepathology has the potential to provide specialist support in the clinical management of such cases.

Analysis of telecytology consultations

A total of 46 cases accrued over period of 3 years were analyzed.[9] The cases included 44 FNAC and 2 exfoliative cytology smears. The concordance (absolute concordance, qualified diagnosis or minor, clinically unimportant discrepancies) for telecytology was 91% (39 of 43 cases). The diagnosis was deferred in 5 cases.

The reasons for major discrepancies for both telesurgical pathology and telecytol-ogy were interpretative errors, inadequate sampling, poor-quality sections and images, and inadequate clinical data. We believe that effective use of static telepathology can be achieved by thorough sampling by the referring pathologist, expertise in surgical pathology at the telepathologist's end and effective interaction between the two ends.[3,4,8,9,12]

Conclusion

Telepathology is a powerful technique. To make best use of it, the raw material, i.e. the stained glass slide, must be of optimum quality. We have found that telepathology is valuable in bridging the gap between under-served areas and specialty centres, and can build confidence and capacity in the professionals working in under-served areas. This also reduces professional isolation, as expressed by referring pathologists. Patients from under-served areas receive better professional advice, while saving their travel costs to tertiary centres. Another major advantage of teleconsultation is effective management of turnaround time. In our study, 48% of cases were reported within 8 hours (a single working day) and 91% of cases within 3 days.

It is obvious that telepathology is potentially useful in the developing world. A decision to implement a diagnostic telepathology system in developing countries will be based on numerous factors, but the pivotal factor will be the need for telepathology. A strong impetus to establish communication between distantly located centres can help to establish successful, inexpensive and effective teleconsultation and to transfer knowledge and expertise to medically underprivileged areas and bridge the gap of knowledge and expertise at low cost. I believe that once the advantages of telepathology are visible to pathologists generally, the technique will rapidly gain in popularity.

Acknowledgements

I am grateful to Dr KA Dinshaw, Dr Ashok Mohan, Dr BM Nene, Mr MK Chauhan, Mr TK Ghosh, Mr Manoj Chavan, Mr Amit Satvekar and Mr Bipin Gadhave. I thank Dr Roshni Chinoy, Dr Shubhada Kane, Dr Tanuja Shet and Dr Mukta Ramadwar for reporting telepathology cases and Dr Rajasa Patil and Dr Sanica Bhele for providing logistical support.

Further reading

Arizona Telemedicine Program. Available at: www.telemedicine.arizona.edu/index. cfm.

Armed Forces Institute of Pathology. Department of Telemedicine. Available at: www.afip.org/consultation/telemedicine.

International Union against Cancer (UICC) Telepathology Consultation Center. Available at: pathoweb.charite.de/UICC-TPCC/default.asp.

Kayser K, Szymas J, Weinstein RS. *Telepathology*. Berlin: Springer-Verlag, 1999.

Li X, Gong E, McNutt MA et al. Assessment of diagnostic accuracy and feasibility of dynamic telepathology in China. *Hum Pathol* 2008; **39**: 236–42.

Wells CA, Sowter C. Telepathology: a diagnostic tool for the millennium. *J Pathol* 2000; **191**: 1–7.

References

1. Wootton R. Recent advances: telemedicine. *BMJ* 2001; **323**: 557–60.
2. Weinstein RS, Descour MR, Liang C et al. Telepathology overview: from concept to implementation. *Hum Pathol* 2001; **32**: 1283–99.
3. Desai S, Ghosh TK, Chinoy R et al. Telepathology at Tata Memorial Hospital, Mumbai and Barshi, a rural centre in Maharashtra. *Natl Med J India* 2002; **15**: 363–4.
4. Desai S, Patil R, Chinoy R et al. Experience with telepathology at a tertiary cancer centre and a rural cancer hospital. *Natl Med J India* 2004; **17**: 17–19.
5. Cross SS, Dennis T, Start RD. Telepathology: current status and future prospects in diagnostic histopathology. *Histopathology* 2002; **41**: 91–109.
6. Weinstein R, Descour MR, Liang C et al. An array microscope for ultrarapid virtual slide processing and telepathology. Design, fabrication, and validation study. *Hum Pathol* 2004; **35**: 1303–14.
7. Doolittle MH, Doolittle KW, Winkelman Z, Weinberg DS. Color images in telepathology: How many colors do we need? *Hum Pathol* 1997; **28**: 36–41.
8. Desai S, Patil R, Kothari A et al. Static telepathology consultation service between Tata Memorial Centre, Mumbai and Nargis Dutt Memorial Charitable Hospital, Barshi, Solapur, Maharashtra: an analysis of the first 100 cases. *Indian J Pathol Microbiol* 2004; **47**: 480–5.
9. Jialdasani R, Desai S, Gupta M et al. An analysis of 46 static telecytology cases over a period of two years. *J Telemed Telecare* 2006; **12**: 311–14.
10. Frierson HF Jr, Galgano MT. Frozen-section diagnosis by wireless telepathology and ultra portable computer: use in pathology resident/faculty consultation. *Hum Pathol* 2007; **38**: 1330–4.
11. Kalyanpur A, Neklesa VP, Pham DT et al. Implementation of an international teleradiology staffing model. *Radiology* 2004; **232**: 415–19.
12. Bhele S, Jialdasani R, Kothari A et al. Analysis of deferrals on static telepathology consultation service. *Ind J Pathol Microbiol* 2007; **50**: 749–53.

15 Internet-based store-and-forward telemedicine for subspecialty consultations in the Pacific region

C Becket Mahnke, Charles W Callahan and Donald A Person

Introduction

An early form of telemedicine communication in the developing world was the radio-telephone. A series of ham radio operators would establish a schedule of time available for the long-distance communication between remote locations and more centralized locations. During the early 1960s, one of us (DAP) managed distant medical consultations between US military staff in Panama and distant military groups, missions and embassies from Mexico to South America using the Military Affiliate Radio System. At a prearranged weekly time, a radio operator would connect the various organizations together. Medical questions were discussed, which facilitated decisions regarding local medical care versus evacuation. However, radiotelephony was susceptible to problems caused by the weather and sunspot activity, resulting in loss of bandwidth and sometimes loss of signal. During the same period of the 1950s and 1960s, communications within the far-flung US-associated Pacific Trust Territories were handled in a similar manner.[1]

Early telemedicine work at Tripler Army Medical Center

Tripler Army Medical Center (TAMC) was the test site for the Composite Health Care System, a database of the US Department of Defense. It was deployed in the late 1980s, and included modules for order entry, retrieval of radiology and laboratory results, pharmacy, patient administration and coding information. An email function was added in 1995, and this provided the basis for teleconsultations and referrals within the military health care system in Hawaii and ultimately military medical facilities in the Pacific. File attachments, however, were not allowed in the secure

Composite Health Care System, which limited telemedicine to the written word only.

In 1993, telemedicine consultations with TAMC were begun from the US Army Kwajalein Atoll Missile Range in the Marshall Islands. There was an existing AT&T videoconference system at Kwajalein Atoll. About 150 consultations were conducted over 5 years, and a few unnecessary referrals to Honolulu were avoided.[2] The process, however, was difficult to schedule. Expensive computer and video hardware and costly maintenance with special technical support were required. By virtue of the proximity of the Ebeye Island to Kwajalein, a few Marshallese patients benefited from this demonstration project, but it was obvious that such a technology-dependent system was not practicable in the rest of the Pacific.

In 1995, at the inaugural meeting of the Pacific Basin Medical Association held in Pohnpei, the utility of the Picasso still-image telephone was demonstrated by a consultation on a patient in Palau, some 2400 km away. That consultation avoided the evacuation of the patient from Palau to Hawaii (saving at least US$20 000).[1] Four Picasso telephones were donated by AT&T to jurisdictions in the Western Pacific, and over 30 telemedicine demonstration projects were successfully carried out on the island of Pohnpei, between islands in Pohnpei State, and internationally between Alaska, Hawaii, Pohnpei, New Caledonia, Kosrae State and Palau. Several patients were transferred using this process. However, the cost of long-distance calls became prohibitive, and local health budgets could not continue paying such costs (US$5–10 per minute).[3]

Pacific Island Healthcare Project

At about the same time (1989–1990), a programme to benefit the graduate medical education needs of TAMC's residents in training was developed. The Pacific Island Healthcare Project (PIHCP) was developed to facilitate the referral and treatment of indigenous peoples of the former Pacific Trust Territories, now referred to as the US-associated Pacific Islands (USAPIs). The USAPIs include three US territories (American Samoa, Guam and the Commonwealth of the Northern Mariana Islands) and three independent, freely associated states (the Republic of the Marshall Islands, the Federated state of Micronesia and the Republic of Palau) (Figure 15.1 and Table 15.1). The peoples of the USAPIs suffer from diseases such as tuberculosis, rheumatic heart disease, leptospirosis, dengue fever, pyomyositis and leprosy, as well as chronic diseases such as diabetes mellitus, obesity, hypertension, hyperuricaemia and cancer. In addition, there are surgically correctable congenital lesions, such as cleft lip/palate, congenital diaphragmatic hernia, Hirschprung disease and hypospadius.

The challenges of managing consultations with the time differences (five time zones and an International Date Line) and great distances (8000 km between Honolulu in Hawaii and the Republic of Palau) are formidable. The region is extremely remote (Figure 15.1). Some distant islands and atolls are 600–1300 km from the jurisdiction's capital, reachable only by sailing canoe. Prior to the development of the web-based referral system, consultations from the jurisdictions came in the form of

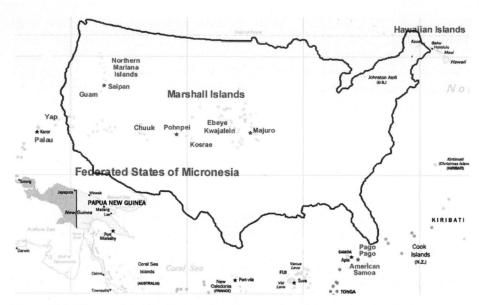

Figure 15.1 US-associated Pacific Islands, with an overlay of the continental USA (to scale) to demonstrate the distances invlolved

Table 15.1 Pacific Island Healthcare Project jurisdictions

Jurisdiction	Population[a] (000s)	Area (km²)	Islands	US Association
Guam	152	1400	1	Territory
American Samoa	64	515	7	Territory
Commonwealth of Northern Marianas	69	1235	21	Commonwealth
Republic of Marshall Islands	66	470	1225	Free association
Federated States of Micronesia	132	1820	607	Free association
Republic of Palau	18	1190	350	Free association
Total	500			

[a]Based on 2000 estimates

letters, long-distance telephone calls, faxes and even the diplomatic pouch. From 1988 to 1997, the PIHCP provided definitive care at TAMC for about 2500 patients from the USAPIs. The web-based system was established in 1997, and in 1998 we were able to demonstrate asynchronous consultations with TAMC.[4]

Since that time, email with attached images has been shown to be an acceptable medium for consultation for almost all patients. Several steps were needed to implement four test sites in Micronesia. First, a consultation web page was created with a request form to ensure that there was sufficient information to allow TAMC specialists to comment. Second, a web page was created to display all current or recent consultations received from the USAPIs. Third, a group of TAMC specialists was trained in the use of a web browser to access the consultations and comment on cases where appropriate. The use of a web-based system provided a flexible approach to patient management discussions. Four sites within Micronesia were selected as test sites: Chuuk, Pohnpei, Palau and Majuro in the Marshall Islands. Each location had relatively inexpensive Internet service providers (ISPs) and 24-hour access to the Internet. Each site was provided with:

- a desktop computer
- a digital camera (D-600L, Olympus)
- a flatbed scanner with transparency adapter (Scanmaker E6 Professional, Microtek)
- a digital video camera (DCR VX-1000, Sony)
- a printer.

In addition, two sites were provided with a digital otoscope and ophthalmoscope (American Medical Devices).

Training was conducted in two phases. First, a group of all interested clinicians at the annual Pacific Basin Medical Association meeting in Chuuk were allowed to test the equipment. Once the equipment had been installed at each site, small groups were trained. For many of the medical officers, this was the first opportunity that they had had to see or use a computer. It should be noted that five senior physicians in Yap, Pohnpei and Palau had access to the web page using their personal computers. Their involvement was important to the success of the programme.[4]

Clinical procedure

The first step in creating an electronic consultation is to gather digital images where appropriate. Even in cases where images do not support the consultation, an image of the patient helps to humanize the electronic process. Images are acquired using a digital still camera, digital video camera or digital medical device camera. Additional images can be acquired using the flatbed scanner (e.g. laboratory results, ECG recordings, photographs and X-ray films). Initially, it proved difficult to produce images of acceptable quality from X-ray films. However, in most cases, careful use of the digital camera to acquire an image on a light box proved satisfactory.[5] Images are annotated using simple image editing software, with date, comments on area of concern and an identifying code as applicable.

Next, the history of the patient must be typed into the computer. This step is often completed before the connection to the Internet is made. The clinicians use a common word-processing program to type the medical history, and then copy and paste it into the website form; we do not use a rigid format for the history. Once complete, the clinician connects to the Internet and submits the case. Depending on the number and size of attached images, this process can take several minutes. The resulting electronic patient record is archived and can be retrieved via the website.

Once a new case is received, an automatic email notification is sent to the PIHCP Director. The Director queries the database to find the case. The information is protected by secure socket layer (SSL) encryption, which meets the current Health Care

Financing Administration guidelines for secure clinical use of the Internet. The consultation is displayed as the provider types it in, with attached images displayed if included. The Director then comments on the case and forwards it to appropriate specialists as required. All comments are stored in the database, complete with time/date stamp and user information.

Specialists are notified of a new case via email. The email message contains a working diagnosis, a case number and a link to the PIHCP website. After reviewing the clinical data and images, the specialist can comment on the case or ask for further information or testing to be done. The remote provider is notified by email of the new comments, and reviews these on the website. If further information is required, he or

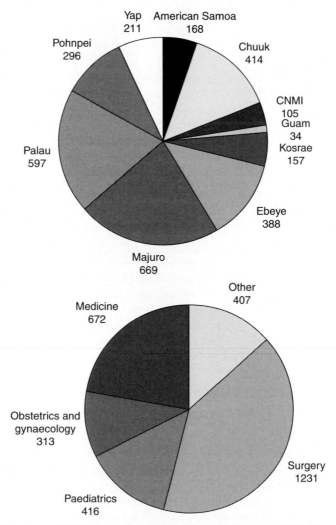

Figure 15.2 Numbers of PIHCP cases (*n* = 3039): (a) origin; (b) type. CNMI, Commonwealth of the Northern Mariana Islands

she can enter the response on the web page. In this manner, a difficult case can be discussed using the website as a discussion group for a specific patient.

Results

By the end of 1999, we had installed 10 workstations in all of the jurisdictions of the USAPIs. More than 3000 consultations and referrals have been submitted in the nearly 10-year history of the telemedicine programme (Figure 15.2). The majority of the cases have come from the Marshall Islands, the Republic of Palau and Chuuk State. The US Congress provides US$2.5–5 million per year to the PIHCP for patient travel and medical care. After an initial investment of approximately US$300 000 to install the workstations and train the local providers, the PIHCP programme has been self-sustaining. The leadership of TAMC has supported the programme and integrated its administration into the hospital's business plan. Administrative support is provided by TAMC's Patient Administration Division and technical support is provided by TAMC's Information Management Division. The Medical Director has provided the direction, leadership and oversight of the PIHCP as a labour of love.

We do not provide a list of indications for telemedicine. The decision to initiate a teleconsultation is left to the referring doctor. The numbers of patients accepted to TAMC for further evaluation and treatment are shown in Table 15.2. With the implementation of the web-based system in the late 1990s, there has been a drop in the

Table 15.2 Pacific Island Healthcare Project: number of patient referrals accepted at TAMC for further evaluation and treatment

Financial year	No. of referrals
1991	326
1992	401
1993	335
1994	462
1995	413
1996	160
1997	228
1998	189
1999	222
2000	225
2001	201
2002	142
2003	154
2004	132
2005	171
2006	139

number of patients brought to TAMC for evaluation and treatment. This has not been due to a decrease in the number of cases submitted to the PIHCP. It has been due to more accurate triage of those who would benefit from transfer to TAMC using the web system. In addition, the web-based system allows many patients to be treated locally with telemedical support from TAMC specialists. Both factors lead to improved health care for a greater number of patients. The costs associated with the care of those patients brought to TAMC are shown in Figures 15.3 and 15.4.

The PIHCP telemedicine system has had a significant effect on medical practice as reflected by the length of stay (Figure 15.5). Prior to the development of the web-based PIHCP system, the average length of stay for Pacific Island patients approached 30 days. Since implementation of the teleconsultation process, the length of stay has fallen, and is currently just over 5 days. This is a consequence of more appropriate triage of patients prior to transfer to TAMC, as well as improved coordination of care once the patient arrives.

Implementation of the web-based consultation system has had other advantages. It has allowed isolated practitioners to stay connected with their colleagues throughout the Pacific and be kept up to date with modern medicine. There has also been educational value for the residents in training at TAMC. Numerous publications have resulted from patient referrals.[5-10] Pacific Islanders have been restored to health, and have returned home to lead normal and productive lives.

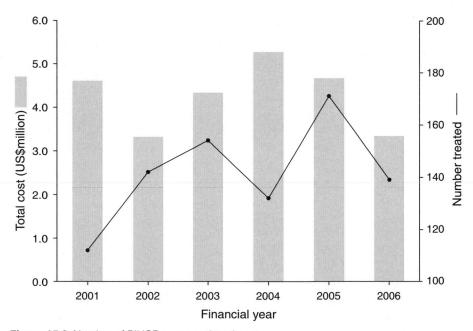

Figure 15.3 Number of PIHCP cases and total costs

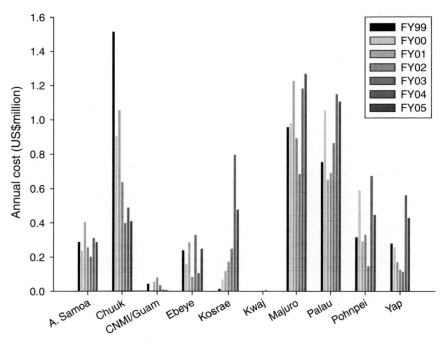

Figure 15.4 PIHCP: total expenditure for all islands. FY, financial year

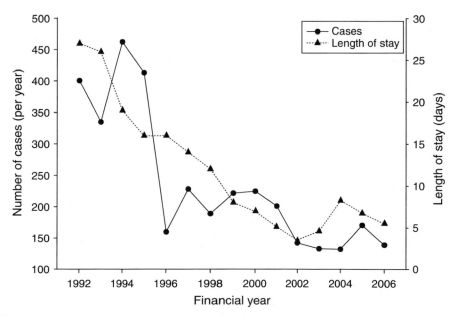

Figure 15.5 PIHCP: number of cases accepted and length of stay

Pacific Asynchronous TeleHealth system

TAMC is the tertiary military medical treatment facility for the US military (active duty staff, retirees and dependants) in the Pacific region. TAMC's area of responsibility includes US military bases in Korea, mainland Japan, Okinawa and Guam (Figure 15.6). These remote military health care facilities are often staffed by relatively junior physicians and have limited access to subspecialty care. Even if subspecialty care is available in the host nation, language and cultural limitations represent significant impediments to providing safe and effective care. A teleconsultation system capable of providing subspecialty services had the potential to improve both access to and quality of health care delivered.

TAMC's asynchronous telemedicine for US military beneficiaries started in 2000, with the Electronic Children's Hospital of the Pacific (ECHO-Pac) asthma intervention. Children with asthma were enrolled from military facilities in Guam, Okinawa, mainland Japan and Korea. Each child was cared for utilizing an asthma clinical pathway with advice from a paediatric pulmonary specialist via the website. All patients experienced an improvement in their asthma. There were fewer emergency room visits and fewer unscheduled acute clinic visits. At the same time, the primary care provider's practice in caring for children also improved as a result of increased use of asthma education and planning.[11]

In addition to the asthma intervention, ECHO-Pac included a general consultation capability modelled on the PIHCP. This feature was far more popular with remote

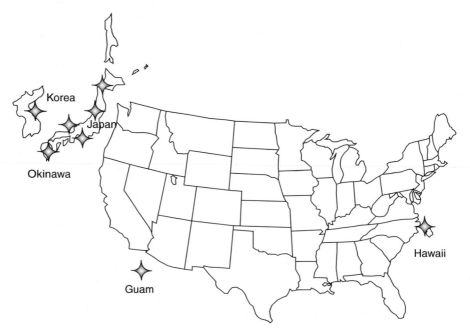

Figure 15.6 US military health care facilities in the Pacific region, with overlay of the continental USA (to scale) to demonstrate the distances involved: Honolulu is closer to Atlanta (7230 km) than it is to Seoul (7320 km) or Okinawa (7480 km)

health care providers than the asthma intervention. From October 2000 until April 2004, a total of 875 teleconsultations were submitted to the ECHO-Pac system from 14 different US military hospitals and clinics throughout the Western Pacific. These consultations included over 1700 images and more than 7000 clinical comments from numerous specialists.

One of the difficulties with technology research is the lack of 'measures of effectiveness' for new initiatives. Technology is often pursued because it can be done, without asking whether it should be done and with no plan to measure whether the technology makes a difference. In 2004, the PacRim Teleconsultation Effectiveness Trial evaluated ECHO-Pac's impact on access to specialty care, the quality of the care provided and the cost savings. A panel of 5 physicians evaluated 267 consultations over a 1-year period. The average time for the consultation to be reviewed and forwarded by the consult manager was 5 hours (SD 3), with a reply from a consultant in an average of 32 hours (SD 14). The diagnosis was modified in 15% of cases, the diagnostic plan was modified in 21% and the treatment plan was modified in 24%. Air evacuation to TAMC for further evaluation was reduced by 30%. Given the significant cost of moving patients (approximately US$5800 per case), use of the ECHO-Pac teleconsultation system demonstrated significant cost avoidance.[12]

As a result of the success of the ECHO-Pac teleconsultation system, TAMC launched the Pacific Asynchronous TeleHealth (PATH) system in 2004. PATH was created with a modular design to expand the capabilities to the care of both paediatric and adult patients. Subsequent modules have included Lightning Med (used by military health care providers in Afghanistan and Iraq) and a module for tele-auscultation development and testing.[13] The secure website allows health care providers at medical treatment facilities throughout the Pacific region to submit cases for subspecialist input. Referring physicians provide clinical information, along with images, video and sound as necessary. At the TAMC, physician managers forward the case to the appropriate subspecialty for comment, and email messages notify all involved in a case when new information or comments have been added.

Differences from the Pacific Island Healthcare Project

Although PATH was modelled on the PIHCP website, it became apparent that the different patient and referring provider populations served would require some modifications to the teleconsultation process. For example, US military beneficiaries have both increased health care options and expectations compared with patients served by the PIHCP. Since use of PATH is not mandatory, referring providers can simply refer the patient for local specialty care (if available) or for air evacuation to TAMC or another tertiary military treatment facility. Our philosophy has been to simplify the teleconsultation process where possible, knowing that many health care providers will opt for the least time-consuming option when sending a patient for subspecialty care. As a result, the processes of teleconsultation submission, administration and multimedia handling have continued to change with technology innovations and provider needs.

Documentation and privacy requirements are demanding in PATH, which must comply with all US regulations. The results of teleconsultation must ultimately reside in the patient record, so we developed a system that allows the consultation notes to be printed onto standard US military health care forms for inclusion in the patient's record. The security is sufficient to comply with the Health Information Portability and Accountability Act of 1996. The password encryption protocols are rigorous so as to ensure security. Although email is used to inform providers of new information regarding a specific case, no individually identifiable health information is included in the messages.

Documentation of services provided in PATH is important. Although few US insurance companies offer reimbursement for asynchronous telehealth, the Surgeon General of the Army grants appropriate workload credits for telemedicine. For this purpose, a billing module was created in PATH allowing for workload capture on the part of the subspecialist. Once a teleconsultation is entered into the PATH system, the patient administrators receive an email message informing them of a new patient requiring registration into the local hospital system. Once a subspecialty provider completes teleconsultation services in PATH, the billing module allows for easy coding of diagnosis. On completion, departmental coders are alerted of the billing form via email and can enter the data into the system. This streamlined approach reduces the extra work required of the consultant (approximately 10–15 seconds to complete and email the workload credit form) while documenting the workload provided by PATH. Accurate documentation is essential to continued funding of the PATH system.

Experience with PATH

Since its launch in October 2004, the number of consultations submitted to the PATH system has increased (Table 15.3). There has also been a 20% increase in the number of images submitted per teleconsultation in just over two years. Since the opening of the adult telemedicine module, nearly one-third of all consultations submitted have been for adult patients. This rapid growth verifies the demand for adult subspecialty teleconsultation services in the region.

The system is designed to accept all types of referrals. When a physician is registered in PATH, and during the consultation process itself, referring providers are reminded that it is not intended to be used for medical emergencies. Currently, there are over 600 registered users from 30 military hospitals and clinics throughout the Pacific. All of this activity has occurred despite the fact that PATH's use is optional,

Table 15.3 PATH teleconsultation workload

	2004	2005	2006
Paediatric consultations	181	259	290
Adult consultations	97	167	117
Total	278	426	407
Number of images	248	353	457
Number of comments	2370	3793	2745

and no formal system training occurs. Since most US military physicians serve for only one to two years in the Western Pacific, there is high turnover among PATH users.

As described above, the PATH system improves subspecialist access and quality of care while reducing health care expenditures from air evacuation or referral to host-nation specialists. Even for patients who are transferred to TAMC for further evaluation, PATH minimizes health care expenditures by reducing test duplication and coordination of efficient diagnostic and therapeutic options, resulting in a more rapid return to duty.

Challenges

Like many telemedicine systems, PATH was initially funded by research and development funds without a clear plan for financial sustainability. Once initial funding had been obtained, we sought funds from referring institutions based on the cost savings from avoided air evacuations. We chose this avenue because of the high cost of air evacuation (US$3000–6000 per patient), believing that the 30% reduction demonstrated in the PacRim Teleconsultation Effectiveness Trial[12] would make the system sustainable. Owing to the financial structure of the US military health care system, however, no single institution was responsible for these expenditures and, although each potential organization felt that PATH was a useful service, none was willing to contribute to its costs. Fortunately, the Army Surgeon General recognized PATH's value and provided funds (approximately US$100 000 per year). Since the initiation of the workload capture function in late 2006, we anticipate that the revenue generated from PATH's teleconsultation services will provide the necessary financial resources for future sustainability.

The US military's transition to an electronic medical record (EMR) has resulted in further challenges for the PATH system. Since the clinical information needed for teleconsultation is already stored in a digital format in one of several computer systems, remote US health care providers have requested system interoperability to streamline the consultation process. In addition, the results of a PATH teleconsultation must find their way back to the patient's EMR so that future caregivers have access to the information. At present, this is a manual process, albeit one under review.

The introduction of telemedicine has provided opportunities to expand PATH's capabilities. We are currently experimenting with a variety of tele-auscultation devices for telecardiology. Although there was initial enthusiasm about using these devices, once the novelty wore off most were abandoned because of the time required and the lack of technical support available. We have learned that, although transmission of useful telehealth information may be possible with these devices, they must first be tested and integrated into PATH for seamless use prior to deployment. This is a challenging task, owing to the range of proprietary software and hardware, and the few interoperability standards.

Improved communications in the Western Pacific, by non-secure email, telephone or fax, has resulted in frequent consultations by health care providers outside the

PATH system. Since these routes allow for easy, rapid consultation, some health care providers prefer this to utilizing the PATH system. However, such consultation routes do not meet privacy requirements, result in little, if any, clinical documentation, and fail to generate workload credit for the physicians involved.

Future work

We continue to develop the PATH system. For example, the tele-auscultation module allows remote digital stethoscopy. This includes a digital heart sounds recording system, which can be operated via a graphical user interface. Using this system, paediatric cardiologists can differentiate normal from abnormal heart sounds with a high degree of accuracy.[13] We are also beginning to use the PATH system for tele-education. This will provide continuing medical education to staff distributed throughout the Pacific region.

Acknowledgements

The views expressed here are those of the authors and do not reflect the official policy of the Department of the Army, Department of Defense or the US Government.

Further reading

Mahnke CB, Mulreany, MP. PacRim Pediatric Heartsounds Trial: store-and-forward pediatric telecardiology evaluation with echocardiographic validation. In: Klapan I, Poropatich R, eds. *Remote Cardiology Consultations Using Advanced Medical Technology – Applications for NATO Operations*. NATO Science Series, I: Life and Behavioural Sciences, Volume 372. Amsterdam: IOS Press, 2006: 65–72.

Swinfen R, Swinfen P. Low-cost telemedicine in the developing world. *J Telemed Telecare* 2002; **8**(Suppl 3): 63–5.

Tripler Army Medical Center. *Pacific Island Healthcare Project (PIHCP)*. Available at: tamc-tmed.tamc.amedd.army.mil/pihcp.

Wootton R, Youngberry K, Swinfen R, Swinfen P. Referral patterns in a global store-and-forward telemedicine system. *J Telemed Telecare* 2005; **11**(Suppl 2): 100–3.

References

1. Yano V, Finau SA, Dever G et al. The PBMA and telemedicine in the Pacific: the first steps. *Pac Health Dialog* 1997; **4**: 81–4.
2. Delaplain CB, Lindborg CE, Norton SA, Hastings JE. Tripler pioneers telemedicine across the Pacific. *Hawaii Med J* 1993; **52**: 338–9.
3. Person DA, Whitton RK. An Internet based consultation and referral network between Tripler Army Medical Center and hospitals in the Western Pacific. In: *Proceedings of Pacific Medical Technology Symposium*, 1998: 132–8.

4. Person DA. Pacific Island Health Care Project: early experiences with a web-based consultation and referral network. *Pac Health Dialog* 2000; **7**: 29–35.
5. Ruess L, Uyehara CF, Shields KC et al. Digitizing pediatric chest radiographs: comparison of low-cost, commercial off-the-shelf technologies. *Pediatr Radiol* 2001; **31**: 841–7.
6. Person DA. The Pacific Island Health Care Project: easing the cancer burden in the United States associated Pacific Islands. *Pac Health Dialog* 2004; **11**: 243–7.
7. Person DA. The Republic of Palau and the Pacific Island Health Care Project (PIHCP). *Pac Health Dialog* 2005; **12**: 132–40.
8. Hensel KS, Person DA, Schaefer RA, Burkhalter WE. An internet-based referral/consultation system for the US-associated Pacific Islands: its contribution to orthopedic graduate medical education at Tripler Army Medical Center. *Mil Med* 2005; **170**: 214–18.
9. Belnap CP, Freeman JH, Hudson DA, Person DA. A versatile and economical method of image capture for telepathology. *J Telemed Telecare* 2002; **8**: 117–20.
10. Meza-Valencia BE, de Lorimier AJ, Person DA. Hirschsprung disease in the US associated Pacific Islands: more common than expected. *Hawaii Med J* 2005; **64**: 96–101.
11. Malone F, Callahan CW, Chan DA et al. Caring for children with asthma through teleconsultation: 'ECHO-Pac: The Electronic Children's Hospital of the Pacific'. *Telemed J E Health* 2004; **10**: 138–46.
12. Callahan CW, Malone F, Estroff D, Person DA. Effectiveness of an Internet-based store-and-forward telemedicine system for pediatric subspecialty consultation. *Arch Pediatr Adolesc Med* 2005; **159**: 389–93.
13. Mahnke CB, Abbas M, Mulreany MP. PacRim Pediatric Heartsounds Trial: asynchronous pediatric cardiology evaluation via tele-auscultation. Presented at the 2nd Annual Pediatric Telehealth Colloquium, San Francisco, CA, 6–8 September 2007.

16 Telemedicine support for a global network of Italian hospitals

Gianfranco Costanzo and Paola Monari

Introduction

In 2002, the Italian Ministry of Health began a project to support Italian hospitals around the world. This was driven by an ad hoc governing body, the Alliance of Italian Hospitals Worldwide. The IPOCM (Integration and Promotion of Italian Hospitals and Health Care Centres Worldwide) project originated from a census of Italian hospitals abroad conducted by the Ministry of Foreign Affairs. By using an elastic definition of the term 'Italian', hospitals were identified in most developing countries. The hospitals included those with Italian ownership, Italian management or Italian physicians and health staff, and also those managed or owned by Catholic religious orders.

In the initial census, there were 41 Italian hospitals or other health care centres. Almost immediately, another hospital was added to the list (Table 16.1), and after the First Conference on Italian Hospitals Worldwide, which was held in Rome, other Italian health care centres applied to be included. At present, there are 79, and the number is expected to increase in the future.

The project's vision was of a new kind of international health cooperation that was able to keep results locally, for use by health providers who are committed to improving the health status of the population. In other words, the intention was not to adopt a spot approach to health cooperation, which might alleviate the specific health needs of certain population groups, but rather to share with local staff the most appropriate methodologies for attaining ambitious and sustainable targets.

Within this framework, telemedicine was considered as one strategic factor in the structure and organization of the health care network. Since telemedicine facilitates diagnosis, medical consultation and assistance using the resources of centres of excellence, it could therefore improve both medical and administrative support for Italian hospitals abroad. A model based on the use of the Internet[1-9] which is autonomous and cooperative at the same time would conform with the principle of subsidiarity, i.e. decisions would be taken at the nearest level of responsibility.

At the 2003 conference in Rome, Italian hospitals abroad made the request to be part of a democratic organization. The Alliance of Italian Hospitals Worldwide was

Table 16.1 Italian hospitals

Country	Hospital
Albania	Poliambulatorio Padre Luigi Monti, Tirana
Angola	Hospital da Divina Providencia, Luanda
Argentina	Ospedale Italiano di Buenos Aires
	Ospedale Italiano Garibaldi, Rosario
	Ospedale Italiano Monte Buey
	Ospedale Italiano di Cordoba
	Associacion Hospital Italiano Regional Del Sur
	Ospedale Italiano De La Plata
Armenia	Ospedale Redemptoris Mater, Ashotsk
Brazil	Poliambulatorio Nossa Senhora Aparecida, Foz do iguaçu
	Hospital Italiano di Rio de Janeiro
Burkina Faso	Centro di Accoglienza Notre Dame de Fatima – CANDAF, Ouagadougou
	Centre Médical avec Antenne Chirurgicale St Camille, Nanoro
	Centro di Salute e Promozione Sociale Suore Figlie di San Camillo, Ouagadougou
	Centro Medico St Camillo, Koupela
	Centro Medico St Camillo, Ouagadougou
Canada	Ospedale Italiano Santa Cabrini Montréal
Côte d'Ivoire	Centro Don Orlone, Bonoua
Democratic Republic of the Congo	Hôpital Général Conventionné Catholique, Kimbau
	Hôpital de Mokala, Kinshasa
	Hôpital Txingudi, MC Lumbi
Egypt	Ospedale Italiano Umberto I, Cairo
Ethiopia	HEWO Hospital – Quihà, Mekele
	Italian Dermatological Centre IISMAS, Mekele
Jordan	Ospedale Italiano – ANSMI, Amman
	Ospedale Italiano – ANSMI, Kerak
India	Indian Spinal Injuries Centre, New Delhi
Israel	Ospedale Italiano – ANSMI, Haifa
	Holy Family Hospital, Nazareth
Kenya	Piccola Casa della Divina Provvidenza, Chaaria
	Tabaka Mission Hospital, Tabaka
	St Camillus Mission Hospital, Karungu
	Consolata Hospital Nkubu, Meru
Morocco	Ospedale Italiano – ANSMI, Tangier
Paraguay	Sociedad Italiana de Socorro Mutuo, Asuncion
Syria	Ospedale Italiano – ANSMI, Damascus
Sudan	Mary Immaculate Hospital. Mapourdit
Tanzania	Mbweni Hospital 'Santa Maria Nascente'
Uganda	St Mary's Hospital di Lacor

Table 16.1 Italian hospitals (contd)

Country	Hospital
Uruguay	Ospedale Italiano Umberto I, Montevideo
Venezuela	Policlinico Santa Ana, Ciudad Bolivar
Zambia	Italian Orthopaedic Hospital, Lusaka
	Ospedale Mtendere Mission, Chirundu
Zimbabwe	St Michael's Mission Hospital, Ngezi
	Luisa Guidotti Hospital, Mutoko

then formally established. The founding partners were a number of government ministries. Immediately afterwards, certain centres of excellence in Italy were invited to join the Alliance. It was agreed that all partner hospitals in Italy and abroad would cooperate on health by supporting the network. The strategic objective was to contribute expertise from Italy to increase the quality of health care in Italian hospitals abroad.

Policy-making process

Under normal circumstances, a distinction can be made between the different phases in the policy-making process.[10] Accordingly, the Italian Ministry of Health began a public policy cycle. The phases were agenda setting, policy formulation, policy implementation and policy evaluation, i.e. those of classical public policy research.

The agenda setting was established on the basis of the wishes of the Italian hospitals abroad, which expressed a need for diagnostic support and organizational assistance. Within the Ministry of Health, a group of experts who later on would be working for the IPOCM project started studying the problem, using systematic methodologies and tools. Five objectives resulted:

1. To connect the Italian hospitals abroad with centres of excellence in Italy and the Secretariat for Technical Assistance (STA) in Rome
2. To reduce diagnostic and organizational shortcomings among doctors working in Italian hospitals abroad, through a teleconsultation service
3. To increase the individual and collective skills of the health personnel through an e-learning service
4. To facilitate twinning arrangements between hospitals and facilitate government agreements with the countries hosting Italian hospitals abroad
5. To find out more about the health needs of Italian hospitals abroad in order to provide better cooperation and sustain the acquisition of medical equipment.

Task environment

Since the IPOCM participants and activities were functionally interconnected, actions of any one could potentially affect the others.[11] Given this complex framework for

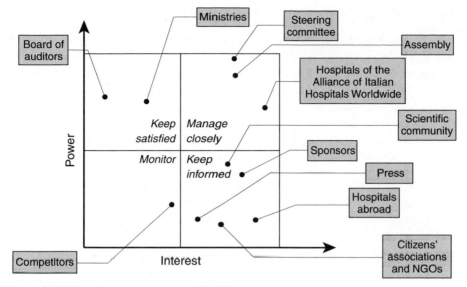

Figure 16.1 The Alliance's power-interest grid

action, an assessment of stakeholders and their relevance was undertaken. The relevant internal stakeholders were the founding ministries and the associated hospitals in Italy and abroad. The relevant external stakeholders were the hospitals in the developing countries, the scientific community, citizens' associations and the press.

Observation of the policy arena requires accurate management of all stakeholders. They can be prioritized using the power versus interest grid.[12] Figure 16.1 shows the power–interest grid of the project stakeholders.

The task environment of the Alliance describes the ideal area occupied by its stakeholders, such as clients, providers, competitors, unions, employees, financiers, institutions and scientific organizations. It is also a place in which the Alliance operates intense and continuous relationships.[13]

In order to pursue the project's objectives, telemedicine instruments and political levers were identified, all of them designed to empower health professionals abroad. Medical teleconsultation and e-learning services were designed. In addition, an inventory of health equipment was set up in order to allow hospitals abroad to benefit from health equipment donated by institutions in Italy. (A complete description of the Alliance's services and user manuals is available at the Ministry of Labour's website.[14])

Teleconsultation

Various telemedicine approaches have been used over the last few years.[15–17] In particular, those of medium or low cost that use customized computer applications have been found to be best for developing countries. This is confirmed by the extensive use of the Internet[18,19] and email in low-resource settings,[20] on the basis of cost–benefit considerations, high availability of connection services and common knowledge about their use.

The methodology adopted for the network was to assess first the technological need expressed by each Italian hospital abroad. As a consequence of this, all information from the different countries was collected and studied by the Secretariat in order to identify those that were viable. The availability of local Internet connectivity was examined, and standard contracts to be signed by hospitals with Internet service providers (ISPs) were developed. All this work was designed to allow all hospitals to have similar connectivity. The best approach for about 30% of the hospitals, most of them in the sub-Saharan area, was a satellite connection through individual contracts with a non-profit-making provider. To improve interoperability, the hospitals were equipped with similar workstations. Finally, software specifications were produced.

The Alliance's network is based on access to the Internet via ADSL, HDSL (high-bit-rate digital subscriber line) or full-duplex 256 kbit/s K_u-band satellite communication. The satellite connections are mainly used by hospitals in sub-Saharan Africa. Workstations are PCs equipped with peripheral devices such as a digital cameras, printers and A4 scanners. The teleconsultation architecture is based on a Management Centre (MC) located at the Secretariat in Rome. The client software allows either an asynchronous telemedicine interaction or a real-time videoconference.

Two different types of users are involved. The referring doctors are located in 45 hospitals abroad and the specialists are located in 34 hospitals in Italy. The choice of specialist for a given teleconsultation is not made at the referring site. Instead, the teleconsultation allocation is performed by the MC. This guarantees the same quality to all referring doctors. The MC allocates the request to the most appropriate specialist based on a routing matrix. The MC can monitor the process until the teleconsultation is completed (the target is to complete consultations within 72 hours). The Alliance's database contains 86 disease code groups, according to the *International Classification of Diseases*, 9th revision, *Clinical Modification (ICD9-CM)*,[21] which expand into 8500 single disease codes. Each specialist centre is responsible for negotiated code groups, and organizes itself to satisfy the service workload within the established targets for reply time and performance quality. Most specialist centres decided to concentrate the incoming referral traffic on a single workstation.

The referring doctor uses the client software to generate an email message containing clinical case data, or to access a videoconsultation if necessary. When compiling the fields on the electronic form, structured XML messages are created. Since both enquiry and reply are managed by the same client software, any health centre is able to act as a referral or a specialist site. The referring doctor, in addition, can invite a close examination of a clinical case by sending a videoconsultation invitation to the specialist.

International standard medical terminology is supported by the system, as well as five different languages (Italian, English, French, Portuguese and Spanish). Diseases are codified according to ICD9-CM and drug names are taken from a standard reference work.[22] The interface collects all relevant data for the teleconsultation request or reply into encoded fields, in order to allow later textual retrieval and statistical analysis. ICD9-CM codes and the patient's gender and age are the relevant pieces of information for the routing function performed at the MC, and they are put into the form by the referring doctor through multi-option lists. Most attached files are captured by digital cameras, and are usually sent after compression (i.e. with a .zip extension). Some attached files are taken directly from diagnostic equipment where feasible.

The database does not store any patient identity information, and therefore the system complies with Italian privacy law. The message reaching the MC contains a teleconsultation identification number, which is automatically generated by the software, as well as the hospital and workstation identifiers. Request and reply data are stored in a teleconsultation record in the database (Microsoft Access), which also holds diagnostic attachments and other information, such as the time of the request delivery at the MC and the time of the reply being forwarded to the referring doctor. Attachments are classified by content (e.g. patient pictures, reports, images or chart recordings). The attachment extension is automatically captured by the system, allowing the MC to detect possible mismatches between the number of attachments that are sent and those actually received. Transfer protocols between the PC and mail server are SMTP and POP.

In addition, a videoconsultation can be requested by a referring doctor in relation to a clinical case where a reply has already been delivered. It can also be requested by a specialist when sending the reply. The MC manages the videoconsultation requests until the referring doctor and the specialist reach an agreement about the date and time. The MC's main functions allow clinicians to contact hospitals in different time zones while they are not online and allow clinicians to handle requests for videoconsultation. Once the meeting has been agreed, the MC notifies the caller, and those involved are sent an invitation message that contains a link to the web portal. Finally the system sends an alert message some minutes before the scheduled time to ensure that both doctors are available in front of their PCs. Doctors can therefore launch the session from any workstation with a browser that accepts ActiveX controls and discuss the case with the help of the relevant documentation.

E-learning

Global support to health personnel includes the provision of an e-learning service oriented to the needs of doctors and health staff abroad. This facility is provided in addition to training events on specific topics of common interest.

Assessment of training needs

One main problem was to understand as accurately as possible the scale and quality of the training required. The Secretariat reviewed various information sources. The first was the declaration given by the hospital at the time of application to the Alliance. They are required to complete a health personnel training requirement form for each of their health staff. This information is then stored in a database ready for analysis.

A second source was the registration of doctors and health staff with the Alliance e-learning platform. Potential users are asked to give information about their professional and training profile, curriculum and career expectations. They are also requested to state their training need in terms of medical disciplines. This information is also stored in the database and used for subsequent analysis.

A third source, although an indirect one, is the medical teleconsultation service itself, with a database that provides statistics about the most commonly used ICD9-CM codes. The teleconsultation data therefore identifies disease areas that deserve particular attention and thus training support.

Other aspects that are taken into consideration are the hospital resources and the sociopolitical framework. Developing countries, especially the least developed countries, have their own agenda on health topics.

Production of learning content

Most of the learning materials that have been produced are the result of an assessment of the training needs expressed by the hospitals. Each centre of excellence selected its own production materials and made them available to the Secretariat. These materials were optimized for uploading and organized by training area and by an assigned ICD9-CM code.

Other important data accessible via the platform come from the medical teleconsultation reports. In fact all teleconsultations result in reports that are classified by ICD9-CM code, and therefore a referring doctor can consult this archive before making a new teleconsultation request. The teleconsultation service therefore has substantial training benefits.

In addition to all this, the Secretariat has produced 18 new learning courses in response to identified training needs:

1. Oral urgent treatment protocol
2. Infectious disease prevention
3. Disorders of growth
4. Periodic fevers in the child
5. Chronic diarrhoeas
6. HIV/TB comorbidity
7. Clinical and biochemical ART monitoring
8. Hypertension in pregnancy
9. Post-partum haemorrhage and puerperal infections
10. Ectopic pregnancy
11. Ovarian tumours and their complications
12. Menorrhagia
13. Lung TB radiological diagnosis
14. Hospital infections
15. Biological risk and vaccine prevention for health personnel
16. Low economic impact reconstructive prosthesis techniques
17. Pharmacological and surgical therapy in acute oral infections
18. Infectious diseases in pregnancy.

The courses were produced by teams that are facilitated and monitored by the

Secretariat for Technical Assistance. The MC looks after the whole production process with an expert who manages relations with the external producer company. The role of the MC's expert is essential in monitoring the timing, given the complexity of the multiple production processes.

Health equipment inventory

In response to requests for new equipment coming from doctors working abroad, the Secretariat produced a web-based inventory for health equipment that was being donated. In 2005, Italian law provided the legal framework for public health centres to give notice to the inventory of the planned disposal of functioning health equipment. Thus, the inventory allows a centre to make the equipment available for an interested hospital abroad. Hospitals can see all equipment on the inventory and reserve items according to their need. This system, which matches offer and demand, improves the efficiency of the donation process and provides a picture of the entire donation cycle, which is useful for a better cooperation policy.

An ontology for the Alliance

Classification of diagnoses and other statistical data is fundamental to the work of the Alliance. This led to an ontological definition of the Alliance's services.[23,24] ICD9-CM codes are ontology agents of the teleconsultation routing matrix. Doctors can scroll through the list of training materials and cross-link the interservice ontology agent, taking advantage of different databases. The same thing is possible when using the web-based inventory of donated medical equipment (which is the third service of the Alliance), where the agent is hospital structure, as well as when talking of teleconsultation, where both ICD9-CM and hospital structure are considered (Figure 16.2).

Quality control

Customer satisfaction

In 2005, a survey of service satisfaction was carried out among teleconsultation users. The areas investigated were technology, communication and organization. The results of the survey showed that 89% of specialists expressed positive judgements, and 86% of referring doctors. There were only a small number of negative judgements (about 9%). Criticisms were discussed subsequently with specialist and referring centres in order to improve service quality.

The Secretariat urged the MC to intervene on a few points related to technological and organizational matters. In about 10% of the hospitals, the MC detected transcoding actions on teleconsultation messages operated by some Microsoft Exchange mail servers, as well as difficulties related to internal security policies. These

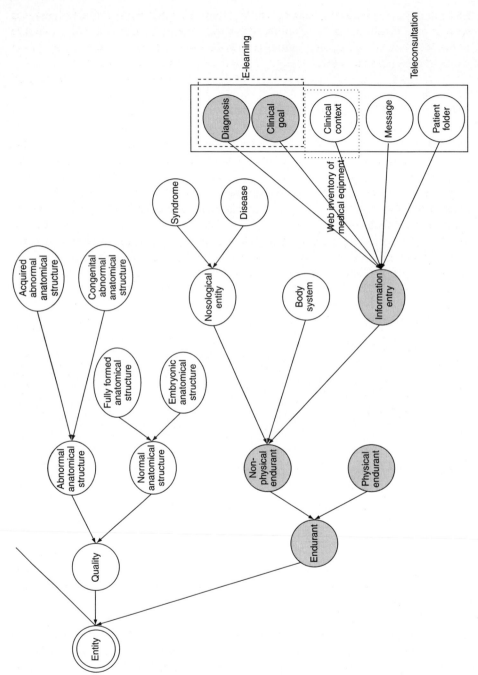

Figure 16.2 The first implementation of the Alliance's reference ontology. (Adapted from *Top Level Concepts of the Reference Ontology of Medicine*. Laboratory of Applied Ontology of Rome, National Research Council.)

problems were overcome by helping the hospital IT departments to properly configure their internal mail servers and security systems. The automatic alarm facilities at the MC helped to identify the problem of lost attachments and to solve it.

As far as the service organization at the health centres is concerned, after experiencing some mismanagement of time and allocation of requests, hospitals were advised by the Secretariat to install the teleconsultation workstation in the health directorate in order to manage the incoming flow of enquiries centrally. Some teleconsultation forms were not properly filled in by the referring centres in terms of completeness of medical data for diagnosis, so the Secretariat intervened in order to improve the request quality and speed up the processing. This represents a global process of optimization.

In 2006, a second survey on satisfaction was carried out. The results were positive in relation to the national health centres and to the Italian hospitals worldwide. For the latter, a slight decrease of service satisfaction was recorded in comparison with the previous survey. The reasons are essentially due to the 'distance' of some physicians who in Italy are far from the day-to-day problems of hospitals in other countries. As far as the specialists are concerned, communication can sometimes be difficult (mostly because of the use of the English and Spanish languages on the form, rather than Italian, and the lack of clinical data).

Manual of procedures

The total quality management approach adopted by the Alliance includes a manual of procedures. Procedures are planned for each of the Alliance's services with the help of the relevant people in the operational management. This is an attempt to standardize actions in a conceptualized framework. It helps operators to manage routine and unexpected events. Procedures are revised either periodically or when needed.

Insights

Common difficulties experienced during the first years of the project included a shortage of local infrastructure and a lack of financial resources. War conditions in some of the countries hosting the Alliance's hospitals provided additional problems. Planning and implementation activities were therefore very important, and the Secretariat accomplished these tasks successfully. We concentrated on finding technical solutions tailored to the *micro* dimension of each problem, since it was impossible to act with a country-level approach. The motivation and cohesion of the hospitals were continuously supported by the Secretariat, and there was public–private sponsorship for some technical solutions. After four years of experience, it is clear that success is mainly due to the strong organizational framework provided by the Secretariat, in terms of methodologies and procedures. This has made it possible to produce better results than are common with telemedicine projects in developing countries, where simple email is the usual medium of communication. Key factors in our success were a telecommunication network, specialized software for teleconsultation, an organized database and ad hoc ontologies.

There were other components that were also essential for the success of the initiative. The hospitals in Italy provided valuable expertise, both in teleconsultation and in distance learning. In addition, it should be mentioned that free-of-charge participation of hundreds of specialists would be simply inconceivable if done outside the public health system.

Finally, all doctors of Italian hospitals worldwide have left their own mark in strengthening the mission of the Alliance, which is both ethical and cooperative. The mixture of all these things has made the programme effective, and now partnership appears to be a main asset.

Conclusion

The IPOCM programme is rather different from other telemedicine work recorded in the literature. Although it shares some elements with other telemedicine initiatives in developing countries, it has relied on a solid organizational element as well as standardized procedures. Institutional support, in terms of resources and know-how, was crucial in ensuring sustainability and high service quality. Furthermore, good governance was required to keep all these elements together. Appropriate resources and good governance are therefore important components for a public policy focused on health partnership in developing countries.

Further reading

Aas IH. The future of telemedicine – take the organizational challenge! *J Telemed Telecare* 2007; **13**: 379–81.

Geissbuhler A, Bagayoko CO, Ly O. The RAFT network: 5 years of distance continuing medical education and tele-consultations over the Internet in French-speaking Africa. *Int J Med Inform* 2007; **76**: 351–6.

References

1. Vassallo DJ, Buxton PJ, Kilbey JH, Trasler M. The first telemedicine link for the British Forces. *J R Army Med Corps* 1998; **144**: 125–30.
2. Vassallo DJ. Twelve months' experience with telemedicine for the British armed forces. *J Telemed Telecare* 1999; **5**(Suppl 1): 117–18
3. Edejer TT. Disseminating health information in developing countries: the role of the Internet. *BMJ* 2000; **321**: 797–800.
4. 4. Fraser HS, McGrath SJ. Information technology and telemedicine in sub-Saharan Africa. *BMJ* 2000; **321**: 465–6.
5. Vassallo DJ, Swinfen P, Swinfen R, Wootton R. Experience with a low-cost telemedicine system in three developing countries. *J Telemed Telecare* 2001; **7**(Suppl 1): 56–8.
6. Vassallo DJ, Hoque F, Roberts MF et al. An evaluation of the first year's experience with a low-cost telemedicine link in Bangladesh. *J Telemed Telecare* 2001; **7**: 125–38.

7.   Graham LE, Zimmerman M, Vassallo DJ et al. Telemedicine – the way ahead for medicine in the develop-ing world. *Trop Doct* 2003; **33**: 36–8.

8.   Wootton R. Design and implementation of an automatic message-routing system for low-cost telemedi-cine. *J Telemed Telecare* 2003; **9**(Suppl 1): 44–7.

9.   Cone SW, Carucci LR, Yu J et al. Acquisition and evaluation of radiography images by digital camera. *Telemed J E Health* 2005; **11**: 130–6.

10. Anderson JE. *Public Policy-Making.* New York: Praeger, 1972.

11. Kirsh D. Adapting the environment instead of oneself. *Adaptive Behavior* 1996; **4**: 415–52.

12. Eden C, Ackermann F. *Making Strategy: the Journey of Strategic Management.* London: Sage, 1998.

13. Johnson G, Scholes K. *Exploring Corporate Strategy.* Englewood Cliffs, NJ: Prentice-Hall, 1993: 75–114.

14. Ministero del Lavoro, della Salute e della Politiche Sociale: Settore Salute. Available (in Italian) at: www.ministerosalute.it.

15. Mitka M. Developing countries find telemedicine forges links to more care and research. *JAMA* 1998; **280**: 1295–6.

16. Strode SW, Gustke S, Allen A. Technical and clinical progress in telemedicine. *JAMA* 1999; **281**: 1066–8.

17. Rodas EB, Latifi R, Cone S et al. Telesurgical presence and consultation for open surgery. *Arch Surg* 2002; **137**: 1360–3.

18. Fisk NM, Vaughan JI, Wootton R, Harrison MR. Intercontinental fetal surgical consultation with image transmission via Internet. *Lancet* 1993; **341**: 1601–2.

19. Kuntalp M, Akar O. A simple and low-cost Internet-based teleconsultation system that could effectively solve the health care access problems in underserved areas of developing countries. *Comput Methods Programs Biomed* 2004; **75**: 117–26.

20. Zolfo M, Lynen L, Dierckx J, Colebunders R. Remote consultations and HIV/AIDS continuing education in low-resource settings. *Int J Med Inform* 2006; **75**: 633–7.

21. National Center for Health Statistics, US Centers for Disease Control and Prevention. *International Clas-sification of Diseases*, 9th revision, *Clinical Modification (ICD9-CM)*. Available at: www.cdc.gov/nchs/icd9.htm.

22. *Martindale: The Complete Drug Reference*, 35th edn, London: Pharmaceutical Press, 2007.

23. Gruber TR. Toward principles for the design of ontologies used for knowledge sharing. *Int J Hum Comput Stud* 1995; **43**: 907–8.

24. Eccher C, Purin B, Pisanelli DM et al. Ontologies supporting continuity of care: the case of heart failure. *Comput Biol Med* 2006; **36**: 789–801.

17 Telemedicine in Nepal

Mohan R Pradhan

Introduction

Telemedicine is the process of providing medical expertise remotely with the help of telecommunication. It is particularly valuable in remote areas, and is therefore useful in Nepal, where the few specialists are separated from most of the population. Nepal has one of the lowest gross national products (GNPs) (US$300) per capita[1] and one of the lowest literacy rates (50%)[2] of the South Asia Region. These factors have contributed to the prevalence of communicable, respiratory and nutrition deficiency diseases, which are among the most common disorders seen in hospital outpatient departments. Telemedicine is therefore an attractive potential means of improving health services. In industrialized countries, real-time telemedicine is commonly used. However, this modality is not applicable in a developing country, like Nepal, because of the high cost of bandwidth and the poor telecommunication infrastructure.

The alternative modality, more suitable for a developing country, is store-and-forward telemedicine. In a store-and-forward interaction, the referring doctor usually enters the clinical information and digital images in a computer. The information can then be transmitted via a dial-up Internet connection as an email attachment to a central computer. The expert doctor can access the data independently at a convenient time. The size of the images attached to email messages is a potential problem with this technique, which may necessitate some degree of image compression.

HealthNet Nepal

HealthNet Nepal is a non-governmental organization (NGO) that provides affordable Internet services to the Nepalese health community, access to health information and technical support for various regional information-sharing initiatives. It has developed its own software, called Hnet telemedicine.

Development of the software

When we examined the available telemedicine software, we found that open source software was not suitable for our purpose[3] and that commercial software could not be easily modified. It was therefore decided to develop software suitable for telemedicine in the context of Nepal.

The local system collects a clinical history and images, which are then transmitted to a specialist for diagnosis. For the clinical history, both general information and discipline-specific information are collected. The general information includes the following:

- patient information
- basic information
- personal history
- past medical history
- family history.

There is also discipline-specific information for the following specialties:

- pathology
- radiology
- dermatology
- cardiology.

In acquiring digital images, the following components were considered.

Pathology
Images were obtained using a digital camera (Nikon CoolPix 4500). This type of camera is suitable for pathology. It has a resolution of 4 megapixels (Mp), which is sufficient for telemedicine according to the recommendations of the American College of Radiology.[4] An additional advantage of this camera is that it can be easily mounted on a microscope with a 30 mm eyepiece adapter.

Radiology and dermatology
It was found that using the same camera for pathology was not practical. The camera used for radiology and dermatology was a Nikon CoolPix P4, which has a higher resolution (8 Mp). An additional feature of this camera is its vibration-reduction ability, which makes it suitable for taking pictures in shaky conditions.

Cardiology
For cardiology, an ECG machine was used (ECG 9620L, Cardiofax) that directly transfers an ECG image to a computer. Thus, there is no need to use a digital camera to photograph ECG recordings.

Software for data transfer and security

The software ensured data security during transfer in the following ways.

Image processing
Once images have been stored in the computer, they need to be cropped to reduce the file size and annotation has to be provided for better description of the clinical problem. A simple graphics package was developed for this purpose and incorporated into the client software of the Hnet telemedicine system. This graphics package allows

cropping, annotation, rotation, colour balance and conversion to black and white. In addition, the free image-viewing software IrfanView was used.[5]

Compression
Image compression was used to reduce the quantity of memory required to store an image. For example, an image that has a resolution of 640 × 480 pixels with 24-bit colour requires 900 kbyte of storage. If this image can be compressed at a compression ratio of 20 : 1, the quantity of storage required is reduced to about 45 kbyte. Hnet has used the camera's built-in JPEG image compression at a ratio of 16 : 1. It has been found that image compression of 60–80% can be achieved without significant loss of diagnostic quality.

Security and confidentiality
Data stored in a computer must not be read or compromised by unauthorized users. The Hnet software uses password-level encryption. The passwords are stored in MD5-encrypted format for security. Without an authorized login, no one can run the application.

Receiving and reviewing cases
After logging on to the Hnet system, the two physicians concerned, typically a remote physician or health worker and a medical specialist in a hospital, communicate by email. After uploading a case, the server selects a doctor on a simple round-robin basis from the names listed in the roster. The server regularly watches for a reply from the doctor. If a doctor does not reply to a case within 12 hours, then the case is automatically assigned to another doctor listed in the roster. Doctors are categorized into groups, such as dermatology, radiology, cardiology and pathology. These specialists can view only their own cases.

Digital photography guides

A technical manual was developed as a basic guide for non-medical professionals and general practitioners on how to take clinical photographs in radiology, pathology and dermatology using a digital camera.

Pilot project

The pilot telemedicine network was implemented from July 2004 to December 2006. The project was financed by the PAN Asia programme of the IDRC, Canada (see Chapter 7). The following hospitals referred cases for telemedicine:

- AMDA Hospital, Damak (eastern region)
- Siddhartha Children's and Women Hospital, Butwal (western region)
- Siddhi Memorial Hospital, Bhaktapur (central region).

Specialist expertise was provided from the following central-level hospitals:

- Teaching Hospital, Tribhuvan University (Department of Radiology and Dermatology)
- Kathmandu Medical College (Department of Pathology and Department of Dermatology)
- Sahid Ganga Lal National Heart Centre.

The medical experts located at the medical colleges and special hospitals of the central level (capital city) were chosen because the doctors there had better knowledge of IT and were willing to participate in the project. The local hospitals were chosen based on the size and location of the local population.

It was found that the availability of telemedicine increased the volume of teleconsultation and provided exposure to a rural community for the medical interns of medical colleges. It also provided continuing education and reduced the professional isolation of health professionals working in rural areas. All these factors improved the quality and efficiency of the health service. With the use of telemedicine, access to the literature through the HINARI system of the World Health Organization increased. The observations below are based on informal communication with the referring physicians.

Study

A study was conducted in Nepal to assess whether telemedicine based on store-and-forward technology would be satisfactory for the diagnosis of cases sent from remote rural areas in the specialties of dermatology, radiology, pathology and cardiology. There were two components to the work: a basic component and a clinical component.[6] The basic component was to define the minimum technical specifications to ensure that diagnostically important information could be captured through a clinical history and digital image. This component also included an investigation of the medical expert's ability to make an accurate diagnosis based on digital images and clinical history. The second component was to evaluate whether the technology would improve the process of health care delivery by increasing information flow and reducing professional isolation.

For inclusion of cases, data were collected from the field sites. These cases were entered into the computer of the client site and uploaded to the server. On the server, the specialist doctors completed their perception of the image exposure and diagnostic quality using a binary scale (0 = poor or 1 = adequate). At the second stage, the specialist doctors recorded their confidence in the presence of each diagnostic indicator on a five-point scale (1 = definitely absent to 5 = definitely present). The ratings from these scales were used for receiver operating characteristic (ROC) analysis. The ROC analysis was used to determine whether the image quality was sufficient for diagnosis.

A two-step rating method was used to plot the ROC data. First, a dichotomous variable indicating quality of image (0 = negative or 1 = positive) was used. Second, the dichotomous variable based on the quality of the image was further rated based on a five-point scale (1 = definitely negative to 5 = definitely positive. The use of five categories is a reasonable compromise between the needs of ROC analysis and the precision with which the observers can be expected to reproduce their ratings. The five-point rating scale was used to calculate predicted probability. This predicted probability along with the dichotomous variable can be used to plot an ROC curve in order to provide a visual impression of the reliability of the points. The statistical package SPSS 11.5 was used for calculating predicted probability using a logistic regression model. Based on the dichotomous variable, a predicted probability ROC curve was plotted.

Similarly, provisional diagnosis by primary care physicians and diagnosis by clinical experts was used for comparing baseline medical knowledge of primary care physicians with clinical experts. These data were used only in dermatology.

Study findings

A total of 218 cases were observed:

- dermatology: 75 cases
- radiology : 90 cases
- histology : 34 cases
- cytology: 19 cases.

The gold standard for any specialist referred remains the traditional method of consultation, i.e. in the case of radiology, it is the viewing of an X-ray film; in the case of pathology, it is viewing through a microscope; and in the case of dermatology, it is face-to-face consultation.

We adopted an affordable system that was appropriate to our needs.[7] Compared with real-time systems, store-and-forward systems are more practical and less expensive. Store-and-forward methods allow the use of low-cost equipment, low-bandwidth connections and asynchronous consultation. This approach has been used successfully in industrialized countries where high-quality images are transmitted via telemedicine networks for consultation.[8]

Digital cameras are an efficient method of obtaining digital images. Krupinski et al[9,10] evaluated the effectiveness of digital photography for dermatology and bone trauma diagnoses, and found that digital camera images were of satisfactory quality. Piccolo et al[11] found high diagnostic concordance between telepathology and histopathology diagnosis. Lim et al[12] and High et al[13] evaluated a digital camera for teledermatology, and also found high concordance with face-to-face diagnoses.

For determining the quality of images sufficient for diagnosis, a ROC analysis was performed. It has been suggested that qualitative conclusions can be drawn from ROC experiments performed with at least 100 observations.[14] In our example, all four tests (dermatology, radiology, histology and cytology) had low p values ($p < 0.5$).[15] Figure 17.1 shows the ROC curve for dermatology. It can be concluded that the images had the ability to detect disease.

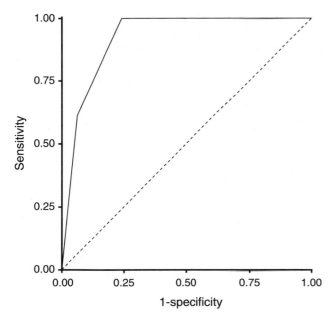

Figure 17.1 ROC curve for dermatology (the broken line represents no discrimination, i.e. a random guess)

Willingness to participate in the telemedicine project

In Nepal, there are few doctors. There is only one doctor for 6000 people (the doctor-to-population ratio is 1 : 6000). Our study showed that practising doctors usually did not use IT for knowledge updating. The reasons given for not using IT were that most of the doctors were busy practitioners and they perceived that they could manage communicable, respiratory, tropical and nutritional deficiency diseases without recent information. Another reason was the heavy patient workload.

However, the circumstances are different in medical colleges, since doctors are required to update their knowledge in order to teach students. IT has become a useful medium for updating their knowledge. So, doctors working in medical colleges and special research institutes are chosen as experts for the diagnosis of certain cases. Another reason is that doctors working in medical colleges and research institutes feel comfortable in using IT.

Age of users

All the users were aged 31–50 years. This included participants from both central and local hospitals. The reason may be that the younger generation grew up with computers, witnessing developments in computers and the Internet first hand.

Gender

Only one (10%) female was involved in a telemedicine project, and she was a health professional from a central hospital. In Nepal, medicine has been and still is a male-dominated profession. Nurses were not involved in telemedicine in the local hospital. The reason is that consultations are like a second opinion, which exclude nurses' participation because they do not have the doctors' level of competence.

Organizational position

With reference to the organizational position of participants, it was found that staff involved in the telemedicine project were doctors or technicians responsible for the technical part of the project.

Users' attitudes to telemedicine

The technical components of telemedicine were related to the computerization process of central and remote sites. The problems related to the computerization process were related to low computer literacy and the absence of reliable communication infrastructure. In this context, the users' attitudes depended on their general knowledge and familiarization with computer technology. All participants in the project from local hospitals and central hospitals felt comfortable with IT as a whole and telemedicine in particular. Telemedicine gave them an opportunity to enhance their efficiency and distance learning and to minimize professional isolation. With the help of telemedicine, they were able to create databases for various diseases, their forms and methods of treatment. Doctors perceived that the databases helped to improve their efficiency.

Consultation areas

Telemedicine was used for the purpose of general guidance, assessment of diagnosis, treatment and examinations. It was also found that confidence between local and remote hospitals was crucial to achieve and maintain a fruitful dialogue. Often it is difficult to state the diagnosis from the first information transferred. For this, two-way communications in the form of chat is provided to make a precise diagnosis.

Collaboration between doctors at local and central level

The users in the telemedicine project noted that their collaboration with professionals changed with the help of telemedicine. Doctors become more open to advice from their colleagues and specialists. Doctors came to believe that the process of patient care could be enhanced through telemedicine, and their trust in information technology increased.

Exposure to rural areas

In Nepal, most doctors are reluctant to work in rural areas owing to professional isolation, lack of facilities to update their knowledge and lack of continuing education. In medical colleges, as a part of an internship programme, a doctor has to work in rural areas. The telemedicine process minimized the gap of professional isolation and gave the opportunity for continuing education in rural areas. This first-hand experience in rural areas with telemedicine may motivate doctors to work in rural areas when their medical courses are completed.

Drawbacks

Although telemedicine clearly has a number of potential benefits, it also has some disadvantages. The main drawbacks are a potential breakdown in professional relationships and a number of organizational problems.

Breakdown in the relationship between health professionals

Skilled staff at the remote site sometimes perceive that their autonomy is threatened by the use of telemedicine, or, worse still, think that they will become no more than technicians, acting solely at the guidance of the remote specialist.[16]

Organizational problems

The following organizational problems were identified in Nepal:

- Fear of the unknown. Nepal remained poorly networked because of inertia, fear and technical inexperience of higher management personnel in government and NGOs.
- Lack of trained manpower. In spite of widespread enthusiasm about IT, there are very few local facilities for higher-level technical training.
- Possessiveness. In a country with the lowest GNP in the region and having few opportunities, people, including higher-level management, tend to hoard everything. They do not hesitate to break contracts, even for minor financial benefits. This attitude runs counter to networking and information sharing.

Economic evaluation

An analysis was carried out to compare the cost of telemedicine with the cost of traditional methods of providing health care services (Table 17.1). Only variable costs were considered. The cost charged by the remote site was approximately 50% less than the charge to be paid in city areas. However, the patient need not bear the cost of transportation and lodging. The telemedicine service charge would be sufficient to

Table 17.1 Comparison of variable costs (1 US$ = Rs0.65)

Type of service	Charge through traditional method (Nepalese Rs)	Charge through telemedicine (Nepalese Rs)
Radiology (plain X-ray)	15	15
ECG	400	200
Pathology (cytology)	500	250
Dermatology	200	50
Transportation (nearest city)	200	—
Lodging	200	—

cover the fixed costs and to pay the fees of the expert. Thus, only the cost of the expert's Internet connection would have to be borne by the remote centre. It is too early to calculate all the costs (fixed and variable) in order to estimate whether telemedicine could become financially sustainable.

Research findings

We also compared the baseline medical knowledge of primary care physicians with clinical experts. Here, we also found that there was no difference in the diagnosis among primary care physicians and expert doctors. This supports the view that textual information supplemented by images is sufficient for diagnosis.

The telemedicine system helped primary care physicians to interact with medical experts. This, in turn, helped to reduce the professional isolation of health care staff working in rural areas.

At the start of the project, we found technophobia among health professionals working in rural areas. To reduce this, we provided IT training courses to all the health professionals working in rural areas. These training courses helped rural health workers to become familiar with IT. These health workers also found that IT could enhance their efficiency. The technical knowledge encouraged staff to use IT in other areas such as hospital information systems, to improve the efficiency of the hospital and to provide access to the health literature to update their knowledge.

Future developments

In our research project, we found that there was potential for telemedicine in Nepal, especially in rural areas, but also in urban areas. It was also found that textual information with images was sufficient for diagnosis in many cases. Telemedicine helped medical education, medical care and collegial support. However, continuation of the work after the project has finished will depend on how the local health professionals and medical experts support the services. To support and continue the telemedicine work, there should be other computerized health services, such as distance education, digital libraries and computerized hospital information systems. That is, telemedicine cannot develop in isolation. These types of activities will encourage rural health workers and medical specialists to continue the telemedicine work. As users become more comfortable with the technology, they are inclined to experiment with new applications. These activities help to enhance their efficiency, update their knowledge and reduce professional isolation.

Low-cost telemedicine based on store-and-forward systems has also been carried out in other developing countries. For example, the Swinfen Charitable Trust established a telemedicine link to support the Centre for the Rehabilitation of the Paralysed (CRP) in Savar, near Dhaka in Bangladesh, in July 1999[17] (see Chapter 19). Based on the success of the Bangladesh project, the Swinfen Charitable Trust supplied digital cameras and tripods to more hospitals in other developing countries. These included the Patan Hospital in Nepal (March 2000), Gizo Hospital in the Solomon Islands (March 2000), Helena Goldie Hospital in the Solomon Islands (September 2000) and LAMB Hospital in Bangladesh (September 2000). In South Africa, the technique has been used for referrals from remote clinics. The US Armed Forces have made use of store-and-forward telemedicine for telepathology (see Chapter 15), and a link has been established between Italian hospitals worldwide (see Chapter 16).[18] Store-and-forward teledermatology has been used in linking remote parts of Africa to teaching hospitals in the USA and Europe.

Suggestions were invited from the users in Nepal for improving the telemedicine service. The following were the main suggestions:

- Include separate funding for telemedicine in hospitals with telemedicine units and in central hospitals providing expert advice.
- Improve the technology for telemedicine from still images to videoconferencing.
- Increase the frequency of consultations and organize videoconferences.
- Define a list of cases for mandatory advice apart from emergency cases.
- Computerize the hospital information systems, which will help to follow up patients treated earlier.

It is not easy to answer the question whether telemedicine in a developing country is cost-effective, since this requires evaluation in a properly controlled, scientific trial. Unless this can be done, the answer to the question whether telemedicine represents an appropriate use of resources will remain unknown.[19]

Further reading

Blanchet KD. Innovative programs in telemedicine. *Telemed J E Health* 2008; **14**: 318–22.
Clarke M, Thiyagarajan CA. A systematic review of technical evaluation in telemedicine systems. *Telemed J E Health* 2008; **14**: 170–83.
iPath Association. *Telemedicine in Developing Countries*. Available at: ipath.ch/site/node/19.
Latifi R, ed. *Establishing Telemedicine in Developing Countries: From Inception to Implementation*. Amsterdam: IOS Press, 2004.
Wurm EM, Campbell TM, Soyer HP. Teledermatology: how to start a new teaching and diagnostic era in medicine. *Dermatol Clin* 2008; **26**: 295–300.

References

1. United Nations Development Programme. *Nepal Millennium Development Goals (MDG): Progress Report 2005*. Available at: www.undp.org.np/publication/html/mdg2005/mdg2005.php.
2. World Health Organization. *Country Health System Profile: Nepal*. Available at: www.searo.who.int/en/Section313/Section1523_6870.htm.
3. Carnall D. Medical software's free future. *BMJ* 2000; **321**: 976.

4. American College of Radiology. *ACR Standard for Teleradiology, 1998*. Available at: imaging.stryker.com/images/ACR_Standards-Teleradiology.pdf.
5. IrfanView. Available at: www.irfanview.com.
6. Perednia DA, Brown NA. Teledermatology: one application of telemedicine. *Bull Med Libr Assoc* 1995; **83**: 42–7.
7. McGee R, Tangalos EG. Delivery of health care to the undeserved: potential contributions of telecommunications technology. *Mayo Clin Proc* 1994; **69**: 1131–6.
8. Szot A, Jacobson FL, Munn S et al. Diagnostic accuracy of chest X-rays acquired using a digital camera for low-cost teleradiology. *Int J Med Inform* 2004; **73**: 65–73.
9. Krupinski E, Gonzales M, Gonzales C, Weinstein RS. Evaluation of a digital camera for acquiring radiographic images for telemedicine applications. *Telemed J E Health* 2000; **6**: 297–302.
10. Krupinski EA, LeSueur B, Ellsworth L et al. Diagnostic accuracy and image quality using a digital camera for teledermatology. *Telemed J* 1999; **5**: 257–3.
11. Piccolo D, Soyer HP, Burgdorf W et al. Concordance between telepathologic diagnosis and conventional histopathologic diagnosis: a multiobserver store-and-forward study on 20 skin specimens. *Arch Dermatol* 2002: **138**: 53–8.
12. Lim AC, Egerton IB, See A, Shumack SP. Accuracy and reliability of store-and-forward teledermatology: preliminary results from the St George Teledermatology Project. *Australas J Dermatol* 2001; **42**: 247–51.
13. High WA, Houston MS, Calobrisi SD et al. Assessment of the accuracy of low-cost store-and-forward teledermatology consultation. *J Am Acad Dermatol* 2000; **42**: 776–83.
14. Metz CE. Basic principles of ROC analysis. *Semin Nucl Med* 1978; **8**: 283–98.
15. Zweig MH, Campbell G. Receiver-operating characteristic (ROC) plots: a fundamental evaluation tool in medicine. *Clin Chem* 1993; **39**: 561–77.
16. Hjelm NM. Benefits and drawbacks of telemedicine. *J Telemed Telecare* 2005; **11**: 60–70.
17. Vassallo DJ, Swinfen P, Swinfen R, Wootton R. Experience with a low-cost telemedicine system in three developing countries. *J Telemed Telecare* 2001; **7**(Suppl 1): 56–8.
18. Della Mea V, Beltrami CA. Telepathology applications of the Internet multimedia electronic mail. *Med Inform (Lond)* 1998; **23**: 237–44.
19. Wootton R. The possible use of telemedicine in developing countries. *J Telemed Telecare* 1997; **3**: 23–6.

18 Telemedical support for surgeons in Ecuador

Stephen Cone, Edgar J Rodas and Ronald C Merrell

Introduction

A surgery project for the isolated and under-served in Ecuador, which began more than 25 years ago, has matured into a fixed element of service delivery. Telemedicine was first applied to support the surgery programme in 1995.[1] Ecuador has characteristics that make it highly suitable for telemedicine.

Ecuador (more properly called the Republic of Ecuador) has a population of 13 million.[2] They are a mixture of European heritage and indigenous peoples, and occupy three distinct geographical zones.[3] The westernmost zone is the coastal region. The central zone is the highlands (the Sierra). The easternmost region (the Oriente) marks the beginning of the Amazonian rainforest.

The majority of the population work in the service industry, many being employed in eco-tourism.[3] However, the unemployment rate is 10.6%, with poverty affecting 39% of the population.[3] The gross national product (GNP) for Ecuador is US$4070 per capita.[2] The average per capita expenditure for health care is US$127.[2] Total health care spending for the country is 5.5% of the gross domestic product (GDP).[2]

Health concerns in Ecuador

Ecuador has certain medical problems that are common to much of the rest of the world, some that are common to tropical regions and some that are common to developing countries. These three categories are important in considering illness in Ecuador. Like the world in general, Ecuador is facing changing illness patterns that reflect the emergence of chronic conditions, rather than the acute, infectious diseases more common in earlier times. There is also increasing interpersonal violence and trauma (mainly due to increased motor vehicle activity) and tropical disease. As a developing country, Ecuador has the common problems of sanitation, nutrition and access to health care.

Despite these challenges, life expectancy in Ecuador is similar to that in industrialized countries, with recent data predicting 70 years for males and 75 years for females.[2] Infant and child mortality are high, at 22 and 25 per 1000 live births, respectively.[2] Compared with 10 years ago, non-communicable diseases have increased in importance (up to 42% of deaths), as have injuries (21% of deaths), while communicable diseases have declined as a measure of the burden for mortality (down to 37% of deaths).[4]

Medical system in Ecuador

Ecuador has developed a health care system based on a combination of public, private and volunteer support. In 2000, the total health workforce (physicians, nurses, midwives and dentists) numbered 41 000.[2] There were 18 000 physicians (or 1.5 per 1000 people).[2] These numbers do not include the traditional tribal healers, once an important part of the culture of the indigenous peoples. With 39% of the people living in rural areas, and up to 30% of the population classified as Amerindian,[3] the role of the 'curanderos' in health care is still significant.

The more common, Western-style practitioners study in a traditional style of medical education, modelled on the European system. The national government supports the education of doctors (six years of medical school followed by a one-year internship), in return for which the doctors are expected to provide a year of service, typically in rural/under-served areas.

The national government is also responsible for 41% of total health spending, of which about 15% is from social security funds, the rest coming from the Ministerio de Salud Publica (MSP), the public health ministry.[2] In many cases, the patient's family is responsible for providing meals, medicines and some materials during the course of care. Despite the efforts of private payers, and government support for health care, about 25% of the population do not have access to health care.[2]

For people in rural areas and the poorest sections of urban areas, care may be non-existent or may come from volunteer providers. Many providers in the country are philanthropic organizations, such as the Fundación Cinterandes (Cuenca, Ecuador). Many health care workers are volunteers from the USA and elsewhere. Interplast and Operation Smile are two examples of plastic surgery missions well established in many developing countries, including Ecuador.

Intermittent surgical services

Volunteer organizations, such as those mentioned, provide intermittent surgical services to meet the surgical needs of under-served populations. This has previously been decried as poor-quality care, since the surgeon does not follow the care of the patient directly throughout the process of healing. However, intermittent surgical services are becoming recognized as part of a comprehensive system of health care delivery.[5] With the use of telemedicine, the distance between patient and surgeon becomes less of a problem and, with a system of integrated providers (primary care and specialist), the patient need never be without expert opinion.

The original intention of the mobile surgery programme of the Cinterandes Foundation was to use Ecuadorian and international volunteers to provide intermittent surgical services to under-served populations. The system has subsequently expanded to become a more inclusive, integrated part of a continuum of care.[1] Since 1994, the Cinterandes Foundation has been providing surgical care to remote populations, decreasing the need for patient/family travel (and travel-related expenses), reducing delays in treatment, and the associated mortality and morbidity.[1]

The mobile surgery programme is based on a truck with an operating room built on it (Figures 18.1 and 18.2). There is a small permanent staff, which is supplemented with volunteers and students. However, even from the beginning, it was apparent that the role of local providers would be essential. The local primary providers supply initial contact with the population in need, and act as the continuing contact for follow-up care. In many ways, the mobile surgery programme operates like the typical specialist practice, depending on primary care for patient referrals, and then proceeding through preoperative care, the operation and the immediate postoperative care. Local surgeons lend support and participate when the mobile programme is in their community. Thus, the programme is properly integrated into a model of continuous care.

Prescreening evaluation is extremely important in the mobile surgery programme. It is during this period that the primary care providers in the region, working under strict protocols, recruit patients with surgical problems for further evaluation. Cinterandes personnel then travel to the area to evaluate the patients, decide which patients are appropriate for the mobile surgery programme, which of them have priority needs, which patients have disqualifying comorbidities and which patients need medical treatment before surgical consideration.[1,6-8] This careful prescreening has

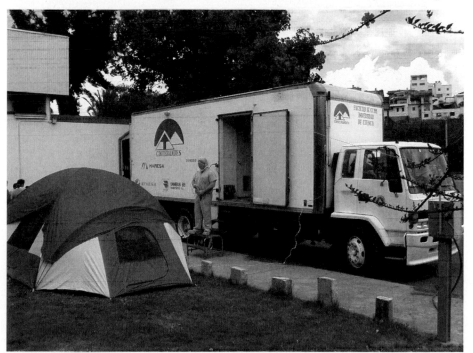

Figure 18.1 Operating room on the truck with tents for patient preparation and recovery

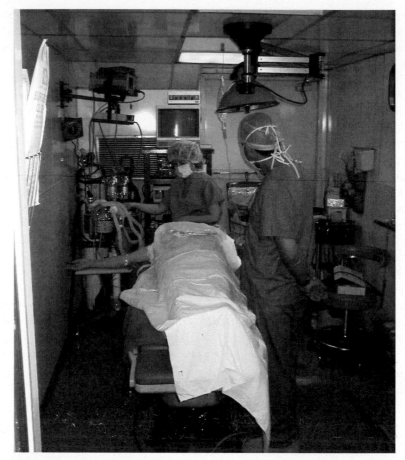

Figure 18.2 Interior view of the operating room, showing the induction of a patient. Note the laparoscopic equipment in the background

been important to the success of the programme. Patients with additional illnesses or infections may be referred to definitive facilities or may be excluded, to avoid unnecessary complications. Those who are accepted into the programme must be followed using existing local resources after surgery.

Prior to the day for surgery, the truck arrives on location, and parks outside the local health care facility. On the day of surgery, patients are re-examined in the local facility or in a Cinterandes tent (when local facilities are lacking).[1,7,8] After surgery, while the patient is recovering from anaesthesia, he or she is transferred to the recovery area, either in the local facility or in a recovery tent. During this time, postoperative care is arranged and ambulatory patients are discharged to home.

Cinterandes personnel provide the initial postoperative care.[1,7,8] Generally, doctors and students/residents see any patients still in the facility on the morning of the first postoperative day, returning to base in the afternoon. For those ambulatory patients sent home on the day of surgery, the postoperative plan has already been discussed with the patient and local provider. For those patients spending the night in the facility, postoperative plans are decided upon and communicated prior to discharge.

Although the initial postoperative evaluation is performed by the Cinterandes personnel, continuing care requires the support of the local caregivers. Continued postoperative care generally consists of visits at one week, one month and six months after surgery – or more frequently in the case of complications or suture removal. While these visits are performed by the local providers, the Cinterandes personnel remain available for consultation by telephone, advising about wound care and providing guidance about transferring patients in need of more advanced care.[7]

Understandably, this interdependence has made the interaction with local providers an important part of the success of the intermittent surgical service in Ecuador. Local providers and patients need the additional services provided by the intermittent surgical service to avoid costly alternatives or increased morbidity/mortality. The mobile surgery programme depends on the local providers to find suitable patients, arrange preoperative evaluations, assist with surgical scheduling and provide postoperative care to the patients.

In addition, the mobile surgery programme has come to develop an interaction with local and international medical education. The local schools in the Cuenca region provide students and residents to help with the surgery programme, in turn gaining a unique educational experience.[1] With this success, the Cinterandes Foundation has expanded the educational role to include students from foreign medical schools, who also gain valuable experience in learning about a new culture and medical system.

Programme activity

The Cinterandes Foundation has been operating the mobile surgery programme in various areas of Ecuador since 1994.[1] In that time, the programme has visited 15 of the 22 provinces in the country, performing approximately 40–50 surgical trips per year, i.e. each location generally receives more than one visit per year.[5] Thus, the surgical truck is in operation almost every week.

The programme has performed over 4500 operations in general surgery and specialties such as gynaecological and paediatric surgery.[1,5] Even with this patient volume in a small, mobile operating room, there has been no recorded mortality, and only four major complications (bleeding, cardiac arrest, pulmonary embolism and gastrointestinal injury).[5] A complication rate of less than 1% is similar to that of sophisticated US surgical centres. At this workload, the average cost of an operation performed by the mobile surgery programme is less than US$100.[5] These costs are met by the programme, so the service is free to patients.

Telemedicine to support surgery

Telemedicine has made a strong contribution to the intermittent surgical service. The first step was to apply digital records and review the management of the programme.

Next, the primary care, Foundation and international consulting sites were connected by dial-up Internet connections for email (Figure 18.3). Then the needs of the programme were assessed. The telemedicine stations were installed, personnel were trained in their use, and all participants were encouraged to practice protocols and use the Spanish-language electronic health record (EHR) before programme implementation. Both store-and-forward and real-time telemedicine were used.

Telemedicine support is, of course, limited by the telecommunications available. The rate that data (bits) can be transferred between sites is known as bandwidth. Table 18.1 shows the bandwidths of some of the different means of connectivity. All around the world, telecommunications continue to improve. However, in remote areas of the developing world, slower-speed connections remain the most robust medium for telemedicine.

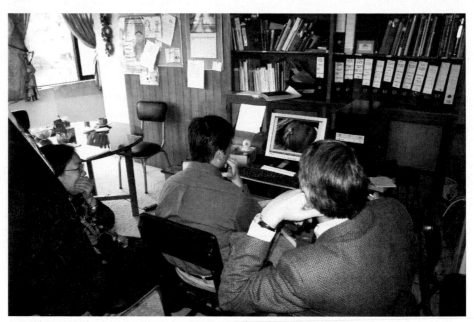

Figure 18.3 Cinterandes Foundation headquarters in Cuenca, during review of patient postoperative records. The images shown on the computer screen were collected during the postoperative care of a patient following a laparoscopic cholecystectomy

Table 18.1 Common connectivity modalities and associated bandwidths

Modality	Bandwidth
Ordinary telephone network (PSTN)	Up to 56 kbit/s
Integrated services digital network (ISDN)	64–128 kbit/s
Digital subscriber line (DSL)	256 kbit/s–2 Mbit/s
Cable modem	512 kbit/s–8 Mbit/s
Ethernet	10 or 100 Mbit/s

In developing a telemedicine system in such areas, it is often necessary to use connections of limited bandwidth.[6,9] Satellite transmission could certainly be employed, but the high cost usually makes this impractical. The ordinary telephone network (PSTN) is available in most of Ecuador, so that dial-up modems permit connection to an Internet service provider (ISP).[6,8,10] A technician may operate the equipment for the clinician, while attempting to familiarize the local providers with the use of such technology.[6]

The procedure for telemedicine to support mobile surgery begins with patient registration and the creation of an EHR. The data can be text, pictures (e.g. JPEG images), video or voice recordings. Registration includes the medical history and demographics, and can be longitudinal for primary care management. When surgical consultation is needed, there are, by protocol, strict criteria for acceptable patient risk for comorbidity and scope of surgery. The record is forwarded to the Foundation in an email attachment with a question. Staff at the Foundation assess the problem, recommend further diagnostic tests if necessary, order preoperative measures and, if appropriate, schedule the surgical procedure. Videoconferencing between the Foundation and patient is an option. This has been done using Microsoft NetMeeting. By this screening mechanism, the requests for surgical care are managed promptly and efficiently. Prior to telemedicine, large surgery consulting clinics took up enormous amounts of time, with little patient care offered. After operation, the same EHR keeps the surgeons apprised of the patient's progress and any complications, for care continuity. This postoperative phase can also use videoconferencing.

The telephone network can also be used during the operation to allow distant surgeons to advise (telementoring) or to educate (distance education).[10] Better-quality video and audio during surgery has been achieved with higher-bandwidth connections, for example using a satellite link from time to time. While an intraoperative videoconference is certainly improved with increased bandwidth, the pre- and postoperative visits are also better with the use of improved video. Low-bandwidth video transmission results in lower-resolution images or slower frame rates, or both, which may be unacceptable.[11] However, in increasing the bandwidth, the biggest problem is the cost. None the less, clinically acceptable transmission has been consistently achieved at 56 kbit/s using the ordinary telephone network.[6-10]

Videoconference consultations can run as smoothly as in-person examinations. Telemedicine establishes a sense of continuity in the care of the patient, and a link between the patient, primary provider and surgeon, despite the distances and intermittent services. The cost of telemedicine in Ecuador has been low once computers (US$1500) and digital camera (US$250) have been supplied. Training is provided by volunteers, and the only ongoing cost is for telecommunication. The cost of a local ISP is quite affordable in Ecuador.

The cost of telemedicine should be compared with that of on-site screening and consultation. In general, telemedicine allows time savings in a three-day surgical mission. For the cost of the ISP, there is a 25% increase in efficiency. The impact on patient safety is difficult to quantify, but the rarity of transfers suggests that telemedicine is at least as good as conventional management.

Experience in Ecuador

The role of the primary caregiver in the use of intermittent surgical care cannot be overemphasized. Likewise, the role of the primary caregiver in supporting the use of telemedicine should not be underplayed. The equipment used in primary care centres must be familiar to the providers, with utility beyond the support of intermittent surgical services. The equipment should be used daily and computer skills should be encouraged on a regular basis. This daily practice, along with curiosity and an interest in providing better care for their patients, prompts primary caregivers to seek additional skills with computers. Databases can provide a good means of storing patient data, allowing both archiving and retrieval. Spreadsheets simplify the process of calculating statistics. The addition of a digital camera to the equipment available in the clinic allows for digital image documentation of lesions, radiographs and the general appearance of patients. Digital cameras are now reasonably easy to use. One primary care doctor in the eastern rainforest region of Ecuador computerized his entire clinic, networking five computers (Figure 18.4) in different treatment areas, sharing the same database, and integrating images from a handheld digital camera, a video camera, a microscope eyepiece camera and an ultrasound scanner.[12] He has even employed the equipment in remote areas.

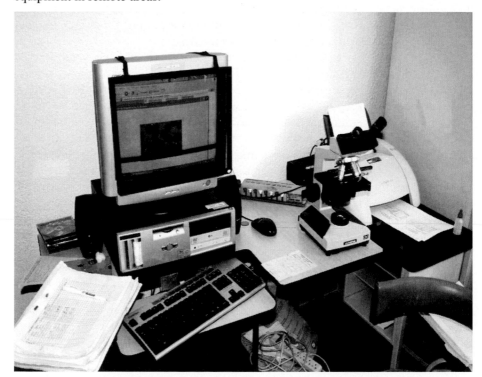

Figure 18.4 Primary care site in Macas. Computers are connected via a local area network (LAN). The unit shown is stationed in the clinic's laboratory, and can import microscopic images into the EHR, via an eyepiece camera

Early on, the surgeons in the Cinterandes Foundation recognized the importance of the role of primary care providers in supporting the continued intermittent mobile surgery programme. Using existing communications systems in rural areas of Ecuador, the surgeons have been able to integrate the primary providers into the prescreening process of surgical care. Store-and-forward telemedicine, i.e. asynchronous transmission of information, provides the basis for this support. As in work done in Kenya,[9] primary care providers can send information via email to the surgeons for review prior to a surgical trip.[6-8,10] With this advance information, surgeons are able to make better decisions about appropriateness for surgery. Equally important, the surgeons may use this opportunity to address the problems that made the patient inappropriate for surgery, and may direct further care for the patient. In Ecuador, the programme has sent students and junior surgeons to the field areas to set up and perform the remote clinics. Local providers have been enlisted to conduct the prescreening clinics, and have networked with permanent telemedicine stations in primary care clinics in three areas of Ecuador.[7] These connections employ computers with telephone dial-up modems that deliver, at best, 26 kbit/s bandwidth. Yet the system has prospered and continues to function (see Figure 18.3). The ISP may not have a fixed Internet Protocol (IP) address for the subscriber, and this can be very frustrating. Furthermore, the ISP's servers have limited capacity, and there is a consistent decline in quality and reliability during business (high-traffic) hours.

Prescreening of patients only needs store-and-forward telemedicine. However, video interaction by NetMeeting is possible. For the prescreening work, the videoconferencing may elicit further information and support informed consent. Low bandwidth may be used intraoperatively, sometimes with the additional transmission of high-quality still images.[13] As considerable image compression is required at these low bandwidths, higher-bandwidth transmission is certainly easier and faster for video-intensive applications.[11] A hand-carried, portable satellite communications system provides 64 kbit/s connectivity, while larger models and vehicle-mounted models provide even greater bandwidths. Using two 64 kbit/s satellite channels in parallel (i.e. a total of 128 kbit/s), transmission of live surgical images from the mobile surgery equipment can be performed at 30 frames per second with little image degradation.[14] Using a computer, rather than a videophone, allows sharing of email messages and forwarding of still images and other data. A full record of the surgical procedure is possible with video recording into a computerized database complete with patient and procedure information.[14]

Anaesthesia may also make use of telemedicine. In addition to using store-and-forward technology to share a patient's data and develop an anaesthetic plan, higher bandwidth allows transmission of live anaesthetic images and data. A single 64 kbit/s satellite connection provides enough bandwidth to transmit images, including endotracheal intubation via a fibre-optic intubation system, along with physiological data during the surgical procedure.[16]

Following surgery, the patient recovers in a familiar locality with familiar caregivers. It is important in this setting to provide a means for the concerns of the patient and the health providers to reach the intermittent surgery team. The telemedicine systems in place can provide support for postoperative care. Wound images and data may be sent in a store-and-forward manner, unless the surgeon decides that real-time videoconferencing is required. Again, the relationship with the local providers is important to the success of the intermittent surgical service.

The mobile surgery programme in Ecuador has enjoyed clinical success. This has been accompanied by great success in maintaining social support for patients in their communities and solidarity with primary care providers. Telemedicine has made this programme more efficient, and therefore available to more patients. The interactions with consultants outside Ecuador have matured into sound professional friendships.

Further reading

American College of Surgeons. *Operation Giving Back*. Available at: www.operationgivingback.facs.org.
Istepanian R, Laxminarayan S, Pattichis CS. *M-Health. Emerging Mobile Health Systems*. New York: Springer, 2006.
Latifi R, ed. *Establishing Telemedicine in Developing Countries: From Inception to Implementation*. Amsterdam: IOS Press, 2004.

References

1. The Cinterandes Foundation. Available at: www.cinterandes.org.
2. World Health Organization. Ecuador. Available at: www.who.int/countries/ecu/en.
3. Central Intelligence Agency. *The World Factbook: Ecuador*. Available at: www.cia.gov/library/publications/the-world-factbook/geos/ec.html.
4. Pan American Health Organization. *Country Health Profile: Ecuador*. Available at: www.paho.org/English/SHA/prflECU.htm.
5. Rodas E, Vicuna A, Merrell RC. Intermittent and mobile surgical services: logistics and outcomes. *World J Surg* 2005; **29**: 1335–9.
6. Doarn CR, Fitzgerald S, Rodas E et al. Telemedicine to integrate intermittent surgical services into primary care. *Telemed J E Health* 2002; **8**: 131–7.
7. Mora F, Cone S, Rodas E, Merrell RC. Telemedicine and electronic health information for clinical continuity in a mobile surgery program. *World J Surg* 2006; **30**: 1128–34.
8. Rodas E, Mora F, Tamariz F et al. Low-bandwidth telemedicine for pre- and postoperative evaluation in mobile surgical services. *J Telemed Telecare* 2005; **11**: 191–3.
9. Lee S, Broderick TJ, Haynes J et al. The role of low-bandwidth telemedicine in surgical prescreening. *J Pediatr Surg* 2003; **38**: 1281–3.
10. Rosser JC, Bell RL, Harnett B et al. Use of mobile low-bandwith telemedical techniques for extreme telemedicine applications. *J Am Coll Surg* 1999; **189**: 397–404.
11. Broderick TJ, Harnett BM, Merriam NR et al. Impact of varying transmission bandwidth on image quality. *Telemed J E Health* 2001; **7**: 47–53.
12. Cone SW, Hummel R, Leon J, Merrell RC. Implementation and evaluation of a low-cost telemedicine station in the remote Ecuadorian rainforest. *J Telemed Telecare* 2007; **13**: 31–4.
13. Broderick TJ, Harnett BM, Doarn CR et al. Real-time Internet connections: implications for surgical decision making in laparoscopy. *Ann Surg* 2001; **234**: 165–71.
14. Rodas EB, Latifi R, Cone S et al. Telesurgical presence and consultation for open surgery. *Arch Surg* 2002; **137**: 1360–3.
15. Cone SW, Leung A, Mora F et al. Multimedia data capture and management for surgical events: evaluation of a system. *Telemed J E Health* 2006; **12**: 351–8.
16. Cone SW, Gehr L, Hummel R, Merrell RC. Remote anesthetic monitoring using satellite telecommunications and the Internet. *Anesth Analg* 2006; **102**: 1463–7.

19 A low-cost international e-referral network

Richard Wootton, Pat Swinfen, Roger Swinfen and Peter Brooks

Introduction

Telemedicine provides the opportunity of delivering health care at a distance, and reduces the need for a face-to-face interaction. It is often conducted by videoconferencing, which permits a high-quality interaction between the parties concerned, but demands relatively expensive equipment and high bandwidth communications. In the context of developing countries, there has been little use of videoconferencing, for the obvious reason of cost. Most of the videoconferencing work that has been conducted has been for the purposes of education.[1–3]

Although there has been little use of real-time telemedicine, much useful clinical work has been performed in developing countries using store-and-forward techniques, which are less expensive of infrastructure and easier to organize because the interaction between the parties concerned is asynchronous. The two main methods of store-and-forward telemedicine are based on use of web messaging or on email.

Web telemedicine

In web-based telemedicine (for clinical purposes), the referring doctor connects to the Internet and completes a web-based proforma that stores the patient details and any associated images on a remote server. This information is reviewed by a specialist at some later time, and appropriate diagnostic and management advice is provided. The specialist's reply is stored on the web server, from where the referring doctor can access it. To ensure patient confidentiality, the information comprising the telemedicine interaction is normally stored on a secure server and protected by passwords.

The US military had considerable experience with web-based teledermatology in the late 1990s in Europe.[4] They have also operated a web-based teleconsulting system from the main US Army hospital in Hawaii that supports referrers in hospitals (mainly military hospitals) on US-associated Pacific islands.[5,6] Further details are provided in Chapter 15.

Finally, a software package called iPath was developed for telepathology case conferences, and several tens of thousands of case conferences have now been conducted – technically by a number of different organizations who all use the same software. The use of this software for general clinical work (i.e. non-pathology) is more recent.[7]

Email telemedicine

One drawback of web-based telemedicine is that in developing countries there are still places where Internet connections are expensive, and therefore web access in particular is restricted. Almost all health care facilities have, or could have, telephone access to the Internet, so this represents the lowest-cost communications medium for telemedicine.

In email-based telemedicine, the telephone network is used to transmit email messages via a dial-up connection to an Internet service provider (ISP). The referring doctor records the relevant patient information in the body of the email message, and images of patients, or X-ray films, can be attached if required. The specialist can reply by email at a convenient time.

Email telemedicine is cheap, but it has some drawbacks:

- On any significant scale, i.e. with multiple referring doctors and multiple specialists, managing the traffic is a demanding and labour-intensive task. Messages may then fail to be replied to.
- Information sent in an ordinary email message is not secure. Although the case details can be anonymized to protect patient confidentiality, this depends on the message sender, and is often difficult to enforce in practice.
- Because the referring doctor enters free text, it is much harder to ensure that all relevant patient history details are collected.
- Any system of communication that employs email will sooner or later be bombarded with spam or nuisance messages.

Two long-running examples of the use of email for low-cost telemedicine are the work of the Swinfen Charitable Trust and of Partners Telemedicine.

Swinfen Charitable Trust

The British military first used email telemedicine successfully in Bosnia.[8,9] In the 1990s, Lieutenant Colonel David Vassallo, together with Surgeon Commander Peter Buxton and Wing Commander John Kilbey, established a technique in which a digital camera was used to capture images, which were then downloaded to a laptop computer. The images were attached to an email message and then sent to the Royal Hospital Haslar in the UK for evaluation and advice. A commercial INMARSAT satellite telephone link was employed for communication in the field. The system proved useful when a Czech Forces Helicopter crashed in Bosnia in January 1998, severely injuring five crew members.[10] David Vassallo and Peter Buxton generously shared information about the system with Lord and Lady Swinfen, enabling them to start a pilot project at the Centre for Rehabilitation of the Paralysed in Bangladesh. This began in 1999 (see below).

Partners Telemedicine

Since 2001, email consultations have been used to support health workers at a rural clinic in northern Cambodia. The email advice comes from specialists at a tertiary hospital in Phnom Penh and from the Massachusetts General Hospital in Boston. In

2003, a second site at a small hospital in northern Cambodia began referring cases.[11] Further details are provided in Chapter 13.

Start of the network, 1999

The Swinfen Charitable Trust was established in 1998 to assist poor, sick and disabled people in the developing world. It is an apolitical, non-religious organization, registered as a charity in the UK. The Trustees decided to provide medical specialist advice, free of charge, to assist doctors caring for poor patients, as they were unaware of any such service at the time. In July 1999, an email telemedicine link was established for a hospital in Bangladesh, the Centre for the Rehabilitation of the Paralysed (CRP). The CRP, which is located near Dhaka, is a specialist spinal injury unit that services a large region of South-East Asia. Email referrals thus concentrated mainly on orthopaedics and neurology problems.

The email referrals were received by the administrators of the charity and sent on for reply to members of a small panel of medical specialists who had kindly offered to provide advice free of charge. This was a pilot study and, after a year of email referrals, a paper was published demonstrating that the system worked satisfactorily, and provided patient benefit and medical education to the referring doctors.[12]

The CRP has continued to refer cases to the Swinfen Charitable Trust network. At the time of writing, 182 cases have been referred in 10 years (Figure 19.1).

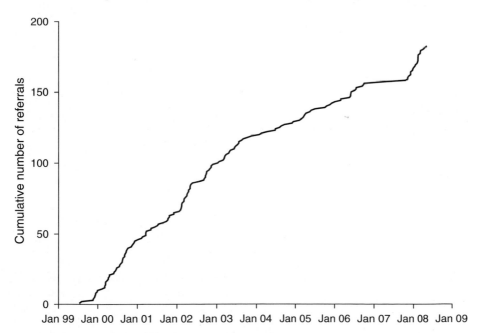

Figure 19.1 CRP referrals, July 1999–June 2008 inclusive

Growth of the network, 1999–2004

Although the initial telemedicine link to the CRP was a pilot study, word of its value quickly spread and, by the end of its first year of operation, two other telemedicine links had been requested. These were established at hospitals in Kathmandu, Nepal and the Solomon Islands. From then on, the numbers of links requested and set up grew rapidly.[13]

Manual management of the messages by the charity (e.g. forwarding a new referral message to an appropriate specialist, forwarding the resulting reply to the referrer and dealing with any subsequent dialogue) was satisfactory for a single hospital, but rapidly became unmanageable as the number of hospitals and the email workload increased. It was also difficult to extract statistics about the operation of the network, since plain email provides a poor archive, because it is 'unthreaded'. An automatic email message-handling system was therefore developed by the Centre for Online Health at the University of Queensland.[14] This came into operation in 2002, and solved several of the problems associated with manual message management.

From July 1999 to March 2003, the network grew to 17 hospitals. As well as more referring hospitals, more volunteer specialists were recruited.[13] Many were from the UK and Australia. The Swinfen Charitable Trust continues to be indebted to the consultant specialists and others who contribute voluntarily to the operation of the network.

Iraq and the Middle East

The Iraq war began in March 2003 with the invasion of Iraq by a multinational coalition of troops from the USA and the UK, supported by smaller contingents from Australia, Poland and other nations. In 2004, the administrators of the Swinfen Charitable Trust visited Basra as part of a British medical mission. During that visit, contact was made with doctors from several Iraqi hospitals, who subsequently joined the email referral network (Figure 19.2). This led to a jump in the number of cases referred from Iraq in particular, and from other parts of the Middle East generally (Table 19.1).

A review conducted in 2007 showed that there was evidence of improved management of cases as a result of email telemedicine.[15] The review also showed that the case mix from countries of the Middle East was different from that from the rest of the world (although, technically, the difference was not significant at $p < 0.05$). There was more obstetrics and gynaecology, and less medicine and radiology (Table 19.2). Despite the majority of Middle Eastern cases being referred from Iraq, relatively few were the direct result of conflict, and there were fewer trauma and fracture cases than from the rest of the world. There were also comparatively fewer referrals in infectious and tropical diseases. The relative absence of trauma cases can perhaps be explained by well-developed local expertise in trauma care. This local expertise was honed during the Iraq conflict, during the eight years of the Iraq–Iran war and during the internal troubles of the Saddam Hussein regime.

Table 19.1 Origin and numbers of cases referred from July 2002 to June 2008

Middle East		Rest of World	
Afghanistan	85	Antarctica	2
Iraq	311	Bangladesh	254
Kuwait	1	Bolivia	15
Pakistan	28	Cambodia	16
Uzbekistan	31	China	2
		East Timor	27
		Ethiopia	28
		Gambia	2
		Guinea	12
		Laos	2
		Lithuania	1
		Madagascar	1
		Malawi	9
		Mozambique	7
		Nepal	272
		Papua New Guinea	59
		Russia	1
		Sierra Leone	2
		Solomon Islands	93
		Sri Lanka	23
		St Helena (UK)	24
		Sudan	28
		Tibet	10
		Tristan da Cunha (UK)	34
		Uganda	20
		Yemen	2
		Zambia	15
Total	456	Total	961

The U21 consortium

The Universitas 21 (U21) is an international grouping of 21 leading research-intensive universities in 13 countries from around the world. The purpose of the consortium is to facilitate collaboration between the member universities and to create opportunities for them on a scale that none of them could achieve by operating independently or through traditional bilateral alliances. The U21 consortium has a strong health sciences group, led by the deans of medicine, nursing, dentistry and rehabilitation sciences of the various member universities.

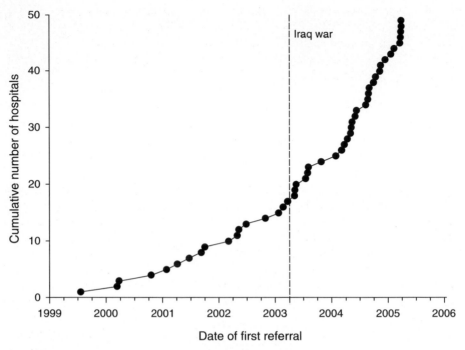

Figure 19.2 First-referral dates for Iraqi hospitals (*n* = 49)

Table 19.2 Types of queries for the cases referred from July 2002 to June 2008

	Middle East		Rest of world	
	n	%	*n*	%
Allied health	2	0.2	12	0.9
Anaesthetics	19	2	3	0.2
Emergency medicine	5	0.6	4	0.3
General practice	1	0.1	0	0.0
Internal medicine	227	27	456	33
Mental health	5	0.6	10	0.7
Nurse	4	0.5	11	0.8
Obstetrics and gynaecology	159	19	66	5
Other	19	2	23	2
Paediatrics	168	20	260	19
Pathology	23	3	36	3
Radiology	15	2	94	7
Surgery	203	24	392	29
Total	850	100	1367	100

At the suggestion of the health sciences group, a Memorandum of Understanding was signed between the U21 consortium and the Swinfen Charitable Trust in 2006. The main objective of the Memorandum was to advance the aims of the Swinfen Charitable Trust by drawing on U21 resources, such as consultants, medical students, nursing/allied health students and other support.

The first pilot project involved U21 universities providing support to an under-served health facility in a developing country.[16] The initial aim was to assist local doctors via information and communications technology – telemedicine – and to involve U21 medical students on elective placements. As well as establishing low-cost telemedicine networks in developing countries, a long-term aim was to gather data about their effectiveness.

The project began in mid-2005. In the first two years, a total of eight medical students from four U21 universities spent their electives at hospitals in Pakistan, Papua New Guinea and Sri Lanka. Most electives lasted about four weeks. Most of the students were in their final year.

A total of 49 cases were referred either directly by the students or indirectly by the medical staff with whom they worked (i.e. after the students had left).[17] The students were responsible for a total of 49 e-referrals, which resulted in 67 queries in a wide range of specialties. The median response time was 20 hours (interquartile range 5–85). Follow-up data were obtained in 14 of the 30 cases from one hospital (47%). The major categories of the 67 queries were internal medicine, paediatrics and surgery, and in very similar proportions to the 785 queries managed by the Swinfen Charitable Trust over the same period.

Before the project began, some initial concerns were expressed by certain consortium members about possible medicolegal risks, and whether students would feel superfluous in a local health care environment. Happily, none of these matters turned out to be real problems. Indeed, the students reported that the U21 project gave a purpose to their placement. One student expressed it as follows: 'often students don't always have a "role" other than to sometimes feel as though you are hanging around as the silent observer. This way you could feel as though you were contributing.' [17]

The presence of a medical student facilitated e-referrals by relieving the pressure on the local doctor to undertake the necessary clerical and technical work. The students reported a rewarding elective experience, which appears to have the potential to increase the ease with which heavily burdened medical staff in developing countries can make use of e-referrals.

The future

Over the first 10 years of its operation, the Trust has established telemedicine links for 135 hospitals/clinics in 34 countries and dealt with over 1700 referrals (Figure 19.3). How do we rate the success of this international e-referral network after 10 years of operation? There are many indicators that could be employed to measure success in telemedicine.[18] These include longevity and clinical outcomes.

If longevity is the criterion, then the Swinfen Charitable Trust is doing pretty well

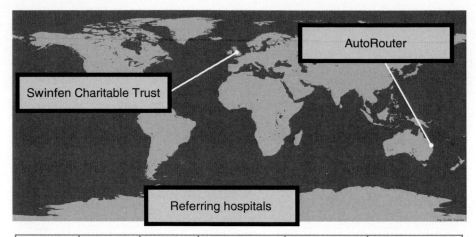

Afghanistan, 5	Colombia, 1	Guyana, 1	Madagascar, 1	Russia, 1	Tibet, 1
Albania, 1	DR Congo, 1	Iraq, 40	Malawi, 4	Sierra Leone, 1	Tristan da Cunha (UK), 1
Antarctica, 1	East Timor, 2	Kenya, 1	Mozambique, 1	Solomon Islands, 5	Uganda, 2
Bangladesh, 6	Ethiopia, 5	Kuwait, 3	Nepal, 10	Somalia, 1	Uzbekistan, 2
Bolivia, 1	Gambia, 5	Laos, 2	Pakistan, 9	Sri Lanka, 5	Yemen, 1
Cambodia, 2	Ghana, 1	Liberia, 1	Papua New Guinea, 3	St Helena (UK), 1	Zambia, 2
China, 1	Guinea, 1	Lithuania, 1	Philippines, 1	Sudan, 1	

Figure 19.3 Swinfen Charitable Trust Network (July 2008)

for a telehealth operation, many of which – as has been observed elsewhere – blossom on a wave of initial enthusiasm and then wither when the seed funding runs out. However, if clinical outcome is the criterion, then the operation represents a failure at present, because there are no formal follow-up data. This is due to the fact that the majority of patients, once treated, return home, and do not come back to the hospital for follow-up appointments. This occurs because of travel distance, time and cost, including loss of income. However, one of the aims of the U21 involvement is to obtain follow-up information, and the medical students in Papua New Guinea have begun providing it (and it is showing useful outcomes).[17]

It is also worth pointing out that the Swinfen Charitable Trust must be providing a clinically useful service to the referrer doctors, or they would not continue to use it. This was confirmed in a survey of referrers conducted in 2004.[19]

Ultimately, sustainability probably depends on scaling up the size of the present operation, which in turn requires the real costs to be met, i.e. when operating on a large scale, depending only on volunteers would be difficult. This would mean paying for the medical time involved in answering the referrals, for example, which in turn would require an income stream. Charities may have difficulty in operating in this environment, i.e. where there are pressures to increase in size to make things financially sustainable, with simultaneous counter-pressures to reduce in size because things depend on volunteers.

The work of the Swinfen Charitable Trust (and others) demonstrates that low-cost telemedicine in the developing world is feasible, clinically useful, scalable and apparently sustainable. However, telemedicine is not yet being used on a significant scale.

What then is the right strategy? The sensible approach appears to be to build intra-country telemedicine networks as soon as practicable. That is, we need telemedicine networks that rely largely on within-country resources. Such telemedicine networks might need to begin with support from outside the country, but they should become independent of outside resources as quickly as possible.[20]

Further reading

Swinfen Charitable Trust. Available at: www.swinfencharitabletrust.org.
Universitas 21 Health Sciences Group. Available at: www.u21health.org/index.html.

References

1. Geissbuhler A, Bagayoko CO, Ly O. The RAFT network: 5 years of distance continuing medical education and tele-consultations over the Internet in French-speaking Africa. *Int J Med Inform* 2007; **76**: 351–6.
2. Vincent DS, Berg BW, Hudson DA, Chitpatima ST. International medical education between Hawaii and Thailand over Internet2. *J Telemed Telecare* 2003; **9**(Suppl 2): 71–2.
3. Ozuah PO, Reznik M. The role of telemedicine in the care of children in under-served communities. *J Telemed Telecare* 2004; **10**(Suppl 1): 78–80.
4. Pak HS, Welch M, Poropatich R. Web-based teledermatology consult system: preliminary results from the first 100 cases. *Stud Health Technol Inform* 1999; **64**: 179–84.
5. Callahan CW, Malone F, Estroff D, Person DA. Effectiveness of an Internet-based store-and-forward telemedicine system for pediatric subspecialty consultation. *Arch Pediatr Adolesc Med* 2005; **159**: 389–93.
6. Person DA. Pacific Island Health Care Project: early experiences with a Web-based consultation and referral network. *Pac Health Dialog* 2000; **7**: 29–35.
7. Brauchli K, Oberli H, Hurwitz N et al. Diagnostic telepathology: long-term experience of a single institution. *Virchows Arch* 2004; **444**: 403–9.
8. Vassallo DJ, Buxton PJ, Kilbey JH, Trasler M. The first telemedicine link for the British Forces. *J R Army Med Corps* 1998; **144**: 125–30.
9. Vassallo DJ, Buxton PJ, Kilbey JH. Telemedicine made easy – the British way. *Mil Med* 1998; **163**: iii.
10. Vassallo DJ, Klezl Z, Sargeant ID, Cyprich J, Fousek J. British–Czech co-operation in a mass casualty incident, Sipovo. From aeromedical evacuation from Bosnia to discharge from Central Military Hospital, Prague. *J R Army Med Corps* 1999; **145**: 7–12.
11. Heinzelmann PJ, Jacques G, Kvedar JC. Telemedicine by email in remote Cambodia. *J Telemed Telecare* 2005; **11**(Suppl 2): 44–7.
12. Vassallo DJ, Hoque F, Roberts MF et al. An evaluation of the first year's experience with a low-cost telemedicine link in Bangladesh. *J Telemed Telecare* 2001; **7**: 125–38.
13. Wootton R, Youngberry K, Swinfen R, Swinfen P. Referral patterns in a global store-and-forward telemedicine system. *J Telemed Telecare* 2005; **11**(Suppl 2): 100–3.
14. Wootton R. Design and implementation of an automatic message-routing system for low-cost telemedicine. *J Telemed Telecare* 2003; **9**(Suppl 1): 44–7.
15. Patterson V, Swinfen P, Swinfen R et al. Supporting hospital doctors in the Middle East by email telemedicine: something the industrialized world can do to help. *J Med Internet Res* 2007; **9**: e30.
16. Wootton R, Jebamani LS, Dow SA. E-health and the Universitas 21 organization: 2. Telemedicine and underserved populations. *J Telemed Telecare* 2005; **11**: 221–4.
17. Wootton R, Swinfen PA, Swinfen R et al. Medical students represent a valuable resource in facilitating telehealth for the underserved. *J Telemed Telecare* 2007; **13**(Suppl 3): 92–7.
18. Wootton R, Hebert MA. What constitutes success in telehealth? *J Telemed Telecare* 2001; **7**(Suppl 2): 3–7.
19. Wootton R, Youngberry K, Swinfen P, Swinfen R. Prospective case review of a global e-health system for doctors in developing countries. *J Telemed Telecare* 2004; **10**(Suppl 1): 94–6.
20. Wootton R. Telemedicine support for the developing world. *J Telemed Telecare* 2008; **14**: 109–14.

20 Telemedicine in China: Opportunities and challenges

Jie Chen and Zhiyuan Xia

Introduction

China is a large country, with a huge population and poor telecommunications infrastructure (although communications are being improved rapidly). The level of social and economic development differs greatly between the coastal areas of the country and the rural areas in the west. Health resources are relatively well developed and easily available in the coastal areas, while there are shortages of medical care and drugs in the poor and rural areas. Patients in rural areas often experience difficulties in accessing medical care. If they travel long distances to access higher-quality medical care, they incur a heavy financial burden.

Telemedicine past and present in China

In industrialized countries, the concept of using communications technology to distribute medical expertise is not particularly new. However, the development of telehealth is relatively new in China. The earliest telehealth activities began in the late 1980s. An emergency consultation in 1986 that was provided for a ship's crew via radiotelegrams is recognized as the earliest telehealth activity in China. In 1988, the General Army Hospital in Beijing carried out a neurosurgery case discussion with a German hospital. Shanghai Medical University developed one of the earliest telemedicine systems in China. In September 1994, they succeeded in performing a teleconsultation between the Huashan hospital and staff at the Shanghai Jiaotong University.[1]

The first generation of telemedicine systems in China was based on videoconferencing via the telephone network (PSTN). In 1995, with the support of the Shanghai Education and Research Network, Shanghai Medical University launched a pilot telemedicine project and established a telemedicine centre.[2] At about that time, people began to employ the Internet to search for medical help. One of two well-known cases occurred in March 1995: a girl named Yang Xiaoxia in Shandong Province had an unidentified disease and asked for help through the Internet. The disease was finally diagnosed as a phagocytic bacterial infection in her muscles. The other case was in the same year. A student named Zhuling at Beijing University was sick for unknown reasons. After searching for help via the Internet, more than 1000 reply emails helped her to prove that she had heavy-metal poisoning.[1]

At this stage, a few health-related institutions began to develop experimental telehealth systems. The authorities noticed this trend, and began to support these telehealth activities.

In 1997, the telemedicine system of Shanghai Medical University obtained the recognition of the country leaders at the national IT exhibition. This boosted interest in telehealth. Various organizations and institutions began their telehealth programmes. The late 1990s was a period of rapid progress for telehealth in China. The Jin-Wei (Golden Health) Telemedicine Network began operation in July 1997, and many national-level hospitals in Beijing and Shanghai were included in this network. The network provided remote consultation and remote education services for hospitals in 21 provinces, including Yunnan, Sichuan, Tibet and Xinjiang, via satellite communication. In the same year, the International Medical Network Committee of the China Medical Foundation established their telemedicine network. Following these two large telemedicine programmes, many others emerged. The Shuang-wei (Satellite Health Education Network of the Ministry of Health) network was sponsored by the Ministry of Health, and the MediChina BYL telemedicine network was sponsored by the Shanghai municipal government. There were also many telehealth programmes initiated in other areas, including Guangdong, Sichuan, Fujian and Yunnan provinces.[3] When telehealth activities began to grow in China in the late 1990s, the national health authority recognized the importance of supervising them, and the Ministry of Health established a set of rules for telehealth in 1999.[4]

The rapid development of telecommunications infrastructure in the late 1990s helped to make telehealth a routine activity in China. The ordinary telephone network, the ISDN network, satellite communications and the Internet were all employed for telehealth purposes. Many different organizations, including the government, medical universities, hospitals and even some private companies, built telehealth networks and made telehealth a routine application. Generally, they provided remote consultations and remote education services for users of their networks.

Telehealth programmes in China

Since 1997, many different telehealth programmes have been conducted in China. These programmes have been sponsored by different entities, have employed different telecommunication means and have operated at different scales. Some programmes have built large telehealth networks and connected many different health organizations.

One of the most well-known telehealth programmes was the Jin-Wei Telemedicine Network (the Golden Health Medical Network). This network was established with the support of the Ministry of Health. The network operation centre was located in Beijing and was a satellite network covering the whole country. Many national-level and lower-level hospitals from more than 20 provinces were included in this network.

The satellite communication allowed an 8 Mbit/s upload speed and 2 Mbit/s download. Between 1997 and 2003, the Jin-Wei Telemedicine Network provided remote consultation services for more than 1000 patients, and provided remote education services for more than 50 000 doctors and nurses. The Jin-Wei organization also developed a website to provide health-related information services for users. However, the high cost of satellite devices and communications prevented many low-level hospitals from connecting to this network. Subsequently, the Jin-Wei network began to employ ISDN as a second telecommunication method to cover more hospitals.[3,5]

The CMF (China Medical Foundation) Telemedicine Network was also a large-scale telemedicine programme. It was supported by a non-profit-making organization, the International Medical Network Association. It began in 1997. From the start, several different methods of telecommunication were employed. First, telephone lines were used to establish a network covering basic level hospitals, then ISDN and the Internet were used to connect higher-level hospitals, and eventually satellite communication was used to connect national-level hospitals. The aim of the CMF Telemedicine Network was different from that of the Jin-Wei network, in that it mainly provided telehealth services for basic-level hospitals. It used telephone line communication and desktop videoconferencing.[3,5]

The aim of the Shuang-wei (Satellite Health Education Network of the Ministry of Health) network was to provide remote medical education services for doctors and nurses all over the country. It was supported by the Ministry of Health and began routine operation in 2001. Satellite and optical fibre were employed as the major telecommunication means. The network supported different kinds of remote education, such as live broadcasting, video on demand, the interchange of online education materials, and point-to-point or multipoint videoconferencing.[3,6]

The BYL Telemedicine Network was a branch of the China Social Development Network. It was supported by the Shanghai municipal government and connected Shanghai and western areas of China. Various telecommunication media, including satellite, fibre-optic cables, the Internet and telephone lines, were employed in this network. Specialists in Shanghai provided an image consultation service for patients in other areas. When Shanghai provided telehealth services for western areas via this network, they also provided business information services.[3]

A Chinese Traditional Medicine Telemedicine Network was established by the Chinese Academy of Traditional Chinese Medicine in 1997. It employed ISDN for telecommunication to provide a traditional Chinese medicine consultation service for international and domestic patients.[3]

Several other telehealth programmes were set up in China in the late 1990s. These included the Sino-Japanese Telemedicine Collaboration for high-resolution medical image consultation, the Sino-Russian Satellite Telemedicine Collaboration, and the telemedicine programmes of the Sun Yet San University, the Shanghai Second Medical University and the Western China Medical University. The Shuang-wei and BYL networks are still in operation. The programmes had different purposes, employed different technologies and telecommunication media, and were supported by different organizations.[3] Since 2003, some provinces have established their own regional telemedicine networks: the Fujian Province Telemedicine Network was set up in late 2003 and the Gansu Province Telemedicine Network in late 2007. All these regional telemedicine networks are supported by local government and are still in operation.

Telehealth programme of Shanghai Medical University

Shanghai Medical University (SMU) provided medical services, teaching and research, and had about 5000 students. It had an excellent technical reputation in China. Many departments in SMU-affiliated hospitals were well equipped, and some departments were ranked the best in the country. In 2000, SMU was merged with Fudan University to set up a new Fudan University.

SMU was a pioneer of telehealth in China. In 1994, it began a telehealth pilot project. It developed the first general telehealth system in China, which was based on low-bandwidth videoconferencing over the telephone network. Through this system, a surgeon in Huashan Hospital (an affiliated hospital of SMU) succeeded in providing a remote consultation service for a patient in Shanghai Jiaotong University. In 1995, with the support of the Shanghai Education and Research Network, SMU launched a pilot telehealth programme and established a telemedicine centre. It began to develop telehealth systems conforming to international standards. In 1996, SMU began cooperation with the telecommunications authority in Shanghai. Various telecommunication companies began to establish different telecommunication connections for the telemedicine centre.[2,7]

In 1997, SMU established a telehealth network based on the telemedicine centre. The telehealth service providers were 7 affiliated hospitals of SMU, and the telehealth service users were more than 20 hospitals from remote and rural areas. The task of the telehealth centre was to act as the administrative and telecommunication centre. All the service providers were connected to the telemedicine centre by optical fibre. The service users were connected by the ordinary telephone network, the ISDN network or satellite, according to cost. The network connected hospitals from 21 provinces, including Xinjiang, Tibet, Yunnan, Sichuan, Heilongjiang, Jiangsu and Zhejiang. In the telemedicine centre, there were nurses for remote consultation administration and technical staff for support. Each hospital of the service providers and service users had its own operation staff. Figure 20.1 illustrates the structure of the network.[8]

The SMU Telemedicine Centre developed many administrative rules for remote consultation in China. Only professors or associate professors were eligible to provide telehealth services. The operation staff had to have completed special training in the network. When the service users requested a remote consultation, they had to submit full information about the patients. Because most of the hospitals in the network from remote and rural areas lacked digital devices, they often needed to digitize images using a digital scanner. The Telemedicine Centre provided a set of operational guidelines for the service users after their research in this field. The Telemedicine Centre also designed a procedure for remote consultation administration. In 1999, it developed a web-based remote consultation administration database. By using this

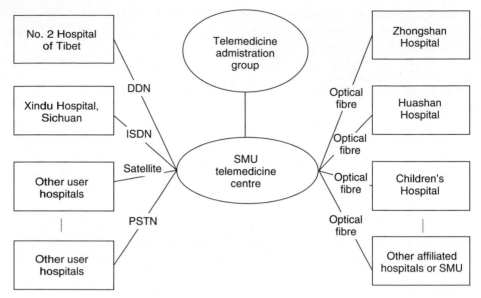

Figure 20.1 The structure of the SMU Telehealth Network

database, the service users could apply for remote medical consultation services via the network, and the Telemedicine Centre could despatch remote consultation requests to the appropriate service providers. Also, the consultation providers in Shanghai could schedule the remote consultations via the network. As a multimedia database, it could accept data in the form of images, video and audio information relating to the remote cases that needed consultation.[8]

In 1996, the SMU Telehealth Network began to experiment in distance medical education. It provided distance education services for the doctors and nurses in the hospital on Chongming Island. Subsequently, the SMU Telemedicine Centre developed a remote education system. This comprised two parts. One was a videoconference system, by which teachers and students could have real-time discussions. The other part was a media system, which could be used for media broadcasting, video on demand, recording and editing. By using this system, teachers could finish their own tasks via the Internet.

The SMU Telehealth Network (now part of Fudan University) is still in operation. It has provided remote consultation services for more than 2000 patients in remote and rural hospitals. These patients have been from various specialties, including cardiology, oncology, surgery, neurology and paediatrics. In their remote consultations, the specialists only provide a second opinion or suggestion for the doctors in the user hospitals, because of the absence of legislation that would permit them to make a diagnosis. The network has also provided more than 1000 hours of distance medical education for the Dali Medical College in Yunnan province and other hospitals in the network.

After they began providing telehealth services for remote and rural users, the specialists received much feedback about the services. A letter from the hospital of Xindu,

Sichuan province described how patients benefited from telehealth. For example, one patient with colon cancer made a full recovery after the operation, following the advice provided in the teleconsultation. She was the oldest patient to have recovered following such an operation at that hospital. Another patient with colon cancer recovered fully without requiring chemotherapy following the advice provided in the teleconsultation. One patient with heart disease avoided an operation to implant a pacemaker.

Video and audio quality varies, depending upon how the rural sites are connected with the telemedicine centre. The best quality is achieved with a digital connection (DDN), followed by ISDN and satellite; unsurprisingly, the quality is quite low via an ordinary telephone line. In China, when providing a telehealth service via telephone line, it can be expected to be interrupted every 5–10 minutes because of connection problems. The quality of the consultation service is therefore poor, and remote education cannot easily be delivered via telephone line.

The costs of the different communication methods also differ greatly. Satellite communication is the most expensive, followed by DDN and ISDN. Telephone line and Internet communication are the cheapest.

Satellite communication is not suitable for a remote consultation service, because of the time delay. However, it is suitable for a unidirectional broadcast service, such as that required for remote education.

When considering all the factors relating to the quality of the system, cost and breakdown rate of the service, it appears that ISDN communication is the most appropriate means of communication for telehealth services in China at present. Internet communication can be used in non-real-time applications, for example to access databases and to apply for remote consultations. Because the bandwidth of Internet communication has been much improved, it can also be used for videoconferencing and remote education, for example video on demand and broadcasting for distance education. Thus, Internet communication has great potential as a communications method for telehealth in China.

Opportunities for telehealth in China

China has the largest population in the world: at the end of 2005, it was 1.3 billion. Health expenditure in China is rising: in 2004, it was 75.9 billion RMB, and accounted for 5.6% of the gross domestic product. In 2004, the per capita expenditure in urban areas was about 4.2 times that in rural areas.[9]

The health sector in China faces two opposing demands: first, it must provide expanded and equitable access to high-quality health care services; second, it must reduce, or at least control, the rising costs of health care. Telehealth offers the promise of giving people equal access to high-quality medical care at affordable cost.

As in most other countries, the highest concentration of medical resources (personnel, information and facilities) in China is in the major cities, so telehealth could be a useful mechanism to balance the differences in the level of access to medical resources.

Information technology in China has grown very rapidly in the last few years. There has been rapid expansion of the telecommunication market and very fast diffusion of the Internet. By December 2007, there were 210 million Internet users in China.[10] Health IT is also developing very rapidly in China: many hospitals have developed a hospital information system, and now health information-sharing networks are developing in many cities. This will facilitate the development of telehealth in China.

The large population and relatively insufficient health resources have produced demands for China to develop telehealth, and the rapid development of IT has provided the opportunities to do so. In 2003, China formulated its national strategy in e-health. The plan outlined the strategy and activities for China to develop e-health in 2003–2010. The plan described the background information, the principles, the goals and the main tasks for China to develop e-health.[11] Telehealth development is part of this plan.

Challenges for telehealth in China

Although there are undoubted opportunities, telehealth also faces many challenges in China.[12] Despite the successes of early telehealth systems in China, not many of them were self-sustaining, and few are still in operation today. A number of implementation barriers remain to be overcome. These include the following.

A lack of understanding of telehealth by society

Often, telehealth is perceived by health authorities as a low spending priority. Because telehealth is not clearly defined, there are different definitions of telehealth, which makes it difficult for patients to understand its potential. Telehealth might adversely affect the relationship between health professionals and patients compared with normal face-to-face consultations. The reasons include physical and mental factors, depersonalization, different process of consultation, reduced confidence of patients and health professionals, different knowledge and skills required of health professionals, and ergonomic issues. There are also various factors that prevent health professionals from accepting telehealth, including too much change, lack of a user-friendly interface, failure to collect the most important information, inadequate training of physicians to use the system, and lack of control by the organization over physician practices. Factors such as doubt about the quality of the telehealth and conflicts between the telehealth procedure and traditional clinical schedules will prevent patients and health professionals from accepting the new system.

Incomplete telehealth organizational structure and lack of human resources

In many health institutes that conduct telehealth programmes, there are no special telehealth departments or staff. Lack of organizational and personnel resources is a major constraint on telehealth development.

Lack of standards

In China, the telehealth systems and services are developing very rapidly, but the standardization of telehealth lags behind. Standardization of telehealth system components and services is an important element for integration of heterogeneous systems. There are no standards for telehealth in China, and this has restricted developments. For example, in the rural hospitals, there is no digital X-ray equipment, so, when they need to transmit X-ray images to specialists in the cities, the X-ray films are often digitized using a scanner. In practice, poor-quality images result, which would be much improved if there were standards to control the digitization process.

Absence of legislation and regulation

Lack of legislation and regulation is also a major barrier to telehealth development and deployment. There are some national regulations for telehealth, such as regulations governing remote consultation administration. But the work on regulation lags far behind the development of telehealth. There are also some legislative barriers. There is no related law focusing on telemedicine, electronic signatures and patient privacy protection. There are problems with medical malpractice liability, because of legal uncertainties.

High cost and insufficiency of funds for telehealth development

Telehealth depends on new technologies. The devices are often relatively expensive. Also, telecommunication costs can be high. However, funds for telehealth are insufficient, because the benefits of telehealth are mainly realized by the patients. Thus, investors do not have a great interest in this field. Another problem is that hospitals in remote and rural areas have a higher demand for access to telehealth services, but also have smaller budgets.

Unbalanced development in different areas in China

Because of unbalanced development, many hospitals in remote and rural areas cannot apply telehealth, owing to limitations of equipment, human resources and telecommunications.

Lack of reimbursement for telehealth services

In China, health insurance does not cover expenditure on telehealth services. Thus, patients need to pay for telecommunications and specialists' fees themselves. This represents a major economic burden for patients.

Lack of evaluation of telehealth programmes

Policy makers lack evidence from evaluation research to help them to decide how to support the development of telehealth.

Policy recommendations

China can learn from experiences in industrialized countries.[12] This suggests that, for the development of telehealth in China, it is necessary to do the following:

- **Strengthen the leadership of government in telehealth development**. The government should establish a special organization to lead telehealth development and promote a government focus on telehealth.
- **Strengthen the supervision of telehealth development**. In China, many different organizations are involved in telehealth activities. Many of these organizations are not health related. It is important to strengthen the supervision of telehealth and prevent unqualified organizations from taking part in telehealth.
- **Promote the development of telehealth standards**. Health authorities should promote the development of telehealth standards with users, researchers, technical and scientific bodies, and industry. Establishing national standards and adopting international standards will be important tasks for China.
- **Develop a legal and regulatory infrastructure that will facilitate telehealth**. Legislation related to telemedicine, electronic signatures and patient health information protection should be constituted.
- **Increase the investment in telehealth**. The government should strengthen its financial support for telehealth development. Also, other sources must be attracted to invest in telehealth. In China, there is a high demand for telehealth services, especially for remote medical education services. Many early distance medical education programmes are still in operation today.
- **Train health professionals and technical staff in telehealth**. Training will help health professionals to understand telehealth, and will also promote the efficiency of telehealth systems.
- **Promote international collaboration, sharing and learning experiences from industrialized countries**. This will help China to develop telehealth.

Telehealth is relatively new to China. It can overcome geographical barriers and make high-quality services available without regard to location. This can help to reduce the unbalanced distribution of health resources. Because telecommunications are developing rapidly in China, there are many opportunities to develop telehealth. There are also many challenges for telehealth to overcome. If the importance of telehealth for China is widely recognized, it will have a better future in China.

Further reading

Fujian Province. [*Telemedicine Network of Fujian Province*]. Available at: www.thydmed.com.

Hsieh RK, Hjelm NM, Lee JC, Aldis JW. Telemedicine in China. *Int J Med Inform* 2001; **61**: 139–46.

References

1. Zhu SJ, Cai JH, Yang QS. The establishment and development of telemedicine. *Hosp Adm J Chin PLA.* 1998; **5**: 277–98.
2. Zhao JA, Xu YX, Chen J. The implementation of telemedicine network group. *Chin Hosp Manage* 1998; **18**: 27–8.
3. Fu Z, Lian P. *Telemedicine.* Beijing: People's Military Medical Press, 2005.
4. Ministry of Health, People's Republic of China. [*Rules for the Development of Telemedicine*]. Available at: www.moh.gov.cn.
5. Li BZ. The progress and prospect of Jinwei program. *Chin Hosp Manage*1998; **18**: 41–3.
6. Ministry of Health, People's Republic of China. [*Satellite Health Education Network of Ministry of Health. Shuang-wei Network*]. Available at: www.sww.com.cn.
7. Xu YX, Mo MQ, Zhao JA. *New Progress on the Internet and Using It in Medicine.* Shanghai: Fudan University Press, 2001.
8. Xia ZY. The administration of telemedicine. *Medl Inf* 2005; **18**: 907–9.
9. Ministry of Health, People's Republic of China. [Official website]. Available at: www.moh.gov.cn.
10. China Internet Network Information Center. *Statistical Survey Report on the Internet Development in China.* January 2008. Available at: www.cnnic.org.cn/uploadfiles/pdf/2008/2/29/104126.pdf.
11. China Centre for Information Industry Development. [*e-Health Development Plan for China in 2003–2010*]. Available at: industry.ccidnet.com/art/793/20051024/356253_1.html.
12. Xla ZY. Challenges faced for telemedicine development in China and corresponding recommendations. *Med Inf* 2005; **18**: 206–9.

21 Telemedicine in South Africa

Maurice Mars

Introduction

South Africa is similar to most other sub-Saharan African countries in facing a substantial burden of disease with limited human and financial resources. South Africa is a relatively large country of over one million square kilometres, with a total population of 45 million. Its people are almost equally divided between rural (46%) and urban areas. With a gross domestic product of US$200 billion, South Africa has one of the largest economies in Africa and accounts for about a quarter of the entire gross domestic product of the continent. Despite this, it has an official unemployment rate of 26% and an unofficial unemployment rate of 41%. About 50% of its people live below the poverty datum.

Burden of disease

The burden of disease in South Africa is great. Until recently, it had more HIV-positive people than any other nation. HIV prevalence in adults aged 15 years or older is 17% and the incidence of tuberculosis is 1.3%.[1] Data from 2000 show HIV/AIDS as the greatest cause of death (30%), with cardiovascular disease (17%), intentional and unintentional injuries (12%), non-HIV-related infectious and parasitic disease (10%), and malignant neoplasms (8%) as the next major causes.[2]

Health provision

Public health services and budgets are devolved from the national Department of Health (DOH) to provincial Departments of Health, with some primary health care services being provided by municipalities. The annual health care expenditure by the government is US$158 per capita.[1] There is a major inequality in health care funding, with private expenditure per person about six times higher than public sector expenditure per person.[3] By African standards, South Africa is relatively well supplied with doctors, with 77 doctors per 100 000 people,[1] but again the distribution of doctors is skewed, with the provincial hospital sector being served by 24 doctors per 100 000 people and 10 specialists per 100 000 people. On average, 34% of the medical posts in the public health sector are vacant.[3]

Telecommunications

Africa did not benefit from the substantial telecommunication infrastructure roll-out and deregulation that occurred during the dot.com boom. As in most African countries, telecommunication in South Africa is still tightly regulated, with the government following a policy of 'managed liberalization'. There has until very recently been a telecommunication monopoly. A licence for a second service provider has now been awarded, but services have yet to commence. The government has 37% and 30% shareholdings in these two service providers, respectively.[4] International bandwidth is provided by undersea cable (SAT 3) and satellite. Although plans for an additional undersea cable running up the east coast of Africa (EASSY) are well developed, the project appears to be stalled at present. Satellite services are licensed to one company, which is totally owned by the Department of Communications.

Internet access charges in South Africa are relatively high when compared with those in industrialized countries, with 20 hours of Internet access costing US$33 per month, compared with US$15 per month for the USA. Similarly, ISDN costs are high, with a 30-minute ISDN link to the USA (at 128 kbit/s) costing US$15.80.[5] ISDN and ADSL access is available in most cities and towns. Wireless coverage is limited by legislation, but it is hoped that Wimax will be made available by several large municipalities. In an attempt to provide low-cost bandwidth facilities, the government has established a state-owned company, but it has yet to trade.[4]

Mobile phone coverage is good and uptake is high. 3G and HSDP services are available in most cities, and GSM coverage is estimated at 93%. Data for the year 2004 indicate that 36% of South Africans have mobile phone access. Local figures suggest that access to a mobile phone may be as high as 75%.[4]

Lack of bandwidth, especially in rural areas, is a major problem facing telemedicine delivery in South Africa. All provincial hospitals are linked to the government network (Govnet). Access to computers with Internet access for doctors and nurses is limited in many rural hospitals and clinics, with doctors having to send store-and-forward cases from home using local Internet service providers. In KwaZulu-Natal, most hospitals have access to a total bandwidth of 128 kbit/s, which must be shared across all sectors of the hospital. Migrating videoconferencing from ISDN to IP is not feasible as yet, because of the limited bandwidth. ISDN access is not always easy to obtain, and delays of up to a year for installation are not uncommon. Likewise, support from the telecommunication company is poor, and the time from registering an ISDN line problem to a repair visit can be several months. ADSL, while available in most cities and larger towns, is dependent on the state of the local telephone exchanges. A survey conducted in 2006 showed that fewer than half of the hospitals in KwaZulu-Natal could be provided with ADSL if requested.

Telemedicine governance

In 1995, the new government formed the National Health Information Systems Committee of South Africa, tasked with designing a comprehensive national health information system for South Africa. Under the auspices of this Committee, a National Telemedicine Task Team was formed in 1998, to implement a national telemedicine strategy for South Africa. Four technical teams were established to work on telemedicine protocols, network infrastructure, legal licensure and ethical issues, and tele-education. These teams were active until 2001, by which time Phase One of the national telemedicine strategy had been implemented. While the national DOH has a Telemedicine Director, management and implementation of telemedicine services was devolved to provincial level during the Phase One project. In order to coordinate this at a provincial level, the Health Act of 2004 requires Members of the Executive Council at provincial level to form a committee that will '… establish, maintain, facilitate and implement health information in the province'. The provinces have taken different approaches to telemedicine. In most provinces, telemedicine is seen as part of the duties of the provincial representatives attending the National Health Information Systems Committee, who may or may not be interested in telemedicine. As a result, telemedicine activity has been limited or non-existent in some provinces. Other provinces have appointed specific telemedicine committees, some of which have been extended to include academic input from the medical schools. Only a few provinces actually provide a budget and posts for telemedicine, but this is slowly changing.

The national telemedicine strategy planned for three phases of development of telemedicine. Only Phase One was implemented and, after evaluation, it was decided not to continue with the project. However, after several years of relative inactivity, there has been renewed interest in telemedicine. The national DOH is developing a new strategic plan for 2008–2013. The Presidential National Commission on Information Society and Development is working on an e-health White Paper, the Departments of Communications and Trade and Industry have included e-health in their most recent strategic plans, and the Meraka Institute of the Council for Scientific and Industrial Research (CSIR) is developing an e-health strategic plan.

The Medical Research Council (MRC) of South Africa has a Telemedicine Lead Programme tasked with evaluating existing and planned telemedicine systems, coordinating national telemedicine activities and establishing tele-education for health care professionals. The eight medical schools in the country have been slow to participate in telemedicine. The University of KwaZulu-Natal is the only medical school with an academic department of Telehealth, and the Walter Sisulu University has a Telemedicine Unit.

Telemedicine background

Telemedicine in South Africa began in the early 1990s, with: radiologists linking CT scanners in Provincial Hospitals in KwaZulu-Natal to the Academic Radiology Department;[6] neurosurgeons in the province providing a teleradiology-assisted service;[7] rural doctors using email-based store-and-forward telemedicine for dermatology, orthopaedics and radiology; and ophthalmologists linking with Moorfields Hospital in London.[8] At the Walter Sisulu University Medical School, store-and-forward telepathology services have been used since 1995, with links to the Armed

Forces Institute of Pathology in Washington and various pathology departments in Europe.[9]

Phase One of the National Telemedicine Strategic Plan was implemented between March 1999 and September 2000, establishing 28 telemedicine sites in six of the nine provinces. Telemedicine services offered included store-and-forward teleradiology using scanned X-ray films, tele-ultrasonography (both real-time and store-and-forward), store-and-forward telepathology and tele-ophthalmology. Of these projects, only the teleradiology service linking three rural hospitals with the Pretoria Academic Hospital could really be deemed a success. In the first 9 months of the Pretoria service, 264 radiographic studies (10% of all the studies performed) were sent for specialist radiologist reporting.[10] Over the years, this developed into a useful CT scan radiology service with the neurosurgical department, but the service ended when the department moved into a new building with no ISDN line access. Tele-ultrasonography, trialled in the Northern Province and KwaZulu-Natal, was used occasionally and then stopped, and the tele-ophthalmology project in KwaZulu-Natal was beset with software problems and never started.

This lack of success meant that the second and third phases of the project, to expand telemedicine capabilities to 71 and then to 200 sites, was not undertaken. The second phase was then changed to an educational project linking the eight medical schools, with the expectation that they would initiate shared tele-education projects throughout the country. Although the medical schools were supplied with videoconference units, this project lacked the support of the deans of the medical schools, and never started.

Many lessons were learned in this process, and were similar to those experienced by others. These can be summarized as follows:[11]

- Failure to fully appreciate the need for a well-structured change management plan
- Lack of participatory buy-in from doctors at the sending and receiving sites
- Inadequate training and support
- Failure of provincial Departments of Health to take ownership and commit human and financial resources to the devolved project.

At the same time as the telemedicine project was being rolled out, the Nkosi Albert Luthuli Central Hospital was built and commissioned in Durban, KwaZulu-Natal in 2002. It is a paperless hospital, and has exposed its staff to aspects of telemedicine through the use of radiology and pathology PACS.

Telemedicine projects

With the relative inactivity of most of the provincial Departments of Health, telemedicine activity was taken up by other agencies and academia. The South African Defence Force together with the MRC developed a mobile laboratory with satellite communication and telemedicine capability.[12] However, no information has been published about its subsequent deployment. The MRC developed a test bed in Mpumalanga Province, linking two clinics and a hospital to the Pretoria Academic Hospital by videoconference. Limited data are available on its use: in 2002, 78 videoconference sessions took place – 68 teleconsultations and 10 tele-education sessions. This has been extended to a wireless network, and a teleradiology project is planned.

In collaboration with the University of Stellenbosch, the MRC has developed a 'home-grown' primary health care workstation for use in primary health care facilities run by nurses and part-time doctors and dentists. It has been trialled intermittently over the past two years at the Grabouw Community Health Centre, with an ISDN-based link to the Tygerberg Academic Hospital. The unit has been designed to be used by health professionals who have limited or no previous computing experience. Features include:[13]

- removal of the need to interact with the operating system
- a simplified alphanumeric input device
- integrated and intelligent video control
- a document interface that is familiar to the local users
- seamless integration of peripheral devices
- a back-up power source
- use of open-source, loyalty-free software.

The experience has revealed some of the common challenges associated with starting telemedicine services in environments where there is a shortage of staff at both the sending and receiving sites:

- Adequate buy-in has to be obtained from users.
- The service must be integrated into the normal workflow of the hospital.
- Incentives should be offered for already overworked staff to use telemedicine, which is seen as an additional and time-consuming burden.
- There should be a local telemedicine champion to drive the changes.

The unit has been used predominantly for teledermatology and paediatric consultations.

Various other enthusiast-driven telemedicine projects have commenced. At the Walter Sisulu Medical School in the Eastern Cape Province, the telepathology services that started in the 1990s have migrated to the iPath platform, with an iPath server located in Umtata. In the first 4 years, 36 pathology cases were referred for international opinion.[9] This service was then expanded to include a teledermatology project, with a general practitioner in a small town in a rural area sending 110 cases in 6 years.[14] An innovative wireless solution, developed by the CSIR, was piloted in a rural Eastern Cape clinic staffed by a nursing sister. The region does not have telephone coverage, and images are sent via a webcam, with a simultaneous voice link, to a doctor in another town.[15] The activity in the Eastern Cape has resulted in the formation of an active telemedicine committee within their DOH. They have set up an education centre with Internet and videoconference facilities in East London, and they are embarking on a large-scale project linking 23 sites, focusing on teleradiology, teledermatology and tele-spirometry. The project is not yet fully functional, and has yet to be evaluated.

A different approach has been taken in KwaZulu-Natal. In 2002, the University of

KwaZulu-Natal established an academic department of telehealth, with a mandate to assist the provincial DOH in developing telemedicine, conduct research in telehealth, and develop academic programmes in telemedicine and medical informatics. In addition to the long-standing teleradiology and teleneurosurgery services in the province, a store-and-forward tele-ophthalmology service has been running between a peripheral hospital and the academic ophthalmology department for several years. When last audited, this service had referred 282 cases in 18 months and had saved 82% of the patients an unnecessary transfer to the academic unit, 118 km away. Despite efforts, it has not yet been possible to replicate this service in any of the other 64 provincial hospitals. A real-time teledermatology service has been running between one hospital and the medical school for several years. At audit in 2006, 132 patients had been seen over 27 months, with 80% being saved a transfer. This service has been replicated in two other hospitals, and further sites are planned. Store-and-forward teledermatology services have been running in parallel, with cases sent from 23 hospitals.

Fledgling synchronous services have commenced in paediatric surgery, plastic surgery and psychiatry. Store-and-forward burn management and diabetic retinopathy screening programmes have also started. Through various externally funded initiatives, there are now 35 hospitals in KwaZulu-Natal with videoconference facilities, not all of which are currently active. The provincial DOH, while being supportive of these initiatives, has not taken ownership of telemedicine. As a result, it has only provided limited technical support, and has not yet provided a specific telemedicine budget. This has recently changed with the provision of posts for telemedicine, the development of a strategic plan and a budget for telemedicine, and the formation of a joint DOH and university Telemedicine Steering Committee for the province.

The national Department of Science and Technology has funded a consortium of the MRC, the Meraka Institute of the CSIR and the University of KwaZulu-Natal in a major three-year project in KwaZulu-Natal. The project will investigate various bandwidth solutions in rural areas, aiming to achieve a minimum of 512 kbit/s. It will also compare the locally produced primary health care workstation with a Chinese telemedicine workstation that has been acquired through a bilateral government agreement, and will conduct research into the development of appropriate administrative and financial models for the use of telemedicine in the South African public health care sector. Other aims are to investigate cultural and ethical matters relating to the use of telemedicine in rural communities, to conduct telemedicine training, to develop a telemedicine hub site and establish a virtual hospital to support the hospitals in the province, and to develop capacity in telemedicine through masters and PhD programmes. It is hoped that this project will result in a sustainable model for telemedicine in South Africa.

The Free State, Northern Cape and North West Province were the other three provinces that received telemedicine infrastructure in Phase One of the national telemedicine project. Their services in teleradiology and tele-ultrasonography have stopped. The Free State is actively investigating the establishment of telemedicine in the province, and has been considering a web-based PACS system for province-wide teleradiology.

The three provinces that were not part of Phase One were Gauteng, the Western Cape and Limpopo. In Limpopo, a telemedicine steering committee was established in June 2006. Videoconferencing was set up between four hospitals. With the assistance of the MRC and the University of KwaZulu-Natal, an ambitious telemedicine and tele-education programme began in the third quarter of 2007. The project includes dermatology, emergency medicine, psychiatry, dentistry, ENT, orthopaedics and surgery.

In Gauteng, work is under way to develop teleradiology in the provincial hospitals. In the Western Cape, an email-based store-and-forward telemedicine project has been running for several years between three district hospitals and the Tygerberg Children's Hospital.[16] A pilot store-and-forward teledermatology project has been started by the MRC and the University of Cape Town, with nursing sisters at four rural sites sending images and case histories back to a dermatologist in Cape Town.[17]

Telemedicine in the private health sector has not been well documented. One large hospital group and some large radiology practices use teleradiology and commercial PACS to transport and store X-ray images and reports, and pathology practices are following suit. There are several informal reports of images being captured during arthroscopic and endoscopic surgery and being sent by email for another opinion. There is at least one ophthalmologist who is sending photographs of retinal images to a colleague for second opinion.

At present, there are no telepsychiatry services in South Africa, but two services and a psychiatry tele-education programme are planned. With recent changes to the Mental Health Act and the requirement to treat psychiatric patients at district and regional hospital level for at least 72 hours, telepsychiatry may prove to be a major growth area. While videoconferenced patient follow-up is relatively common in the industrialized world, it is not yet being used in South Africa. This may be because of the shortage of doctors and the lack of telemedicine site coordinators.

Some novel applications have been developed in South Africa. Cell-Life is a mobile phone and Internet method of monitoring HIV patient adherence to antiretroviral medication.[18] SIMpill is a device that utilizes mobile phone technology and SMS text messages to monitor patients' medication compliance. When a patient opens the pill bottle to take their medication, an SMS text message is sent to a central server. If the patient fails to open the pill bottle within a defined time, the server sends an SMS message to the patient's mobile phone and, if there is repeated non-compliance, to the patient's physician.[19]

Tele-education

Staffing of rural hospitals has been a long-term problem in South Africa. The Government has had to employ doctors from other countries in order to maintain services in some rural areas. In 2004, there were 240 Cuban doctors working in South Africa. A recent press release reported that 1000 doctors are to be recruited from Tunisia, Cuba, Iran and elsewhere to work in rural areas. Studies of the factors that influence local doctors' decisions to work in rural hospitals have identified salaries and professional isolation as key issues. The government has improved salaries through the provision of a scarce skills allowance. Tele-education and telemedicine have been cited as ways of overcoming professional isolation, and the National Telemedicine Strategy included tele-education as an important component of the strategic plan. The attempt to get the eight medical schools to jointly develop a national teaching programme was not successful, and individual medical schools have undertaken tele-education.

In 2001, as part of an e-health learning initiative, the Free State Department of Health set up an interactive satellite broadcast system, and now offers health care training at 40 venues. Their last evaluation included over 2200 users. After the cessation of Phase One telemedicine services in KwaZulu-Natal, the local university approached the provincial DOH, in 2001, and was given approval to use the videoconferencing infrastructure for postgraduate medical education. Equipment has been upgraded, and postgraduate teaching sessions are multicast from the Nelson R Mandela School of Medicine to four other academic sites. In 2006, 765 hours of tuition in 17 academic programmes were shared by videoconferencing. A total of over 72 000 person-hours of tuition were offered in 2006, with approximately 40% of participants situated at rural hospitals. The medical school also shares its teaching sessions with other provinces, including the Walter Sisulu Medical School and the East London Medical Complex in the Eastern Cape, and the Polokwane Hospital in Limpopo. International teaching has taken place in collaboration with several countries in North Africa, Europe and North America.

The Walter Sisulu University has begun postgraduate teaching by videoconferencing, and the Universities of Stellenbosch and Pretoria have offered postgraduate courses by satellite TV. The University of the Witwatersrand has been funded to start a videoconferenced academic programme in public health. The College of Radiology of South Africa, aware of the extreme shortage of radiologists in the academic sector, funded a pilot project to share postgraduate teaching sessions between all eight medical schools by videoconference. The first four sessions have been completed, and are being evaluated before a decision is made to continue the project.

Mindset Health is a partnership between the Mindset Network, the national DOH and Sentech (the Government-owned satellite information and communication technology service provider), which aims to deliver large-scale health education and health promotion. This is achieved through the development of digital health education material delivered by video, by multimedia computer lessons and print, and by daily satellite broadcast to 200 hospitals in South Africa, with on-demand satellite datacasts for health care staff. The TV receivers for the satellite broadcasts are usually placed in the outpatient departments of rural hospitals. The initial focus has been on tuberculosis and HIV/AIDS.[20]

Telemedicine training

Since the Phase One project, there has been very little formal telemedicine training for health care workers. In Mpumalanga, several members of staff were sent to China to be trained on a Chinese telemedicine unit in expectation of its deployment. In the Eastern Cape, a telemedicine training workshop was arranged under the auspices of the Regional Impact of Information Society Technologies in Africa project. Training has also been provided by the MRC, the Walter Sisulu University and the University of KwaZulu-Natal to specific individuals participating in projects.

At postgraduate level, the principles and potential of telemedicine and medical informatics are included in several Masters in Public Health programmes. Formal training in telemedicine is offered at the University of KwaZulu-Natal, where students can take a Masters in Public Health degree with specialization in telemedicine or a Master of Medical Science in telemedicine.

Legislation and guidelines

The DOH is drafting a Telemedicine Act that will address matters such as licensure, consent, data security and patients' rights. With the shortage of doctors in South Africa, there is a need for a pragmatic approach to the issue of licensure, so that the country can take advantage of international telemedicine services. It is hoped that the Act will be enabling and not restrictive. At the same time, the Health Professionals' Council of South Africa is drafting ethical guidelines for telemedicine. While these initiatives are well intentioned, they may be premature, as there is as yet an insufficient base of physicians and nurses with practical experience in telemedicine in South Africa to fully appreciate and debate the implications of some the proposals in the Act. Legislation that may be appropriate for an industrialized country may not be appropriate in a developing country with a shortage of doctors and nurses, and may indeed obstruct the use of telemedicine.

Conclusions

Telemedicine in South Africa appears to be at a crossroads. While its potential is apparent, it is not yet clear whether the potential can be realized in an environment in which there are human resource constraints at both the sending and receiving sites. Despite several years of activity, the volume of telemedicine use is still very low, and most services must be considered as being still in the pilot phase. Efforts to date have been hampered by several common factors. These include lack of buy-in from provincial governments, lack of support from health professionals, lack of technical support, insufficient training, failure to provide site coordinators, lack of administrative and financial models for the public sector, and failure to understand the complexity of change management.

Videoconferenced tele-education for health professionals has been successful, and demand is growing. Tele-education may prove to be the catalyst for rural practitioners to become involved in telemedicine activity. There is renewed interest in telemedicine in South Africa, and this needs to be well managed and coordinated for telemedicine to succeed. To do so probably requires the formation of a national telemedicine association, bringing together the government and the provincial DOHs, universities, nongovernmental organizations, the private health sector and industry. The aim would be to ensure that mistakes are not repeated, that pilot projects are scaled up through cooperation and that local best practice is shared for the common good. If South Africa cannot make telemedicine work, then other poorly resourced African countries are unlikely to succeed.

Further reading

Mars M, Dlova N. Teledermatology by videoconference: experience of a pilot project. *S Afr Fam Pract* 2008; **50**: 70.

References

1. World Health Organization. *World Health Statistics 2007.* Available at: www.who.int/whosis/whostat2007/en/index.html.
2. Bradshaw D, Groenewald P, Laubscher R et al. Initial burden of disease estimates for South Africa. *S Afr Med J* 2003; **93**: 682–8.
3. Health Systems Trust. *Health Statistics.* Available at: www.hst.org.za/healthstats/index.php?Indtype_Id=004002.
4. Esselaar S, Gilwald A, Stork C. *South African Telecommunications Sector Performance Review 2006.* Available at: link.wits.ac.za/papers/SPR-SA.pdf.
5. World Bank. *ICT at a Glance Tables.* Available at: web.worldbank.org/WBSITE/EXTERNAL/DATASTATISTICS/0,,contentMDK:20459133~menuPK:1192714~pagePK:64133150~piPK:64133175~theSitePK:239419,00.html.
6. Corr P. Teleradiology in KwaZulu-Natal. A pilot project. *S Afr Med J* 1998; **88**: 48–9.
7. Jithoo R, Govender PV, Corr P, Nathoo N. Telemedicine and neurosurgery: experience of a regional unit based in South Africa. *J Telemed Telecare* 2003; **9**: 63–6.
8. Kennedy C, Kirwan J, Cook C et al. Telemedicine techniques can be used to facilitate the conduct of multicentre trials. *J Telemed Telecare* 2000; **6**: 343–7.
9. Brauchli K, Oberli H, Hurwitz N et al. Diagnostic telepathology: long-term experience of a single institution. *Virohowe Aroh* 2004; **444**: 403–9.
10. Gulube SM, Wynchank S. Telemedicine in South Africa: success or failure? *J Telemed Telecare* 2001; **7**(Suppl 2): 47–9.
11. Gulube SM. *Evaluation Report of the First Phase of the SA National Telemedicine System (NTS).* Available at: www.kznhealth.gov.za/telemedreport.pdf.
12. Science in Africa. *Telemedicine Gets Mobile.* Available at: www.scienceinafrica.co.za/2004/september/telemedicine.htm.
13. Abrahams JF, Molefi M. *Implementing telemedicine in South Africa 'A South African Experience'.* Available at: www.hrhresourcecenter.org/node/1265
14. Brauchli K, O'Mahony D, Banach L, Oberholzer M. iPath – a telemedicine platform to support health providers in low resource settings. *Stud Health Technol Inform* 2005; **114**: 11–17.
15. Chetty M, Tucker W, Blake E. *Telemedicine in the Eastern Cape Using VOIP Combined with a Store and Forward Approach.* Available at: pubs.cs.uct.ac.za/archive/00000202/01/Chetty.pdf.
16. Bridges.org. *The Tygerberg Children's Hospital and Rotary Telemedicine Project.* Available at: www.bridges.org/case_studies/353.
17. Colven R, Todd G, Wynchank S et al. *A Teledermatology Network for Underserved Areas of South Africa.* Available at: www.medetel.lu/download/2005/parallel_sessions/presentation/0407/A_Teledermatology_network.pdf.
18. Cell-Life. *Cell-Life.* Available at: www.cell-life.org.
19. SIMpill. *Simpill.* Available at: www.simpill.com.
20. International Marketing Council of South Africa. *Beaming Education to the Nation.* Available at: www.southafrica.info/ess_info/sa_glance/education/mindsetedu.htm.

22 Telemedicine in sub-Saharan Africa

Maurice Mars

Introduction

What is the state of telemedicine in sub-Saharan Africa? There is no single repository of information on telemedicine in Africa, so it is difficult to provide current and accurate information on every country. However, it is apparent that many telemedicine projects in Africa are launched with a fanfare of press releases, but there is little or no information about their subsequent progress.

Demographics

Africa has a land mass of 30 million square kilometres, with a total population of approximately 965 million people, who constitute 14% of the world's population.[1] Health provision in Africa is poor. The difference between Africa and the industrialized world was highlighted in the WHO World Health Report of 2006:[2]

> The WHO Region of the Americas with 10% of the global burden of disease, has 37% of the world's health workers spending more than 50% of the world's health financing, whereas the African Region has 24% of the burden but only 3% of health workers commanding less than 1% of world health expenditure. The exodus of skilled professionals in the midst of so much unmet health need places Africa at the epicentre of the global health workforce crisis.

Sub-Saharan Africa can be defined as that part of Africa lying to the south of the Sahara Desert. This includes five countries whose political boundaries are traversed by the geographical boundary. It is made up of 42 countries and 6 island nations, extending as far east as Mauritius in the Indian Ocean.

Burden of disease and population predictions

The burden of disease is great. Africa has most of the HIV-positive people in the world – approximately 24 million. A million people die annually of malaria, and Africa accounts for over 90% of the half billion new cases of malaria each year. There is a high prevalence of tuberculosis, and poliomyelitis has re-emerged.[3] The leading causes of death in the WHO African Region in 2002, in order, were HIV/AIDS, malaria, lower respiratory tract infections, diarrhoeal diseases, perinatal conditions, cerebrovascular vascular disease, tuberculosis, ischaemic heart disease and measles.[4] While the focus of the industrialized world is on the ageing population and how to keep people out of hospital, average life expectancy is still falling in many African countries. Life expectancy is less than 45 years in 7 countries.[3] For the foreseeable future, there will be a large number of people dying in Africa and a substantial birth rate, both of which place heavy demands on health care providers.

Provision of doctors

The WHO recommends that at least 20 doctors per 100 000 population are required to provide minimum basic health care services. Thirty-eight sub-Saharan African countries fail to meet this standard, 31 countries have fewer than 10 doctors per 100 000 population and 13 countries have fewer than 5 doctors per 100 000. It has been estimated that Africa would require an additional one million doctors to meet this minimum requirement. The shortage of health professionals in Africa is a result of underproduction, loss through migration and, surprisingly, in some countries, unemployment. There are 121 medical schools in Africa, with a ratio of 1 per 7.6 million people, compared with the industrialized world's norm of 1 per 2 million people.[5] The medical schools are not equally distributed, with 87 medical schools in 47 sub-Saharan African countries and 34 schools in 6 Mediterranean-rim countries. Four sub-Saharan countries do not have a medical school. The brain drain of health professionals from the developing world is the focus of the WHO World Health Report 2006, with rates of migration of health workers from African countries ranging from 8% to 60%.[4]

Health care funding

There is extreme poverty, with 41% of people in sub-Saharan Africa living on less than US$1 per day.[6] Funding of health care remains difficult. A realistic estimate of the cost of providing basic health care to people in Africa is about US$34 per person per annum. Based on 2004 data, the governments of 34 sub-Saharan African countries allocate less than US$34 per capita per annum to health; 23 countries spend less than US$10 per capita. The average per capita expenditure on health in sub-Saharan Africa is US$22.

In 2001, Member Heads of States of the Organisation of African Unity signed the Abuja Declaration on HIV/AIDS, Tuberculosis and Other Related Infectious Diseases, in which they pledged to set a target of allocating at least 15% of their annual budgets to the improvement of the health sector. This was re-affirmed by the Ministers of Health in the Gaborone Declaration of 2005. Only two countries have achieved this. By 2004, the average general government expenditure on health was 8.8% in the WHO African Region[3] and, by 2005, a third of the countries had reached 10%. There was also a commitment by developed countries to give 0.7% of their annual income in aid. By 2006, only Denmark, Luxembourg, the Netherlands, Norway and Sweden had honoured this pledge.

Telemedicine as a solution?

Telemedicine has great potential to solve problems such as the shortage of health-workers and the provision of care to underserved rural populations (Box 22.1).[7] The

> **Box 22.1 The plight of many rural patients in Africa[a]**
>
> Patients are referred to the Black Lion Teaching Hospital in Addis Ababa from all over Ethiopia. If they do not die on the way to Addis Ababa, they often face long waiting times once they get there. Under-investment in rural health care facilities, a shortage of doctors and the lack of incentives to retain medical staff in rural areas all serve to increase the problem.
>
> Demissie Sahle is a 68-year-old farmer who lives in Amhara, about 200 km north of Addis Ababa. He was ill for six months, and tried to obtain treatment at the nearest health post, but without success. Together with his son Laike, he raised nearly 4000 birr (US$500) to travel to the capital: 'whatever we could sell, we have sold to get here and to pay for treatment, including our only oxen', said Laike. Father and son embarked on the journey, leaving their families and their land behind, unsure whether anyone would look after them.
>
> Telemedicine, if it were to be rolled out to rural areas, could make Demisse Sahle's journey a thing of the past. This case exemplifies the plight of many rural patients in Africa and highlights the potential for telemedicine in Africa.
>
> [a]Adapted from Abebe S. *Ethiopia: Digital Doctors*. London: Panos.[7]

World Health Assembly Resolution on e-health (WHA58.28) of 2005 called on member nations to develop long term e-health strategic plans, provide the telecommunications infrastructure necessary for e-health and establish national centres of excellence. Several African countries have started to develop strategies.

It is disheartening to note that neither the WHO African Regional Health Report of 2006 nor the 2007 WHO publication, *African Health Monitor*, which was devoted to the crises in Human Resources For Health in Africa, mentions telemedicine as a possible solution to the shortage of health workers or the training of health workers in Africa. The World Health Report 2006 mentions telemedicine/telehealth/e-health once: 'Greater access to education at lower cost can be achieved by regional pooling of resources and expanding the use of information technologies such as telemedicine and distance education.'[2] Similarly, the Africa Health Strategy: 2007–2015, developed by the African Union Ministers of Health in April of 2007, makes no mention of telemedicine, telehealth or e-health.[8] The use of information communication technology (ICT) is mentioned twice, in the context of its lack of use to provide evidence to guide action within a health system, and as an 'ingredient' that makes up a functional health system. Africa's commitment to the use of telemedicine is not clear.

The UN Millennium Development Goals (MDGs) include four relating to health: access to clean drinking water, reduced child mortality under the age of 5 years (currently 16.6%), improved maternal health, and combating HIV/AIDS, malaria and other diseases. It is unlikely that any African country will achieve these goals. In 2007, the UN Secretary General found it necessary to form a Millennium Development Goals Africa Steering Group to help African countries improve their performance in meeting the goals.[9] Forty-one countries have begun developing their national strategies in line with the MDGs, and several have included telemedicine in their plans.

Obstacles to telemedicine

There are many obstacles to the implementation of telemedicine in Africa.

Telecommunication costs

Many barriers to the introduction of telemedicine in Africa centre on telecommunications legislation, infrastructure and costs. Telecommunications are not fully deregulated in Africa, and liberalization of policies is required. In 2003, there were monopolies for local, long-distance and international call services in over 60% of the countries, with 10% of the countries allowing monopolies for mobile and very small-aperture terminal (VSAT) services and Internet service providers (ISPs). This, and the fact that about 70% of Africa's continental Internet traffic passes out of Africa, pushes up Internet cost.[10] In the USA, the average cost for 20 hours of Internet access (10 hours peak and 10 hours off-peak usage), based on the cheapest available tariff and including telephone usage charges, is US$15.[11] The average monthly cost for sub-Saharan African countries is US$55. Twenty hours of Internet access a month, for a year, exceeds the annual gross national income (GNI) per capita, in 26 countries. To put these costs into perspective, the annual GNI per capita is US$41 400 in the USA and the percentage of GNI for 20 hours of Internet access is 0.4%. It is not surprising that fewer than 4% of Africans have Internet access and that broadband access is below 1%.[10]

Because of the cost of Internet access, even simple store-and-forward telemedicine is not always an affordable option in Africa. Videoconferencing via ISDN is also expensive. The average cost of a 30-minute videoconference at 128 kbit/s, from Africa to the USA, is US$48.30.[11] Satellite connectivity is also expensive. While VSAT access is available to all African countries, its use in telemedicine has been impeded by legislative problems, which have tended to restrict private enterprise and have resulted in high costs. The average annual VSAT licence fee in 83 African universities is US$13 553, compared with US$426 for European Union universities.[12] VSAT communication has been widely used in pilot projects, but the associated high costs are a factor in the lack of sustainability of some projects.

There has been rapid growth in the use of mobile phones in Africa. Mobile penetration has risen from 3% in 2003 to 21% in 2007, and is forecast to reach 30–35% by 2011. Costs are also relatively high, averaging 27% of GNI per capita per annum, compared with 0.3% in the USA.

Other obstacles

Other obstacles to the introduction of telemedicine include:

- a lack of telemedicine policies at national and regional levels and, as a result, a lack of budgets
- poor connectivity to the rural areas that are most in need of support
- the shortage of doctors and nurses in almost all countries
- low levels of computer literacy among health professionals
- lack of training in telemedicine
- poor technology support
- continuing regional conflicts in Africa
- the absence of administrative and financial models for telemedicine in the African setting.

The shortage of doctors is a particular problem. Telemedicine requires additional effort and, while its potential benefits are acknowledged by most doctors, many will not participate in telemedicine because of the extra work involved and/or the disruption to their work routine.

International telemedicine services may be a method of addressing the shortage of doctors in Africa. However, in the absence of adequate funding, service providers outside Africa are unlikely to be remunerated at the rates to which they are accustomed, if at all. Also, diagnostic and treatment algorithms used in the industrialized world may not be appropriate in Africa, and pharmacopoeias are likely to differ from country to country. The question of liability is yet to be formally resolved.

What has proved to be effective in South Africa is videoconferenced education, and there is a growing demand from African medical schools to participate in shared education. The provision of education may prove to be the catalyst for developing telemedicine services.

Telemedicine initiatives in sub-Saharan Africa

Telemedicine in Africa is not new. In 1984, doctors in London made a diagnosis of Crouzon's syndrome in a patient in Swaziland, using satellite communication.[13] In 1987, there was clinical case-conferencing between Canada, Kenya and Uganda. This consisted of twice-weekly satellite audio-conferences, with EEGs transmitted from Mulago in Kampala to the Health Science Centre at St John's in Canada.[14] Satellite-based store-and-forward telemedicine was used by the US Army in Ethiopia in 1993.[15]

Pan-African telemedicine initiatives

The African Union is an international organization of 53 member states. The New Partnership for Africa's Development (NEPAD) is a special programme of the African Union. NEPAD has developed a health strategy for the African Union, which does not refer to telemedicine or e-health but does refer to 'the appropriate use of technology'.[16] The NEPAD e-school project makes provision for the incorporation of an 'e-health point'. The first NEPAD e-school was launched in mid-2005 at the Bugulumbya Secondary School in Busobya Village in Uganda, and a consortium of private companies has agreed to sponsor the demonstration project of 6 schools in each of the 16 participating countries.

The former President of India announced the launch of the Pan African Network, which aims to connect 53 African countries by satellite and fibre-optic links, to provide tele-education, telemedicine, Internet access, videoconferencing and voice-over-Internet protocol (VOIP) services. For telemedicine, one remote hospital in each country will have access to 10 specialist hospitals (7 in Africa and 3 in India). The remote hospitals will be provided with email and videoconferencing facilities, and facilities for transmission of ultrasound scans, echocardiographs and ECGs. The project has financial backing for five years, and will be coordinated by the African

Union. While this will not provide a solution to Africa's medical problems, it might serve as a starting point for further development and cooperation.

A workshop sponsored by the European Commission and the European Space Agency was held in Brussels in 2006. It established a Telemedicine Task Team, which has subsequently reviewed telemedicine opportunities in Africa. It will make recommendations for future telemedicine actions in Africa and in particular sub-Saharan Africa, with an emphasis on the use of satellite communications.[17]

International telemedicine initiatives

Some international store-and-forward projects, in which African doctors have participated, have been in operation for several years. However, use of these services in Africa has been limited. Why is this? The obvious reasons include the lack of infrastructure, the shortage of health professionals and the cost of bandwidth. What is often overlooked is the lack of training of African health professionals in simple store-and-forward telemedicine. The assumption is made that everyone knows how to take a photograph and send an email message. Many of the obstacles listed previously are relevant.

The Moorfields Eye Hospital ophthalmology projects have linked three regional hospitals in South Africa to England for second opinion services by videoconference and email,[18] and their web-based second-opinion service is used by doctors in South Africa, Gambia, Tanzania and Ghana. The Orbis Cybersight programme also offers store-and-forward services to ophthalmologists in Ethiopia and Tanzania. The Swinfen Charitable Trust's store-and-forward telemedicine service has been used by doctors in Sierra Leone, Ethiopia, Malawi, Uganda and Zambia,[19] as has iPath, which commenced as a telepathology service and evolved into dermatology and radiology services. Private and multinational companies have also set up telemedicine services, both for their employees and for private patients who are able to afford international service.

In the Francophone African countries, the RAFT (Résau en Afrique Francophone pour la Télémédicine) project, based at the Hôpitaux Universitaires de Genève, has been running at eight sites in Mali since 2001, with additional sites in Mauritania, Morocco, Burkina-Faso, Senegal, Tunisia, Cameroon, Côte d'Ivoire, Madagascar, Djibouti and Niger coming on line in 2005. Over the first 5 years, this project ran 98 webcast teaching sessions (50 from Geneva and 48 from Bamako in Mali). The infrastructure was also used for teleconsultations using the web-based iPath platform and IP-based videoconferencing for remote consultations. Only 14 international teleconsultations, for neurosurgery, radiology and dermatology, were reported by 2005. This project has noted that the 'high expectations of satellite technology are still unmet, as the cost of connectivity remains unaffordable for rural communities'.[20]

The African Medical and Research Foundation (AMREF), based in East Africa, was founded in 1957, and has a long history as a flying doctor and radio doctor service. It is currently involved in developing four store-and-forward telemedicine sites in Kenya and Tanzania.

Projects within countries

As well as the international store-and-forward services, there are several examples of telemedicine projects in sub-Saharan Africa. As stated previously, this summary of activity in sub-Saharan African countries is likely to be incomplete, and may refer to some projects that are no longer active, as failure is not often reported.

In Angola and the Democratic Republic of the Congo, a non-governmental organization (NGO) called Promoting Social Development in Africa ran a trial store-and-forward project in collaboration with Partners Telemedicine. The project was not sustainable, and ended in 2005. Botswana has identified the need to set up telemedicine services, and the Botswana–Baylor Children's Clinical Centre of Excellence has established the first telemedicine site in the country. Benin has a histopathology store-and-forward service with Paris, for the management of Buruli ulcers. Burkina-Faso is part of a tele-epidemiology network with France, and also participates in the RAFT project. Burundi participates in the iPath programme. Chad participates in the RAFT programme.

Anesthesia Overseas is assisting in training nurse anaesthetists in Eritrea, and is setting up a telemedicine distance education resource centre in one of the hospitals. Ethiopia is relatively active, although the country's five-year health sector development plan does not include the use of digital technology to improve rural health. In 2006, an ICT for Health workshop attended by 300 people agreed to set up a working group to formulate an e-health strategy for Ethiopia. Telemedicine activity has been supported by a recent grant of US$2 million from India to fund a telemedicine project between Ethiopia and India for 3 years. There is also a report of 10 local hospitals being linked for telemedicine. Doctors have participated in both the Swinfen and iPath programmes and Johns Hopkins runs biweekly HIV clinical case presentations at the distance learning centre in Addis Ababa.

Gabon has participated in iPath. The Gambia has used the Swinfen Charitable Trust service and has participated in the Moorfields project. Ghana too has participated in the Moorfields and iPath programmes, and Satellife has been very active in the evaluation of personal digital assistants (PDAs) for clinical data capture. Ghana is in the process of expanding its fibre-optic connections throughout the country, which will improve its capacity to offer real-time telemedicine. At the same time, two projects are being piloted in a collaborative programme between the University of California at Berkeley and Intel Research. These are the REACH (Remote Asynchronous Communication for Healthcare) and TIER (Technology and Infrastructure for Emerging Regions) projects. In the latter, 5 WiFi networks covering distances of up to 58 km have been installed in Ghana, for use in education.

Guinea, which had early support from the International Telecommunication Union for telemedicine development, does not appear to have made further advances. Guinea-Bissau is participating in the Spacedream project funded by the European Space Agency, which is investigating how Earth observation, navigation and telecommunication systems can be used to improve access to antiretroviral therapy and health care. Telecommunications will be used to connect health workers in rural areas with a central hospital.

Kenya is working on an e-health initiative. The AMREF group has set up telemedicine pilot projects, and the Agah Khan Hospital group has telemedicine links with North America. They are also investigating the use of videoconferenced education between their centres. The Regenstrief Institute at the University of Indiana has a long association with Moi University in Eldoret and helped to found the Open MRS project, which is developing a framework for electronic patient records in resource-poor areas.

The Malawi Polytechnic is developing a wireless network to be used for telemedicine, and the Baobab Health Partnership has developed a touch-screen clinical workstation in open source software, which captures data in real time at the point of patient contact. The patient management system allows poorly qualified health care workers to provide high-quality HIV treatment.

Mali was an early partner in the RAFT programme and, with the ongoing assistance of the Hôpitaux Universitaires de Genève, has implemented the e-well project, which supplies stable power supplies and Internet connections to six sites to enable telemedicine, primary school education, adult literacy and the development of small business enterprises. In 2005, a store-and-forward teleradiology service was established between four hospitals using open source software via switched telephone links. After a slow start due to technical problems, 338 cases were sent in the first 4 months, a case load of approximately 30 X-rays per hospital per month, or about 1 case per day per hospital.

Mauritania has participated in the Raft and iPath programmes, and a strategy for community access to ICT has been proposed. In 1997, Mauritius – which is classified as part of sub-Saharan Africa – launched its first telemedicine project. The project failed, and a new store-and-forward service for radiology and ECGs between a private hospital and a hospital in India was set up in 2005, with a supplementary videoconference link.

Mozambique had a teleradiology service operating in 1998 between two hospitals, but this project was not sustainable. Namibia is a large country with a small population and no medical school. A nuclear medicine telemedicine link between Namibia, South Africa and the UK was established in 2003. Niger is part of a tele-epidemiology network with France, which monitors infectious disease. Doctors in the country have also made use of the RAFT and iPath programmes. Nigeria has Africa's first and only national telemedicine association. In 2006, the first telemedicine centre was launched with a videoconference-based service between a private hospital and a hospital in India.

Rwanda formally launched its national telemedicine programme in 2007. Videoconference links have been established between three hospitals. An active distance education programme in public health has been running between the National School of Public Health and Tulane University. Sao Tome has sent cases to iPath. Sites in Senegal have participated in the RAFT programme, with reports of videoconferenced consultations with Toulouse and three hospitals with store-and-forward facilities for teleradiology and teledermatology. Sierra Leone and Sudan have sent cases to the Swinfen Charitable Trust.

South Africa has several new and established projects and services, which are described in Chapter 21. Tanzania has a store-and-forward project with the Rikshopitalet in Oslo and the Aga Khan Board of Volunteers in North America. AMREF has linked two sites in Tanzania as part of its four-site pilot project. Healthspan International, an NGO, has been active in setting up telemedicine projects using telephone lines, video cameras and television monitors for both store-and-forward and real-time telemedicine.

Uganda has connected three hospitals, and has been very active in a PDA project to gather health data, using Healthnet and Satellife. Through the International Telecommunication Union, there are several projects providing ICT access to rural communities. Cases have been sent to the Swinfen Charitable Trust service from Uganda and Zambia. In Zambia, two hospitals were recently linked to the University Teaching Hospital through a Swedish International Development agency grant.

Conclusion

While there is an upsurge in telemedicine activity in sub-Saharan Africa, it remains to be seen whether sustainable programmes will emerge. There is a need for telemedicine training throughout Africa, as, without it, telemedicine practice will remain the domain of a few enlightened enthusiasts. The use of international projects such as the Swinfen Charitable Trust, iPath, RAFT and the new Pan African Telemedicine Project will assist the introduction of telemedicine, but, unless substantial use is made of these services, they will not make a major contribution to improved health care in Africa. Problems such as international cross-border practice of telemedicine have not yet been adequately addressed, nor have questions of international and ethical standards for the practice of telemedicine. Africa needs to solve these problems so that they do not impede further progress.

For telemedicine to be of assistance in Africa, there needs to be greater government will to embrace telemedicine, changes in telecommunication policies, provision of affordable bandwidth, and the development of sustainable and affordable rural telemedicine solutions. This will require substantial external assistance, goodwill and perseverance.

Further reading

Heinzelmann PJ, Lugn NE, Kvedar JC. Telemedicine in the future. *J Telemed Telecare* 2005; **11**: 384–90.

Kaplan WA. Can the ubiquitous power of mobile phones be used to improve health outcomes in developing countries? *Global Health* 2006; **2**: 9.

Kirigia JM, Seddoh A, Gatwiri D et al. E-health: determinants, opportunities, challenges and the way forward for countries in the WHO African Region. *BMC Public Health* 2005; **5**: 137.

References

1. United Nations. *World Population Prospects: The 2006 Revision Population Database*. Available at: esa. un.org/unpp.
2. 2 World Health Organization. *The World Health Report 2006 – Working Together for Health*. Available at: www.who.int/whr/2006/en/index.html.
3. World Health Organization. *World Health Statistics 2007*. Available at: www.who.int/whosis/whostat2007/en/index.html.
4. World Health Organization. *The African Regional Health Report*. Available at: www.afro.who.int/regional-director/african_regional_health_report2006.pdf.
5. Institute for International Medical Education. *Database of Medical Schools*. Available at: www.iime.org/database/index.htm.
6. United Nations. *Assessing Progress in Africa towards the Millennium Development Goals Report 2008*. Available at: www.uneca.org/cfm/2008/docs/AssessingProgressinAfricaMDGs.pdf.
7. Abebe S. *Ethiopia: Digital Doctors*. London: Panos. Available at: www.igloo.org/libraryservices/download-nocache/Library/external/gvsubmis/922007to/ethiopia.
8. African Union Conference of Ministers of Health. *Africa Health Strategy: 2007–2015*. Available at: www.africa-union.org/root/UA/Conferences/2007/avril/SA/9-13%20avr/doc/en/SA/AFRICA_HEALTH_STRAT-EGY_FINAL.doc.
9. United Nations. Ban Ki-moon launches 'unprecedented' group to boost Africa's development. *United Nations News Centre*. Available at: www.un.org/apps/news/story.asp?NewsID=23809&Cr=millennium&Cr1=development#.
10. United Nations. Better IT connectivity can unleash Africa's economic potential, UN officials say. *United Nations News Centre*. Available at: www.un.org/apps/news/story.asp?NewsID=23870&Cr=information&Cr1=technology&Kw1=africa&Kw2=connectivity&Kw3=economic+potential.
11. World Bank. *ICT at a Glance Tables*. Available at: web.worldbank.org/WBSITE/EXTERNAL/DATASTATISTICS/0,,contentMDK:20459133~menuPK:1192714~pagePK:64133150~piPK:64133175~theSitePK:239419,00.html.
12. Hawkins R. *Enhancing Research and Education Connectivity in Africa*. Available at: www.aau.org/tunis/presentation/Panel1/NREN%20ATICS%20WSIS%20Nov%202005.pdf.
13. Ojo T. Communication networking: ICTs and health information in Africa. *Inf Dev* 2006; **22**: 94–101.
14. House M, Keough E, Hillman D et al. Into Africa: the telemedicine links between Canada, Kenya and Uganda. *CMAJ* 1987; **136**: 398–400.
15. Crowther JB, Poropatich R. Telemedicine in the U.S. Army: case reports from Somalia and Croatia. *Telemed J* 1995; **1**: 73–80.
16. NEPAD. *The New Partnership For Africa's Development (NEPAD) Health Strategy*. Available at: www.nepad.org/2005/files/documents/129.pdf.
17. Asamoah-Odei E, de Backer H, Dologuele N et al. eHealth for Africa. Opportunities for enhancing the contribution of ICT to improve health services. *Eur J Med Res* 2007; **12**(Suppl 1): 1–38.
18. Kennedy C, Kirwan J, Cook C et al. Telemedicine techniques can be used to facilitate the conduct of multicentre trials. *J Telemed Telecare* 2000; **6**: 343–7.
19. Swinfen Charitable Trust. Available at: www.swinfencharitabletrust.org.
20. Geissbuhler A, Bagayoko CO, Ly O. The RAFT network: 5 years of distance continuing medical education and tele-consultations over the Internet in French-speaking Africa. *Int J Med Inform* 2007; **76**: 351–6.

23 Telehealth for mountainous and remote areas of northern Pakistan

Hameed A Khan and Irfan Hayee

Introduction

Pakistan is ranked 124 out of 191 countries in terms of health care.[1] About a third of the population lives below the poverty line, with unhygienic living conditions, poor health, and food and water insecurity. As a consequence, there is a high burden of infectious and chronic diseases among people in Pakistan, especially women and children. Poor nutrition and repeated infections have aggravated the situation. According to a health assessment conducted by the Aga Khan University, Pakistan ranks 157th in the world in terms of infant mortality, and 39th in child mortality.[2] Moreover, with agriculture being the main occupation in the country, the majority of the population still live in rural and remote areas that are underprivileged in terms of access to basic health care services.

The northern area of Pakistan, comprising five districts (Gilgit, Skardu, Diamer, Ghizer and Ghanche), is one of the most remote and disadvantaged regions of Pakistan. The area has a population of around one million people, who live in more than 600 villages scattered over 72 000 km^2 of rugged terrain. Lack of communications is a major problem.

People in the northern area of Pakistan have long been poorly served in terms of access to health and education services. The area is known for its difficult terrain, extreme climate and geographical remoteness from large cities (Figure 23.1). Baltistan and Hunza, particularly, being remote and underdeveloped mountainous regions, do not have access to high-quality health care services. The health facilities do not have specialists, particularly for women's health care. Major hospital and health facilities are a long way away. For instance, Gilgit is about 800 km away from a tertiary health care facility. Owing to the lack of satisfactory health services, people suffer as a result of late diagnosis and treatment. Furthermore, the rural health centres (most of which do not have doctors) are not linked to the hospitals in the main urban centres, resulting in avoidable mortality and morbidity, especially among women, children and the elderly. Lack of information and communication facilities and the absence of development networking compound the problems.

The Commission on Science and Technology for Sustainable Development in the South (COMSATS) was established in 1994 to promote science and technology in all spheres of life. It has 21 developing countries as its members and there are 16 centres

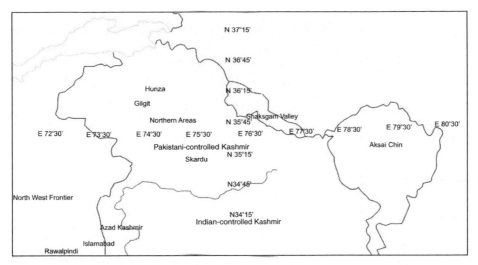

Figure 23.1 Northern area of Pakistan

of excellence. In view of conditions in the northern parts of Pakistan, COMSATS launched a project on telehealth, which went into service in 2005. Its objective was to facilitate access to specialized health services and education, and thereby contribute towards raising the standard of living in the area. The Baltistan Health and Education Foundation, which was working to improve health care services for women in the remote and backward regions of Baltistan, collaborated with COMSATS on the project. The International Development Research Centre (IDRC), a Canadian government development organization, was the principal funding organization (see Chapter 7).

Telemedicine in northern Pakistan

Establishing a telehealth service in the mountainous and remote areas of northern Pakistan required not only having reliable technology but also matching the services to the socioeconomic and cultural environment of the area. This required cultural change, although, after three years, the telehealth service is now well established and accepted by the local communities.

In the rural areas of Pakistan, the lives of people are strongly governed by cultural and traditional norms, which makes introducing change difficult. Women are particularly marked by certain limitations as far as their mobility and interaction with the outside world are concerned. In such a situation, building a rapport with the local people, convincing them to adopt telehealth and interact with people who did not belong to their community, as well as disclosing personal information, especially in the case of women, was a formidable task. However, the COMSATS team was successful in bringing about change in the attitudes of the local people. This meant involving members of the local community in delivering the services, so that patients coming in for consultation did not feel alienated.

The lack of telecommunication infrastructure in the region was a major problem. The government had installed landlines (digital telephone exchanges) to some villages, but these were of poor quality and also expensive for the users. On an experimental basis, the government introduced wireless local loop (WLL) in some villages, but this was not very successful. The only Internet service provider (ISP) in Gilgit was established by COMSATS.

The technology required for the project was installed by COMSATS Internet Services (CIS), the executive agency of COMSATS. The tasks included:

- establishing an ISP at Skardu
- capacity building at the Gilgit node
- training the project staff
- operating the ISP at Skardu
- assisting with procurement of equipment
- documenting the technical aspects of the project.

The equipment for the project is listed in Table 23.1. A major task was obtaining a licence to operate an ISP in Hunza.

Very-small-aperture terminal (VSAT) links between Skardu and Islamabad and between Hunza and Islamabad were established at an initial bandwidth of 128 kbit/s. Internet bandwidth was provided from Islamabad at subsidized rates. Once an ISP had been established at Skardu, surplus money being generated could be invested in the telehealth services.

Project experience

Medical services

During the first phase of the project, a needs assessment was carried out at Skardu. This showed the need for teleconsultations in five medical fields. In order to develop standard operating procedures and to synchronize the efforts of the Telehealth Centre (Skardu) and the Resource Centre (Islamabad), a study was made of various aspects:

- level and type of medical services
- availability of medical specialists
- scheduling of services
- medical equipment required
- clinical requirements of the telehealth service.

The three major areas of focus were:

(1) designing and establishing a telehealth centre
(2) identifying a suitable team of medical specialists
(3) selecting and procuring appropriate medical equipment.

Teleconsultancy services were required in five specialties: general medicine, cardiology, gastroenterology, dermatology and nephrology. After three years of operation, services are now being provided in all fields except nephrology. Services in

Table 23.1 Project equipment

	Quantity
Equipment for the resource centre at Islamabad	
Ethernet switch	1
Videoconference equipment	1
Computer (P -IV, 850+)	1
Printer (HP Laser Jet)	1
Scanner	1
Uninterruptible power supply (3 kViA)	2
Webcam – high-resolution	1
Air conditioners	1
Dish/VSAT equipment	1
Satellite receiver	1
Equipment for telehealth at Skardu	
Videoconference equipment	1
Computers	2
Laser printers	2
Scanner	1
Multimedia projector	1
Generator (25 kViA)	1
Uninterruptible power supply (3 kViA)	1
Interfaces for X-ray and ultrasound	1
Camcorder	1
ECG machine	1
Treadmill stress testing machine	3
X-ray board	1
Ultrasound machine	1
Equipment for the ISP at Skardu	
Generator (25 kViA)	1
Uninterruptible power supply (3 kViA)	3
Server (for authentication, proxy and billing)	3
Networking (e.g. cables and connector)	16
Switch (24 ports)	1
Satellite receiver/modem	1
Dish/VSAT	1
Router	1
HDSL modems	2
Access server	1
Computers	14

psychiatry are being considered. It was initially expected that asynchronous (store-and-forward) telehealth would be used most frequently, but later on, as telehealth came into routine use, the synchronous (real-time) method became common.

Medical equipment

After careful examination it was felt necessary to have similar videoconferencing equipment at both the Telehealth Centre (Skardu) and the Resource Centre (Islama-bad). The equipment chosen (VSX 7000, Polycom) transmitted video calls over an IP connection. The Telehealth Centre was established in the premises of the Abdullah Hospital in Skardu and operated by the collaborating institution, the Baltistan Health and Education Foundation. The hospital is a secondary-level health care unit. The Telehealth Centre is located close to the ultrasound room, reception and the conference room, which makes patient care efficient and reduces teleconsultation times.

To reimburse medical specialists for teleconsultation, it was decided to pay them for each visit to the Resource Centre, and not on the basis of the number of patients seen. Reimbursement for delivering seminars was handled separately. To coordinate a team of medical specialists, it was necessary to have a coordinator between the specialists and the people at the Resource Centre and the Telehealth Centre.

Telehealth Centre at Skardu

Five medical specialists and a telehealth consultant were employed at Islamabad. Teleconsultancy services were operated for a test period, and then later run operationally for patients in Skardu. Training and orientation of staff at the Abdullah Hospital were carried out. Development of a patient information system and linkages with experts and donor and medical organizations were also made.

A total of 361 patients received specialist consultations in the first 4 months of operation. Dermatology was the most common specialty. Women benefited greatly from the service, and showed confidence and satisfaction. In one period, 101 female patients received a specialist consultation, in comparison with 51 male patients. Feedback received from the specialist doctors at Islamabad, as well as project staff at Skardu, called for increased bandwidth to improve the quality of the service.

Experience with the service

The level of trust and confidence of the community grew steadily, as indicated by the steady number of follow-up cases, which ranged between 15% and 20% of the patients each month. A substantial proportion of females benefitted from the service (58% overall).

Despite some problems due to connectivity, infrequent availability of a general practitioner at Skardu and difficulties in data transfer, the telehealth service continued smoothly with minor glitches, and the level of satisfaction of patients and doctors remained satisfactory (on the basis of initial and post-project interviews).

The 1000th consultation was conducted during May 2006. More importantly, women and children (between the ages of a few months and 13 years) were the main beneficiaries of telehealth services. Women account for 61% and children 21% of those receiving specialist consultations from doctors in Islamabad. It was observed that women and children are the ones who suffer the most in the absence of specialized medical services. First, they find it difficult to travel on their own to tertiary care centres in remote areas. Second, it costs them more to travel, since they are dependent on male family members to accompany them because of societal and cultural norms.

Another important fact that indicated the acceptance of the service was that people from rural areas came pouring in to receive specialist consultation. No promotional campaign was run to inform people from outlying areas, and word of mouth seemed to be enough. The consultation data show that in the first few months more consultancies were provided for people from urban areas, while in the later months more consultancies were provided for people from rural areas (Figure 23.2).

Teleconsultations continued as scheduled after the launch of the service in April 2005, i.e. one session a week for dermatology, cardiology, gastroenterology and general medicine. However, the services were disrupted for some time in the wake of the earthquake of October 2005, which caused havoc in the northern parts of Pakistan and killed some 80 000 people.

Although the earthquake did not affect the Baltistan region directly, it made the specialists at the Resource Centre (Islamabad) unavailable for telehealth for most of the consultations in the following month and a half. Most of the medical specialists were engaged in serving a large influx of patients from the earthquake-hit areas at their principal medical facilities, and therefore routine consultations had to be reduced or postponed owing to the emergency situation.

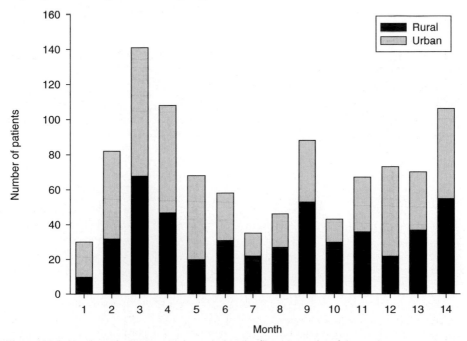

Figure 23.2 Number of teleconsultations during the first 14 months of the project

Problems and corrective measures

Connectivity

Low bandwidth and poor connectivity were the major impediments to telehealth services. Although the telehealth clinic was connected to the ISP through an HDSL modem, the increased clientèle of the ISP at Skardu affected the bandwidth available for data transfer and videoconferencing. Weather conditions and physical damage to copper wires also caused problems.

Various measures were taken to overcome these difficulties. The videoconferencing system was adjusted to make the calls at 128 kbit/s so that packet loss could be minimized. This greatly improved the audio quality during consultations. Separate downlink services were arranged from another service at the ISP in Skardu to make VSAT link bandwidth available for the telehealth project (Figure 23.3). An average of only 32 kbit/s was then used by the COMSATS Internet service from the total 128 kbit/s VSAT link. Fine tuning was done at the ISP to decrease the choking and packet loss.

The graphs of bandwidth usage obtained from the ISP identified the time when the Internet usage was least, and the timings for teleconsultation were adjusted to take advantage of this. The connection between the Telehealth Centre and the ISP was lost twice owing to physical damage to the copper wires between the two sites, which subsequently halted the telehealth service for two or three days each time. Therefore, a second cable link was made available so that it could be used as an alternative connection in case of similar problems in the future.

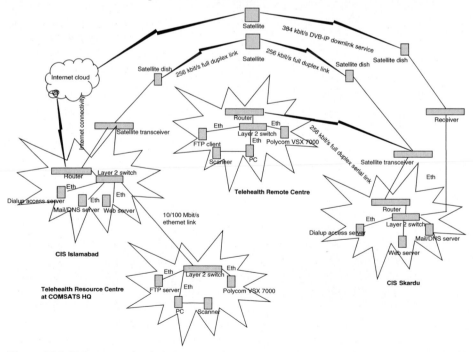

Figure 23.3 Telecommunications

Unavailability of human resources

Infrequent availability of general physicians or well-trained paramedical staff has been one of the major problems in providing the telehealth service at Skardu. Most doctors in Pakistan prefer to work in large cities (either to gain experience or to earn more), and only those who are visiting their families, or female doctors whose spouses are stationed in army units, are available in rural areas. Often, these doctors are available only for a limited period of time, and many leave within a few months. There are few paramedics in the northern parts of Pakistan, and not many are sufficiently trained to provide telehealth services. In view of these problems, the following steps were taken.

A doctor dedicated to the telehealth service at the Abdullah Hospital in Skardu was employed for telehealth. The doctor's role was to present accurate and detailed information about the patients (e.g. the history and basic physical examination results) to the specialist doctors. Having detailed medical data is important for successful teleconsultation. In view of the large number of female patients seen by telemedicine, a female doctor was hired.

All the specialists opined that the quality of consultation was satisfactory when there was a supporting doctor (general physician) present at the remote site to provide the basic data. In the absence of a general physician, it was observed that the consultations were manageable, but did not meet the satisfaction of the specialists.

The computer operator, who was responsible for running the remote Telehealth Centre, gained a lot of experience through hands-on training. He was formally supervised by the doctors at the Telehealth Centre and the Resource Centre, which helped him to gain expertise in delivering services. After training, the computer operator could take a good patient history and perform a general physical examination, e.g. checking blood pressure, pulse and temperature. This was useful if the general physician at the remote centre was not available. Given suitable training, a paramedic or non-medical person can be a useful substitute when a doctor is not available for conducting telemedicine.

Patient information software

The patient information software proved to be of great help in maintaining the medical records of visitors and patients. Initially, the patient information system was developed as a client–server application. The information was thereafter transmitted using file transfer protocol (FTP) servers at both ends. In addition, FTP servers were placed at the ISP to increase the rate of transfer of files, as well as to avoid undue delays in the transfer during power failure or problems in the computers. This option improved the situation to some extent, leaving only the problem that complete data on a patient could not be accessed from one program, making it rather time-consuming. In the light of experience, it was realized that a web-based solution would be a better way in the future of providing similar services from different sites.

It was also realized that there is a need to provide the patient data to the specialists at their workplace and at their homes, so that they can conduct telemedicine without coming to the Resource Centre. Visits of the medical consultants to the Resource Centre could be reduced by using a web portal.

Service methodology

Although the consultations in this project were mainly based on real-time videoconferencing, in a few instances where live consultation was not possible (for technical reasons), the diagnosis and expert opinion were based on store-and-forward information. About 10% of all consultations were performed in this way. It turned out that patient management decisions were easily made in dermatology, while, in the single instance of a cardiology case, it was most difficult. The reason may be that the images in dermatology cases are self-explanatory and require little elaboration, whereas in cardiology there are often many unanswered questions. However, the store-and-forward technique was more time-consuming than live interaction, for both the physician and the patient.

In discussion with the specialists, it appeared that both patients and doctors felt that store-and-forward consultations were inferior to real-time consultations, except in dermatology. In dermatology, a detailed history of the patient along with high-resolution pictures could be sent easily, thus facilitating the correct diagnosis.

Recommendations

Based on our experience, we recommend that careful attention be paid to the design and implementation of telehealth services in underdeveloped areas. It is feasible to utilize relatively inexpensive and robust equipment that is easy to operate and repair. Activities must be chosen that result in benefits for as many people as possible, while the technology chosen should be compatible with immediate health care needs.

As well as support from the government, it is important to persuade private sector and local organizations to participate in planning and implementing telehealth services. The participation of local organizations will not only assist in developing health care services attuned to the local settings, but also facilitate the acceptance of these services in the area. The collaboration between COMSATS and the Baltistan Health and Education Foundation has been a success. It demonstrates how local organizations can catalyze the implementation of telehealth and bring ownership to the community.

Appropriate guidelines need to be developed for establishing high-quality and consistent standards for teleconsultations. Formulating a tele-education strategy and conducting a resource inventory may be helpful in this regard.

An important factor in a successful telehealth service is the information management system. This should be devised in conjunction with the specialists and other doctors who are involved in delivering the telehealth services.

Conclusions

Despite the difficulties, telehealth can be a practical method of providing specialist consultations and supporting other health care services for people in developing countries, particularly those in remote regions. Telehealth can also be used to improve access to the health care providers of these regions and reduce their isolation.

Establishing a telehealth service in Skardu was a difficult task. However, with an enthusiastic team, the project was successful, and it is clear that many patients, especially women and children, have benefited from the service. Those who are unable to travel to cities to obtain specialist advice now have easy access to specialist health care.

Economies may be possible in future by using digital cameras or newer versions of webcams, instead of specialized videoconferencing equipment. In future, the resource centre might be established at a hospital to save time for both the doctor and the patient. While promoting telehealth to doctors, it is important to emphasize that existing health care delivery methods will not be replaced – rather, telehealth will supplement them.

Finally, the general public, patients and health professionals should be informed as much as possible about telemedicine, so that they feel comfortable with the concept. This will mean that future generations will feel at ease in using telehealth to improve traditional methods of health care delivery.

Further reading

Adler AT. A cost-effective portable telemedicine kit for use in developing countries. Thesis, Department of Mechanical Engineering, Massachusetts Institute of Technology, 2000. Available at: www.media.mit.edu/resenv/pubs/theses/AriAdler-Thesis.pdf#search='telemedicine%20problems%20developing%20countries.
Edworthy SM. Telemedicine in developing countries. *BMJ* 2001; **323**: 524–5.
Graham LE, Zimmerman M, Vassallo DJ et al. Telemedicine – the way ahead for medicine in the developing world. *Trop Doct* 2003; **33**: 36–8.
Office of Technology Policy, US Department of Commerce. *Innovation, Demand and Investment in Telehealth.* Available at: www.ncsbn.org/2004Report.pdf.

References

1. World Health Organization. *The World Health Report 2000 – Health Systems: Improving Performance.* Available at: www.who.int/whr/2000/en/whr00_en.pdf.
2. Aga Khan University. *Assessment of Health Status and Trends in Pakistan.* Available at: aku.edu/CHS/pdf/HealthSituationandTrend-Pakistan,2001.pdf.

24 Teleneurology: Past, present and future

Usha K Misra and Jayantee Kalita

Introduction

Telemedicine has been used in many areas of health care. A Medline search for telemedicine papers found 911 articles concerning its use in radiology, 931 in surgery and 735 in pathology (Figure 24.1). There were 69 articles concerning telemedicine in neurology and 19 concerning epilepsy.

The term 'imaging' was found in 710 articles, 'video' in 969 and 'electrocardiography' in 250. 'Electroencephalography', the typical investigation of epilepsy, was found in 27 articles only. The most commonly mentioned aim of telemedicine was consultation (3022), followed by diagnosis (3654) and education (1718). Other

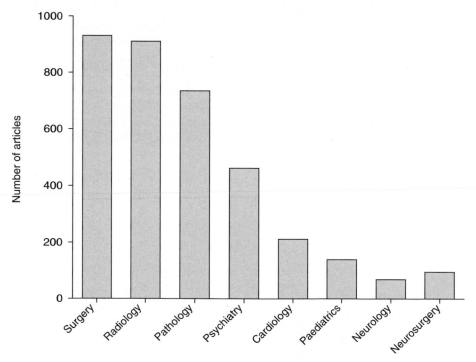

Figure 24.1 The number of telemedicine articles published in different specialities (PubMed search, April 2008)

indications were instrumentation (1729), treatment (2984), cost (2015) and payment (45).

Clinical telemedicine applications can be considered on two axes: a vertical axis representing the level of maturity and a horizontal axis representing the extent of the application. The maturity is based on several factors, including quantity and quality of research pertaining to the application, the degree to which the application has been accepted by the profession, and the development of standards or protocols for its use. The evidence of the application refers to attributes such as technical feasibility, diagnostic accuracy, sensitivity, specificity, clinical outcome and cost-effectiveness. Teleradiology, telesurgery and telepathology rank high on the maturity scale. Psychiatry, dermatology and ophthalmology are regarded as maturing areas of telemedicine, whereas paediatrics and emergency medicine, for example, are emerging specialties with respect to the use of telemedicine (Figure 24.2).[1]

In neurology, real-time telemedicine has the greatest potential in the management of neurological emergencies such as status epilepticus, stroke and movement disorders and in neurophysiology. Status epilepticus and stroke require urgent treatment within the window period for better outcome. Transporting these patients to a specialist centre might take several hours, resulting in high mortality and morbidity. Live demonstration or video recordings of patients with movement disorders and neurophysiological tracings (electroencephalography, nerve conduction studies and evoked potentials) can be transmitted to a specialist centre for expert opinion without physical referral of the patient.

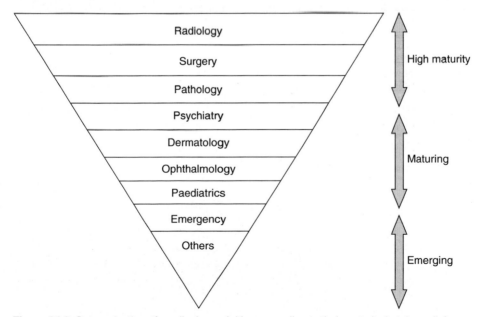

Figure 24.2 Categorization of medical specialties according to their maturity in telemedicine

Epilepsy

Epileptic seizures can be infrequent and difficult to diagnose. The best method of diagnosis is by observation of the seizure episode, and in its absence one has to rely on the description of a bystander. The data concerning seizures are so important that full information should be made available to the physician so as to make or revise the diagnosis. Patients with epilepsy often have travel limitations placed on them, which may cause difficulties with the different centres involved in treatment of multiple handicap. Communication between different hospitals and physicians in difficult-to-diagnose epilepsies can be greatly helped by telecommunication.[2] This can not only avoid frequent and sometimes arduous visits to experts in different hospitals and repeated investigations, but also allow the simultaneous opinion of different physicians to be obtained.

Status epilepticus is an emergency in which seizures recur without the patient regaining consciousness between two discrete seizures, or individual seizures continue for at least 30 minutes. Often, a patient is admitted to a primary centre and is referred to another more specialized centre when the seizure is not controlled. Finally, when the patient reaches an advanced specialized centre, he or she may be have been undergoing status epilepticus for several hours or even longer. This is likely to result in various complications and a poor prognosis. Early diagnosis and prompt treatment would assist with controlling the attack and improving the prognosis. According to a recent study, a telemedicine-based epilepsy service was as safe and effective as conventional face-to-face consultation.[3] In this study, a neurologist was based at a centre and managed epilepsy patients at a rural hospital by video link. Patients were usually accompanied by a family member and always by a trained nurse, who acted as care manager, coordinated medication and ensured compliance, and was able to reinforce what the neurologist said. A comparison was made of patients managed by this method and those managed by a conventional urban clinic. Seizure frequency, emergency room visits and hospital admissions were used as measures of efficacy and safety. No difference was found in these outcome measures between telemedicine and conventionally treated patients.[3]

Acute stroke

Recombinant tissue-type plasminogen activator (rtPA) represents a major break-through in the treatment of ischaemic stroke. If it is administered within 3 hours of onset of stroke, it results in improved survival and outcome.[4] Many institutions lack the specialized personnel and resources necessary to provide the response for acute stroke patients. These institutions depend on the rapid transfer of patients to regional stroke centres for therapy. In practice, the main reason for patients not receiving this therapy is their late arrival after the critical time window of 3 hours. Telemedicine is emerging as an efficient means of making early decisions about therapy.

At the medical centre of the University of Maryland, the tele-stroke service uses videoconferencing and CT image transfer. Between 1999 and 2001, 50 stroke consultations were reviewed. Of these, 23 were managed by telemedicine and 27 by traditional telephone conversation followed by transfer. Two of the 23 telemedicine consultations were aborted because of technical difficulties. Of the patients evaluated by the traditional method, 1 (4%) received rtPA, whereas 5 patients from the telemedicine group (24%) received rtPA and there were no complications due to this therapy. Telemedicine provided a treatment option that was not previously available at the remote hospital. For administration of rtPA, telemedicine was safe, feasible and well received.[5,6]

Assessing the stroke patients and their CT scan by using videoconferencing offers an opportunity to improve stroke care in remote and rural areas. In a study from Swabia, seven rural hospitals were connected to the stroke unit via videoconferencing. One hundred and fifty-three patients were examined by teleconsultation, and a relevant contribution could be made in more than 75% of cases regarding diagnostic work-up, CT assessment and therapeutic recommendations.[7]

Although the number of emergencies is increasing, there is growing anxiety about medical errors and an increasing number of medical negligence cases. Pre-hospital use of telemedicine for stroke is already being piloted, linking patients in an ambulance to the emergency department.[6]

Movement disorders

Telemedicine has been found to be useful for diagnosis, treatment and follow-up of patients with various movement disorders. Live video or prerecorded video clips can be used for these purposes. In a recent study, video clips of normal and abnormal gait disorders were used by a geriatrician for diagnosis and were compared with the diagnosis of the treating clinicians, i.e. the latter was considered the gold standard. The agreement of the video clip examination with the gold standard in identifying abnormal gait ranged from substantial to excellent among assessors, although there was only a low agreement with the gold standard in the detection of specific gait diagnosis. This technique appears to be a valid screening procedure for detecting gait abnormalities, with a sensitivity of 100% and a specificity of 70%.[8]

Telemedicine has also been used to follow up patients with Parkinson's disease in remote areas. Over a 3-year period, 100 teleconsultations were carried out on 34 patients with Parkinson's disease. Each teleconsultation lasted for 30–60 minutes. Patients and providers were satisfied with the consultations, and they reduced the time and cost of travelling.[9]

Neurophysiology

Digital technology for clinical neurophysiology allows teleneurophysiology to be developed. Such a service may improve patient care in remote areas, since the clinician can obtain a second opinion from other centres. The process may even help in education and the creation of a national data bank. A telemedicine facility of this kind has been established in Scandinavian countries.[10]

Neurological outpatients

In remote areas where neurologists are not available, telemedicine has been used for providing outpatient consultations to neurological patients. In a randomized controlled trial, the efficacy of telemedicine consultation was compared with face-to-face consultation, the groups comprising 82 and 86 patients, respectively.[11] The diagnostic categories were similar in the two groups. The patients in the telemedicine group had more investigations, but there was no difference in the number of drugs prescribed. The patients were generally satisfied with both processes, although they were concerned about confidentiality and embarrassment in the telemedicine consultation.

Teleneurology, although feasible in the outpatient setting, is less well accepted than face-to-face consultation, and can lead to over-investigation.[11] However, in a remote area where there are too few neurologists, telemedicine may become a viable option, especially in developing countries.

Mobile phones

The telephone has always been used for consultation between doctors, especially for fixing appointments, calling for home visits or obtaining immediate advice. Following the mobile phone revolution, most urban and even rural people have access to a telephone. This has opened up opportunities for using mobile phones for health care delivery. In developing countries, the doctor:patient ratio is far too low. Specialized and even primary hospitals are overcrowded. The use of a mobile phone can help in obtaining appointments and monitoring therapy, especially in chronic disorders such as epilepsy, migraine, headaches and stroke. Such patients often have to travel long distances, and it may take several hours or even days to obtain a consultation. In such a situation, adjusting the dose of drugs, checking compliance, monitoring side effects and defining the patients who need an early appointment may be done by telephone or mobile phone. The difference between a mobile phone and the ordinary telephone service is not only the former's mobility, but also that mobile phones have additional capabilities, including text messaging, video and Internet facilities.

There is a paucity of randomized controlled trials evaluating the efficacy and satisfaction level of mobile phone consultations in comparison with conventional face-to-face consultations. Psychotherapy delivered by telephone revealed a significant improvement in depression. In telephone-administered cognitive–behavioural therapy, there was an improvement compared with usual care.[12] Patients can often capture an event such as a seizure or movement disorder and present it to a physician for evaluation during consultation.

Medical education

Telemedicine has great potential to transform medical education at undergraduate, postgraduate and professional levels. The educator has to select the appropriate context, content and delivery method to suit the needs of the largest number of the learners. In medicine, education has to continue throughout the professional's career. Learning is greatest when adults act as self-directed, motivated learners, perusing the topics of their interest in the appropriate context, i.e. interactive, practical and self-paced.[13] These principles can be incorporated into a distance education programme.[14] Online continuing medical education (CME) and web-based CME have also provided CME credits for the practising physician. The Internet also has the ability to support the presentation of complex multimedia presentations to augment learning. The Internet has created learning communities.

A survey was conducted regarding the motivation and choice of topics for a journal club and the websites accessed in two institutions. The institutions were the Sanjay Gandhi Post Graduate Institute of Medical Sciences in Lucknow and the King George Medical University in Lucknow. The views of specialty ($n = 58$) and subspecialty ($n = 97$) residents were compared.[15] Most of the residents used Medline and PubMed for choosing their journal club topics. The choice of Google, the Oxford database, Science Direct and the Cochrane Review did not differ between the residents of the two institutions. At the Post Graduate Institute, the choice of articles was based on the availability of good articles, whereas in the Medical College, it was faculty driven. The choice of articles related to patient management and examination were not different between the two institutions. Female residents more frequently selected articles related to patient management or examination, although the difference was not significant.

Internet use by residents and faculty members of the Medical College and the Post Graduate Institute was surveyed by us, and we found that 89% of individuals performed a computer literature search at least once a month. The reason for a computer-based literature search was for presentation in 90% of cases, research in 65% and patient care in 60%. The benefit of literature searching was acknowledged in learning and teaching by 80% of respondents, in research by 65% and in patient care by 54%. Formal training in computer-based literature searching was received by 41%, of whom 80% were residents. Of the participants in this survey, 64% had a home Internet connection and the remainder used the Internet at their workplace or at a cyber café, suggesting widespread use of computers and the Internet by medical personnel.[16]

We have used videoconferencing for neurology teaching in India. We have conducted a neurology educational conference between the Post Graduate Institute and the Medical College. These locations are 1500 km apart. Faculty members and residents of the two departments participated. Desktop videoconferencing systems were connected by an ISDN line at 128 kbit/s. During 2001–2004, there were 30 sessions, 22 of which were successful and 8 partly successful (owing to power and communication failure). In each session, two to four cases were discussed, with clinical pictures, neurophysiological and radiological data as illustrations. Discussions provided inputs for both learning and patient management (Figure 24.3).[17]

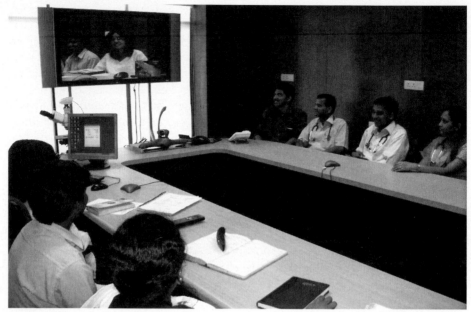

Figure 24.3 A videoconferencing session between the Sanjay Gandhi Post Graduate Medical Institute and a remote centre in India

Telemedicine in India

There are few reports in the literature of the successful use of telemedicine in India. Mahakumbh Mela is a religious congregation that occurs every six years and in which millions of Hindus gather for religious ceremonies and discussions. Such a large gathering of people is associated with inherent health problems, such as infections and accidents, so that health care for the attendees is a major public health problem. The Post Graduate Institute used telehealth to avoid an outbreak of cholera at the Mahakumbh Mela in Allahabad, Uttar Pradesh.[18] Ganapathy[19] took the initiative of providing consultations to distant areas in India in Aragonda and Sriharikota. Desai et al[20] used teleconsultation between a tertiary cancer centre and a rural cancer hospital. Ninety-three cases were analyzed in which static pathology and telepathology were used to obtain a consultation between the Tata Memorial Hospital, Mumbai and the Nargis Dutt Memorial Cancer Hospital at Barshi. A diagnosis was offered in 92 (98%) cases.

Resource availability

In developing countries, an increasing population and a very low doctor:patient ratio represent a difficult challenge for health care. A total of some 800 neurologists in a country such as India with a population of 1.3 billion is inadequate. It will take more than 20 years to achieve a ratio of one neurologist for 50 000 population at the rate of 50 neurologists being produced per year. However, it is not only the numbers that are important. Increasing specialization has reduced the number of physicians who are good at managing emergencies. Although the number of emergencies is increasing, there is growing anxiety about medical errors and increasing number of medical negligence cases.

There is no single solution for upgrading the emergency services, but a favoured model has been a large central hospital with associated local hospitals to which patients are discharged. Unfortunately, this may make the services worse rather than better. Medical emergencies usually occur in a patient's home, and are followed by a journey to the hospital, assessment, admission, treatment and then discharge. A large central hospital means a long journey, which may delay treatment and influence outcome, as in status epilepticus and stroke. In developing countries, roads and transportation are far from satisfactory. Increased distance also causes problems for visiting families, and weakens the link with primary care, which is crucial when discharging patients from hospital. Large numbers of patients in emergency departments lead to long waiting periods. The local hospitals do not share care or staff with large hospitals, and have poor nursing and medical infrastructure. They are uncomfortable about managing seriously ill patients, and thus assume the role of nursing homes, rather than hospitals.

Black et al[21] have proposed a reverse model in which patients are admitted to a local hospital, which acts as the catchment area of a big hospital. The medical and nursing staff would be part of the team working in the central hospital, and would rotate between the hospitals. The local unit would have imaging (CT scanning) and laboratory support (EEG, ECG and biochemistry), as well as high-quality electronic links with the central hospital that would allow the specialists to know almost as much about the patients as if they were examining them directly. Such a system would result in avoiding delay in treatment. Patients who did not need admission could be quickly discharged, perhaps within a single day, and some patients would never need to go to the central hospital at all. Those who went to the central hospital would not need to be assessed again, so that the transfer and admission would be faster.[21]

The cost-effectiveness of telemedicine has been a concern because, in a study of teleneurology from the UK, a comparison of 65 patients in a conventional group and 76 in a teleconsultation group revealed that the telemedicine group needed more investigations and reviews than the conventional group. The average cost of conventional consultation was £49, compared with £72 for the telemedicine group.[22]

Legal questions

The use of telemedicine has raised several legal questions. These include licensing, reimbursement and liability. The question of data security is also a concern in telemedicine. Thus, accidental loss and data corruption must be prevented by providing effective data control management and artefact recognition algorithms. As personal data is involved, the possibility of loss or criminal access must be considered and prevented. Special encryption mechanisms to secure data against unauthorized access or modification are therefore necessary.[12] Patients' right to confidentiality is paramount.

Unless otherwise agreed by both sides, the liability in telemedicine is normally considered to rest with the consulting rather than the advising physician. Procedures for reimbursement of logistical costs in telemedicine need to be developed.

Conclusion

There are concerns that physicians in future may become 'telecarers', at least for part of their working time. A telecarer is a health professional who delivers responsive, high-quality information services, and supports remote patients or clients by using the most appropriate communication technology, such as the telephone, email or instant messaging. The advantages of telecare are the possibility of working from home and better continuity of patient care. However, there are concerns about over-investigation, clinical mistakes and confidentiality. There are also worries about commercial pressures.

A wider market for health service information and products should be welcome. However, the danger of commercial suppliers or cyber-physicians undercutting primary health care services is a possibility, although it may ultimately result in healthy competition. The digital divide in society may also be a concern. People with low education and old age may be excluded from telemedicine, and society must ensure that this does not occur. Telemedicine is a powerful tool, but should be used judiciously and in the interests of society at large.

Further reading

Bashshur RL, Sanders JH, Shannon GW. *Telemedicine, Theory and Practice*. Springfield, IL: CC Thomas, 1997.

Darkins AW, Cary MA. *Telemedicine and Telehealth Principles, Policies, Performance and Pitfalls*. London: Springer, 2000.

Norris AC. *Essentials of Telemedicine and Telecare*. New York: Wiley, 2002.

Wootton R, Craig J, Patterson V, eds. *Introduction to Telemedicine*. 2nd edn. London: Royal Society of Medicine Press, 2006.

References

1. Krupinski E, Nypaver M, Poropatich R et al. Telemedicine/telehealth: an international perspective. Clinical applications in telemedicine/telehealth. *Telemed J E Health* 2002; **8**: 13–34.
2. Elger CE, Burr W. Advances in telecommunications concerning epilepsy. *Epilepsia* 2000; **41**(Suppl 5): 9–12.
3. Rasmusson KA, Hartshorn JC. A comparison of epilepsy patients in a traditional ambulatory clinic and telemedicine clinic. *Epilepsia* 2005; **46**:767–70.

4. National Institute of Neurological Disorders and Stroke rt-PA Stroke Study Group. Tissue plasminogen activator for acute ischemic stroke. *N Engl J Med* 1995; **333**: 1581–7.
5. LaMonte MP, Bahouth MN, Hu P et al. Telemedicine for acute stroke: triumphs and pitfalls. *Stroke* 2003; **34**: 725–8.
6. LaMonte MP, Xiao Y, Hu PF et al. Shortening time to stroke treatment using ambulance telemedicine: TeleBAT. *J Stroke Cerebrovasc Dis* 2004; **13**: 148–54.
7. Wiborg A, Widder B. Teleneurology to improve stroke care in rural areas: the Telemedicine in Stroke in Swabia (TESS) Project. *Stroke* 2003; **34**: 2951–6.
8. Salih SA, Wootton R, Beller E, Gray L. The validity of video clips in the diagnosis of gait disorder. *J Telemed Telecare* 2007; **13**: 333–6.
9. Samii A, Ryan-Dykes P, Tsukuda RA et al. Telemedicine for delivery of health care in Parkinson's disease. *J Telemed Telecare* 2006; **12**: 16–18.
10. Stålberg S. Small bits to big bites. *Muscle Nerve* 2002; **11** (Suppl): S119–27.
11. Chua R, Craig J, Wootton R, Patterson V. Randomised controlled trial of telemedicine for new neurological outpatient referrals. *J Neurol Neurosurg Psychiatry* 2001; **71**: 63–6.
12. Ludman EJ, Simon GE, Tutty S, Von Korff M. A randomized trial of telephone psychotherapy and pharmacotherapy for depression: continuation and durability of effects. *J Consult Clin Psychol* 2007 **75**: 257–66.
13. Knowles MS. *Andragogy in Action: Applying Modern Principles of Adult Learning.* San Francisco: Jossey-Bass, 1984.
14. Ward JP, Gordon J, Field MJ, Lehmann HP. Communication and information technology in medical education. *Lancet* 2001; **357**: 792–6.
15. Misra UK, Kalita J, Nair PP. Traditional journal club: a continuing problem. *J Assoc Physicians India* 2007; **55**: 343–6.
16. Kallta J, Misra UK, G Kumar. Computer based literature search in medical institutions in India. *Ann Indian Acad Neurol* 2007; **10**: 44–8.
17. Misra UK, Kalita J, Mishra SK, Yadav RK. Telemedicine for distance education in neurology: preliminary experience in India. *J Telemed Telecare* 2004; **10**: 363–5.
18. Ayyagari A, Bhargava A, Agarwal R et al. Use of telemedicine in evading cholera outbreak in Mahakumbh Mela, Prayag, UP, India: an encouraging experience. *Telemed J E Health* 2003; **9**: 89–94.
19. Ganapathy K. Telemedicine and neurosciences in developing countries. *Surg Neurol* 2002; **58**: 388–94.
20. Desai S, Patil R, Chinoy R et al. Experience with telepathology at a tertiary cancer centre and a rural cancer hospital. *Natl Med J India* 2004; **17**: 17–9.
21. Black S, Andersen K, Loane MA, Wootton R. The potential of telemedicine for home nursing in Queensland. *J Telemed Telecare* 2001; **7**: 199–205.
22. Chua R, Craig J, Wootton R, Patterson V. Cost implications of outpatient teleneurology. *J Telemed Telecare* 2001; **7**(Suppl 1): 62–4.

25 Telepaediatric support for a field hospital in Chechnya

Boris A Kobrinskiy and Vladimir I Petlakh

Introduction

Emergency situations involving multiple victims require efficient decisions about medical care. The use of modern telecommunications allows improved support for disaster medicine. This includes monitoring of the medical situation, communications about patient transportation problems, and consultative support for the medical stuff working in the disaster area. Teleconsulting may be useful in disaster medicine in a number of ways:

- efficient transfer of information about the nature of the emergency, which is needed to plan the order and scale of evacuation measures
- consultations with medical specialists to support the physicians on site
- optimization of the choice of specialized hospitals for further treatment of the victims.

Modern telecommunications were used for the first time in disaster medicine by the US National Aeronautics and Space Administration (NASA) in 1985 after the earthquake in Mexico City. This allowed better estimation of the medical consequences of the earthquake and facilitated proper rescue measures.[1]

In the former Soviet Union, the first use of teleconsultations in an emergency situation was after the Armenian earthquake of 1988. Telemedical 'space bridges' (i.e. video connections) were established by NASA between Russian and American specialists. This was the first experience of international telemedical collaboration in an emergency situation.[2] The project included audio–video and fax communication between the disaster area in Armenia, clinics in Moscow and four medical centres in the USA.

In 1999, after a train crash in Bashkiria, teleconsultations took place between a hospital in Ufa (Bashkiria), a surgical clinic in Moscow and the Yerevan Diagnostic Centre in Armenia. Dedicated telephone lines were used to provide audio communication and slow-scan black-and-white video images. When connected to the 'space bridge', the system enabled consultations about patients in Ufa with conditions such as burns and psychological trauma, involving specialists at medical centres in Moscow and the USA.

In 1993, the US Department of Defense started using telemedicine to support a peacekeeping force (IFOR) undertaking humanitarian missions in a number of countries. The telemedicine system was called PrimeTime. Physicians at field hospitals in Macedonia, Croatia and Bosnia were connected to hospital specialists in Germany, Hungary and the USA.[3,4]

The most recent use of telemedicine in an emergency situation in Russia was to support the Children's Field Hospital of the All-Russia Centre of Disaster Medicine in the Chechen Republic in 2001. The doctors of the field hospital had to provide care for patients with various conditions resulting from explosion trauma and from firearms, as well as providing diagnosis and treatment for children with a wide range of pathologies, including acute and chronic diseases (e.g. congenital, malignant, neurological and cardiovascular). This situation required distant medical support, which was realized by installing a telemedicine unit at the field hospital.

Remote decision support for the Children's Field Hospital

By 2001, medical services in Chechnya had been almost completely destroyed owing to long-term military conflict. Paediatric care was almost unavailable. The Children's Field Hospital in the Gudermes district of the Chechen Republic included an admission and consultation department, a surgery department, a department of internal medicine and an intensive therapy unit, as well as laboratory and radiology services (Figure 25.1). The hospital was equipped for X-ray imaging, ultrasound scanning and basic laboratory investigations.

The field hospital was admitting not only wounded children, but also children with various diseases from a number of districts of the Chechen Republic. This created serious problems for the relatively small medical staff of the hospital. It was not realistic to refer all the complicated cases to clinics in Moscow or to other Russian cities.

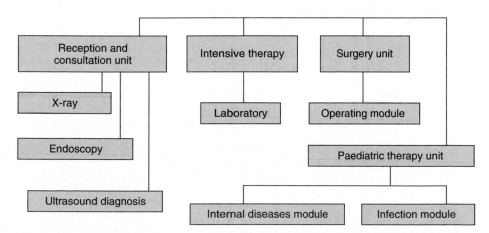

Figure 25.1 Structure of the field hospital

Besides, in a number of cases, urgent consultations with specialists were required, including multispecialist consultations. Therefore, even from the start of the hospital's work, there was a need for support from specialist institutions. Telephone consultations were impractical in Chechnya in 2001, owing to the very poor quality of telephone connections, and their complete absence in a number of areas. An efficient means of communication was required to support the physicians working in emergency situations, including urgent support from specialists. The consultations had to be provided both in store-and-forward mode and in real-time, using videoconferencing.

The implementation of this telemedical support – the first Russian system for disaster telemedicine – was performed by specialists of the Moscow Research Institute for Paediatrics and Children's Surgery, the All-Russia Centre of Disaster Medicine, the Dorodnicyn Computing Centre of the Russian Academy of Sciences, the State Central Air-Carried Rescue Team and a company called Web Media Service.[5]

It was decided that the Medical Centre for New Information Technologies of the Moscow Research Institute for Paediatrics and Childen's Surgery would act as the head telemedicine centre of the system. The telemedicine centre was equipped with a videoconferencing system and modern telecommunication equipment, including fibre-optic cables enabling ISDN connection at 2.048 Mbit/s and IP connection at 1.024 Mbit/s.

Emergency and scheduled teleconsultations were provided by the telemedicine centre, as well as multispecialty videoconference consultations.[6] The Medical Centre for New Information Technologies provided technical support for the field hospital, initially acting as the sole consulting centre. Later on, regular working contacts were established between the field hospital and the Scientific Institute of Medical and Biological Problems in Northern Ossetia, the Fund for Development and Dissemination of New Medical Technologies in Stavropol, the Stavropol Area Hospital and the Republican Children's Hospital in Vladikavkaz.

System architecture

It was clear from the beginning that only satellite communication would be appropriate for telemedicine (Figure 25.2). One satellite channel was used to provide the connection between the consultants in the telemedicine centre and the physicians in the field hospital, and a second channel was used to send requests to the telemedicine centre. Both store-and-forward and real-time traffic were sent by satellite.

Originally, the equipment at the telemedicine unit in the field hospital included:

- a VSAT terminal, including a computer for information transfer at a bandwidth of 1.0 Mbit/s through the satellite system HeliosNet
- a satellite phone system (GlobalStar) to transfer the date to the telemedicine centre at a bandwidth of 9.6 kbit/s
- a videoconference system
- a workstation for the preparation of medical documents (in digital form)

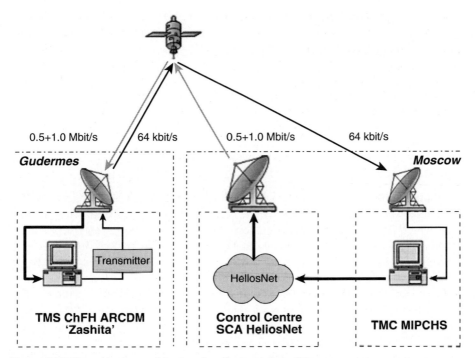

Figure 25.2 Comunication architecture for disaster telemedicine

- peripheral devices, including a digital camera, digital videocamera and flatbed scanner.

The telemedicine unit was set up in one of the tents of the field hospital. The telemedicine unit included work places for videoconferencing and for data preparation (e.g. review of case material and digitizing of documents). A satellite dish was installed near the telemedicine unit tent.

Because of technical limitations on videoconferencing with the GlobalStar communication system, other solutions were sought. A duplex satellite terminal (AT&T) was installed at the field hospital. It provided a bandwidth of 12–16 kbit/s for data transfer. It was also less expensive to use than GlobalTel or INMARSAT.

The satellite link enabled real-time consulting using an asymmetrical IP connection between the field hospital and the telemedicine centre. The experience demonstrated that any reliable communication channel with a transfer rate of 9.6 kbit/s for audio and 56 kbit/s for video could be used as a request channel (provided that no fast movements needed to be demonstrated to the remote party). For the response channel, from the telemedicine centre to the field hospital, a high-rate satellite channel was used.

Experimental use of the telemedicine system began in August 2001. By the beginning of September 2001, operational usage had begun. Between October 2001 and July 2002, the telemedicine system was operational 24 hours a day.

Telemedicine in the field hospital

Teleconsultations were based on asymmetrical access, with a high-speed channel from the telemedicine centre to the field hospital and a low-speed channel in the other direction. The process included:

(1) preparation of the patient's data
(2) digitizing any graphical material
(3) forming the request
(4) transfer of the request and digitized medical documents
(5) real-time consultation.

Receipt of the request and the documents was done by a coordinator at the telemedicine centre, who checked the quality of the received data, referred the documents to a consultant, made journal records about the nature of the consultation and recorded the subsequent consultant's recommendation. The scheme included two main phases: a preliminary phase and the consultation itself.

During the preliminary phase at the field hospital, the patient documentation was assembled and then sent to the telemedicine centre with the consultation request using the low-bandwidth communications channel. The documentation included textual materials and graphical data (e.g. X-ray and ultrasound images and photographs). The total file size was on average about 3–5 Mbyte per patient.

The second phase was information exchange between the telemedicine unit of the field hospital and the telemedicine centre in Moscow using an asymmetrical duplex IP connection. The high-speed channel was used for transfer of large volumes of information, including multimedia data, from the Moscow centre to the hospital, while the low-speed channel was used to transfer relatively limited volumes of information (text, sound, graphical data and, rarely, video data) from the hospital to the telemedicine centre.

On establishing the connection, the participants decided which case to start with. The consultant then opened the relevant document on the screen of a PC in Moscow. Within 5–15 seconds, the same document automatically opened on the screen of the computer in the field hospital. The hospital physician could ask questions orally; if needed, the physician could use a White Board option to show the consultant some part of an opened document (or image). All the consultant's comments (audio, text and graphics) were presented at the field hospital, being transferred via the satellite channel. All the consultations were recorded, which allowed them to be reviewed afterwards, if required.

The subsequent course of a consultation was defined by the situation. Four main variants were possible:

1. A physician could ask another question on the case or document being discussed.
2. The parties could begin the discussion of a new case.
3. The parties could move to a decision about organizational matters.
4. The discussion could be stopped.

Clinical aspects of telemedicine support

During a 14-month period ending in 2002, the Children's Field Hospital delivered care for over 30 000 patients from 17 districts of Chechnya. A total of 2700 inpatients were treated. Telemedicine provided valuable long-term support for the physicians of the field hospital. A total of 179 consultations were conducted (including those in the trial period). The main result was that over 40% of patients were able to continue their treatment in the field hospital after the consultation, instead of being transported to other medical centres. The severity of the conditions of the consulted patients can be seen from the two lethal outcomes in children for whom urgent consultations were requested.

During the period of maximum activity (April–June 2002), there were 64 teleconsultations. The most common consultations (23%) were for children with trauma and orthopaedic problems. Other groups had multiple birth defects (six cases) or congenital hip dislocation (three cases). Trauma consultations were required in six cases: three with complicated ankle fractures, two with leg wounds due to mine explosions and one with hip pseudoarthrosis. Teleconsultations in plastic surgery were required for ten patients: three with cleft palate, three with nerve and tendon trauma, three with burn scar contracture, and one with post-traumatic alopecia. Neurosurgeons conducted consultations for two cases of spinal cord hernia, two of cranial hernia and one of severe cranial trauma. Burn surgeons were consulted about three patients with severe burns. There were teleconsultations in medical genetics: two cases of acrocephalosyndactylia, one of Noonan's syndrome and one of distal acromelia. Cardiologists were consulted about three patients: two with myocarditis and one with rheumatoid arthritis. Two consultations were conducted for children with Hodgkin's lymphoma. Lung diseases were found in two patients: bilateral pneumonia complicated by pyopneumothorax and a severe case of bronchial asthma. Children with portal hypertension and haemocolitis were consulted by a hepatologist and a gastroenterologist.

A number of medical institutions participated in the teleconsultations, including six medical research institutes and five large hospitals. Most of the consultations were conducted by surgical (32) or paediatric (11) departments of the Moscow Research Institute for Paediatrics and Children's Surgery. Ten consultations involved other medical centres of Moscow, while 11 consultations were conducted in the hospitals of the northern Caucasus. The results of teleconsultations during the last three months of the hospital's work are shown in Table 25.1.

The ages and numbers of patients were as follows:

- under 1 year: 11 patients
- 1–3 years: 8 patients
- 4–7 years: 9 patients
- 8–11 years: 10 patients
- 12–15 years: 9 patients
- over 15 years: 8 patients.

Table 25.1 Teleconsultations at the Children's Field Hospital

	Number of consultations
Recommendations about treatment at the field hospital	16
Decision for emergency evacuation	8
Decision for elective transfer outside the Chechen Republic	37
Not completed	3
Total	64[a]

[a]Ten patients had more than one consultation.

During the first months of operation of the telemedicine system, the age distribution of the patients remained similar.

Of the 54 patients who received teleconsultations, 8 were transported to other clinics for further treatment: to Moscow (4), Makhachkala (2) and Stavropol (2). Thirty-seven patients were referred for further examination and treatment. For 16 patients, the treatment initiated at the field hospital was changed. Diagnoses were not made in three cases (one patient died and two consultations were not completed owing to the closure of the hospital). In terms of performance, there were 35 scheduled teleconsultations, 19 deferred and 10 urgent. In addition, five emergency consultations were carried out for critical care.

In summary, telemedicine was highly effective in diagnosis, choice of treatment and transportation of patients to specialized medical institutions in a complicated situation due to the military conflict in Chechnya.

Monitoring during treatment and rehabilitation

In large-scale disasters, disruption of the regional health care system and population migration often occur, which lead to difficulties with patient transfer and medical data recording. Monitoring of the victims during all stages of medical care is essential. In the Russian system, information on the health condition of disabled persons is integrated into a special registry.[7] In the USA, the TRAC2ES system is designed to control the handling of victims evacuated from military operations.[8]

The Russian registry was created for centres of disaster medicine. The users of the registry are health care and social security authorities. Electronic medical records include personal data of a child, data about the parents/guardians, life history, diagnoses, treatment, disability and need for rehabilitation.

The registry was developed to support decision making on the scale and duration of rehabilitation of disabled children involved in disasters, to improve the monitoring of their health status, and rational planning and control of medical and social measures. The database includes:

* assessment of functional capabilities, pathological conditions and social adaptation of the child
* analysis of the child's level of disability

- control of rehabilitation at different stages of medical care
- assessment of the nature of the child's disability
- analysis of the social adaptivity of the disabled child
- the need for prosthetics and special equipment.

Transfer of the information between the centres providing the care for the victims of disasters takes place through the Internet.

Discussion

The experience of regular telemedicine support for physicians at the Children's Field Hospital has demonstrated high efficiency in diagnosis and treatment, as well as in solving the problems of patient evacuation to specialized institutions. Unlike conventional mobile military hospitals, the Children's Field Hospital provided medical care for a wide range of diseases.

It is interesting to compare the results of teleconsulting in the traditional practice of the telemedicine centre and in emergency situations. According to the data from the Moscow Research Institute for Paediatrics and Children's Surgery (2003–2007), transportation from the Russian regions to Federal (Moscow) clinics was required in 17–37% of the consulted patients, depending on the type of pathology. In comparison, 58% of the Children's Field Hospital patients required transportation to specialized clinics in Moscow and other regions. This difference can be explained by the greater severity of the cases and the limited means of diagnosis and treatment at the Children's Field Hospital. Nevertheless, the treatment of 42% of patients was continued in the field hospital, while previously most such patients had to be transported to other medical institutions. The decrease in the need for patient transportation due to the use of videoconsultations has been mentioned previously.[3,4]

Our experience of teleconsultations in Chechnya was somewhat similar to the situation in Somalia during the United Nations humanitarian mission in 1993. During the long civil war in that country, the communication and transport infrastructure was almost completely destroyed. Medical care was limited, and not all medical specialties were represented on the staff of the US military field hospital. However, during 13 months of operation in Somalia, 74 cases involving 248 images were transmitted. For several patients, air evacuation or on-site surgical intervention was avoided because of the teleconsultations.[3]

In other humanitarian operations, a teleradiology (DEPRAD) system was installed by the Georgetown Medical Center to support PrimeTime III.[9,10] In Russia, specialists of the Russian Antarctic Expedition, the Institute of Influenza of the Russian Academy of Medical Sciences, the Baltic Technical University and the company SVIT developed a modular station for diagnosis, the Ambulance-071 YS.[11] The station enables distant delivery of urgent consultations. It enables:

- automatic and semi-automatic recording of electrophysiological, tactile, descriptive and other data
- preparation and transfer of documents

- automatic and semi-automatic processing and analysis of the received data
- expert assessment of patients' functional status
- provision of recommendations for correction of patients' functional status based on expert assessment
- monitoring of patients' functional status.

This station is used in Antarctica. The results obtained demonstrate the value of the approach,[12] which can also be employed in emergency situations.

Although in Chechnya the satellite system provided a relatively simple and reliable connection, this was not mobile communication in the full sense of the term. Recently, fully mobile satellite equipment has become available, and has been used successfully in military and disaster medicine. For real-time consultations, a personal digital assistant (PDA) equipped with a digital camera and telephone has been suggested.[13] Wireless communication for PDAs enables communication between several sites and the centre in the case of multiple victims.[14] Such a situation occurred occasionally in Chechnya, when multiple patients were admitted to the field hospital. A full-scale decision support system for a field hospital could be based on a WiFi network. A wireless network would allow data transfer from the patient's bed, as well as interactive videoconferences directly from the operating room or intensive care unit. Mobile telemedicine of this kind would have been useful during our work in the field hospital.

Limited on-site data collection was possible in the field hospital using a mobile ECG recorder. The American system PrimeTime allowed US physicians to establish video telemedicine sessions anywhere within a war zone and to connect with medical centres in the USA.[4] Direct interactive contacts with rescue teams, using mobile telemedicine systems, by remote consultants would significantly increase the efficiency of decision making in emergency situations.

Prolonged and severe emergency situations often require special provision for psychological support and rehabilitation of the victims. Such support can be provided through telepsychiatry,[15] although this was not available in the case of children treated at the field hospital.

In summary, the challenges faced during the implementation of the telemedicine system in Chechnya were:

- insufficient bandwidth for communications during the first stage of telemedicine work (subsequently overcome by the use of another satellite)
- occasional difficulties in finding specialists in certain areas
- absence of an intra-hospital telemedicine system in the Institute for solving medical problems during videoconsultations
- satellite limitations precluding observation of the dynamics of patients' movements during videoconsultations.

Future disaster telemedicine in Russia

To increase the efficiency of teleconsultations provided for Russian field hospitals, the following are required:

- organization of round-the-clock services in the telemedicine centre
- availability of sufficient medical institutions to provide teleconsulting in emergency situations
- development of the requisite national telemedicine infrastructure and creation of local information systems in disaster medicine centres.

In 2006, successful training exercises of the disaster medicine service were conducted under field conditions using a new, less expensive mobile telemedicine system. This accords with the government's concept of developing telemedicine technologies in the Russian Federation,[16] which provides transition to a new level of information support in disaster telemedicine to enable efficient control over medical care and consultative support for medical teams in emergency situations.

The process of equipping field hospitals with mobile telemedicine units continues. A small Q-band satellite station, developed by Web Media Service, successfully passed testing in 2007. This allows data transfer at 128 kbit/s, i.e. at almost the same rate as via ground communication lines.[5] Mobile telemedicine units have been developed for the needs of space medicine.[17] During the missions of the US Space Shuttle, a mobile set of medical devices for ear, nose and throat and skin imaging, electrocardiography, blood oxygen saturation level, and heart and lung sound auscultation was used.[18] Similar equipment might be used by mobile teams for disaster medicine.

Conclusion

Telemedicine was highly effective in managing paediatric patients at the field hospital in a complicated situation due to the military conflict in Chechnya. The Russian satellite system HeliosNet provided reliable communication, and was not prohibitively expensive. The cost of the equipment in the telemedicine unit of the field hospital was approximately US$5000 in 2001. The cost of operating the satellite system (2008 prices) was approximately US$270 per month (for 10 videoconferences and 15 store-and-forward consultations). In 2001–2002, the estimated cost was some three to four times higher. The costs of the telemedicine work in Chechnya were met by charitable donations from business concerns.

Telemedical support for physicians working in areas of natural disasters, local military conflicts or humanitarian disasters would increase the level of urgent and specialized medical care. An important factor in realizing this will be the presence of a satisfactory telemedicine infrastructure in neighbouring regions and appropriate organization to monitor patients' health during their transportation to hospitals or other specialized medical centres.

Further reading

Hogan DE, Burstein JL. *Disaster Medicine*, 2nd edn. Philadelphia: Lippincott Williams & Wilkins, 2007.

Llewellyn CH. The role of telemedicine in disaster medicine. *J Med Syst* 1995; **19**: 29–34.

Simmons SC, Murphy TA, Blanarovich A et al. Telehealth technologies and applications for terrorism response: a report of the 2002 coastal North Carolina domestic preparedness training exercise. *J Am Med Inform Assoc* 2003; **10**: 166–76.

Teich JM, Wagner MM, Mackenzie CF, Schafer KO. The informatics response in disaster, terrorism, and war. *J Am Med Inform Assoc* 2002; **9**: 97–104.

References

1. NASA satellite aids in Mexico City rescue effort. *NASA News Release* 1985; **85**: 133.
2. Houtchens BA, Clemmer TP, Holloway HC et al. Telemedicine and international disaster response. Medical consultation to Armenia and Russia via a Telemedicine Spacebridge. *Prehosp Disaster Med* 1993; **8**: 57–66.
3. Crowther JB, Poropatich R. Telemedicine in the US Army: case reports from Somalia and Croatia. *Telemed J* 1995; **1**: 73–80.
4. Calcagni DE, Clyburn CA, Tomkins G et al. Operation Joint Endeavor in Bosnia: telemedicine systems and case reports. *Telemed J* 1996; **2**: 211–24.
5. Ehrlich AI, Kobrinsky BA, Petlakh VI et al. Telemedicine for a Children's Field Hospital in Chechnya. *J Telemed Telecare* 2007; **13**: 4–6.
6. Kobrinskiy BA, Matveev NV. Teleconsultations at the Moscow Research Institute for Paediatrics and Children's Surgery. *J Telemed Telecare* 2006; **12**(Suppl 3): 110.
7. Kobrinsky BA. Database of disabled children injured in disasters. *Prehosp Disaster Med* 1997; **12**(Suppl 1): 90–1.
8. Cook R, Woods D, Walters M, Christoffersen K. The cognitive systems engineering of automated medical evacuation scheduling and its implications. In: *Proceedings of the Third Annual Symposium on Human Interaction with Complex Systems*, 25–28 August 1996: 202–7.
9. Levine BA, Cleary K, Mun SK. Deployable teleradiology: Bosnia and beyond. *IEEE Trans Inf Technol Biomed* 1998; **2**: 30–4.
10. Mun SK, Levine B, Cleary K, Dai H. Deployable teleradiology and telemedicine for the US military. *Comput Methods Programs Biomed* 1998; **57**: 21–7.
11. Liaskovik AT, Senkevich YuI, Chasnik VG, Yaschin AV. [The concept of health services in regions with low population density and computer stations in the structure of advisory help.] *Inform Technol Publ Health Serv* 2001; **8/9**: 28–9 (in Russian).
12. Senkevich YuI. [Development of information technologies for medical maintenance of polar expeditions.] *Ukr J Telemed Med Telematics* 2004; **2**: 22–8 (in Russian).
13. Garshnek V, Burkle FM Jr. Applications of telemedicine and telecommunications to disaster medicine: historical and future perspectives. *J Am Med Inform Assoc* 1999; **6**: 26–37.
14. Grasso MA. Handheld computer application for medical disaster management. *AMIA Annu Symp Proc* 2006: 932.
15. Mack D, Brantley KM, Bell KG. Mitigating the health effects of disasters for medically underserved populations: electronic health records, telemedicine, research, screening, and surveillance. *J Health Care Poor Underserved* 2007; **18**: 432–42.
16. [*Concepts of Development of Telemedical Technologies in the Russian Federation.*] Moscow, 2001 (in Russian).
17. Grigoriev AI, Orlov OI. [Telemedicine in Russia.] *Vestn Ross Akad Med Nauk* 2004; **10**: 30–5 (in Russian).
18. Crump WJ, Levy BJ, Billica RD. A field trial of the NASA Telemedicine Instrument Pack in a family practice. *Aviat Space Environ Med* 1996; **67**: 1080–5.

26 Web-based paediatric oncology information and registries: An international perspective

André Nebel de Mello

Introduction

Cancer registration can trace its origins to the first decade of the 20th century, when surveys measuring the point prevalence of cancer were reported from a number of European countries. Permanent registration systems were implemented in Hamburg in 1926, Mecklenburg in 1937 – both discontinued during World War II – Massachusetts in 1927 and Connecticut in 1935. The first national survey on a significant sample of the US population was carried out in 1937–38. By the end of the late 1940s, population-based registries and the survey system (10 metropolitan areas in the USA) had solved most technical problems, and the concepts have been widely used ever since.

The first experiences of using nominal rosters of cancer patients for analytical studies or for linkage with other registries occurred in the late 1940s. Epidemiologists working on those registries realized that incidence and mortality statistics should not be considered as alternatives: the latter are generally valuable, but the former can also provide information on treatment and follow-up. An expert report for the World Health Organization (WHO) concluded that:[1]

> the collection of accurate statistics of cancer incidence and mortality among different … people and … countries may lead to important indications for … studies … [whereas] the information [provided by mortality statistics] … is becoming increasingly inadequate, owing to growing numbers of patients successfully treated and thus not registered in the statistics of death [Thus], we … make the following suggestions:
>
> 1. Great benefit would follow the collection of data about cancer patients from as many different countries as possible.
> 2. Such data should be recorded on an agreed plan so as to be comparable.
> 3. Each nation should have a central registry to arrange for recording and collection of such data.
> 4. There should be an international body whose duty should be to correlate the data and statistics obtained in each country.

In 1950, the WHO created a Subcommittee on the Registration of Cases of Cancer. Within a few years, the Nordic countries, the UK and Canada launched programmes that led to national coverage of registration. The model followed in the USA was different: no national coverage was attempted, and instead a number of county- or state-based registries were created. The surveys on samples of the population were converted in the Surveillance, Epidemiology and End Results (SEER) programme, which produces incidence and survival rates broken down by ethnic groups.

The first worldwide analysis was published in 1966 with the title *Cancer Incidence in Five Continents*.[2] This marked the beginning of a series of publications appearing at five-year intervals, supervised by the International Union Against Cancer (UICC), the International Agency for Research on Cancer (IARC) and the International Association of Cancer Registries (IACR). The data were not simply and passively accepted, but were revised and controlled.[2-4] Two by-products of this strategy have been a worldwide standardization of the activity of registration and the provision through the IARC of technical advice to developing cancer registries.

In 30 years, the number of countries with cancer registries nearly doubled and there was a fivefold increase in both the number of active cancer registries and the total population served by registration (Table 26.1).[4] These increases were concentrated in industrialized countries, whereas in developing countries there was a substantial decrease in registration, attributable to the political and economic situation,[5] leading to the inequalities reported in Table 26.2 and displayed in Figures 26.1 and 26.2.

In the early 1980s, it became apparent that population-based survival rates of cancer patients could be used as an indicator of the quality of cancer care in a given area and that registries could play a major role. The first large-scale international cooperative study, the EUROCARE project, published its first results in 1995,[6] and aimed to increase cooperation between epidemiologists and clinicians in continental Europe and to perform a systematic follow-up of the living status of the registered individuals.

Cancer registries have benefited tremendously from the use of databases and electronic data transfer. The use of the Internet is thus a natural evolution. Most registries

Table 26.1 Coverage in eight volumes of cancer incidence in five continents[4]

Volume	Year of publication	Registries	Populations	Countries	Period (approximate)
1	1966	32	35	29	1960–62
2	1970	47	58	24	1963–67
3	1976	61	79	29	1968–72
4	1982	79	103	32	1973–77
5	1987	105	137	36	1978–82
6	1992	138	166	49	1983–87
7	1997	150	183	50	1988–92
8	2002	186	214	57	1993–97

Table 26.2 Coverage by cancer registries around 1992[3]

Area	Number of registries	Population served by registries (millions)	Total population (millions)	Percentage of population served
Africa	5	0.5	728	0.1
Central and Latin America	11	20.8	482	4
Canada and USA[a]	25	61.9	293	21
European Union	53	119.0	372	32
Other Western European countries[b]	10	8.0	12	67
Other, Europe	10	45.6	344	13
Asia	24	71.4	3458	2
Oceania	9	18.5	29	64

[a]Including Surveillance, Epidemiology and End Results programme, covering approximately 10% of the population.
[b]Norway, Switzerland and Iceland.

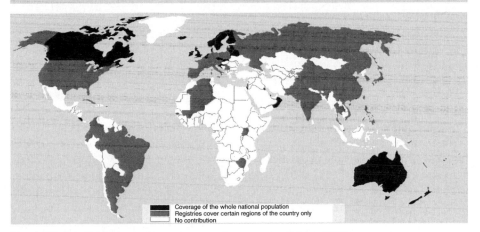

Figure 26.1 Individual countries: coverage by cancer registries 1997[4]

were publishing information online in the early 1990s, and many have already switched to web-based data entry interfaces.

Cancer in children

Cancer is very rare in childhood – it is predominantly a disease of elderly people. In industrialized countries, about 1 in 200 (0.5%) of all cancers occurs in children aged under 15 years. The incidence rate is typically 110–150 per million children per year, equivalent to a risk of around 1 in 500 during the first 15 years of life. Nevertheless, cancer accounts for about 20% of all deaths in children aged 1–14 years, making it the second most common cause of death in children in most of the world (the first is death

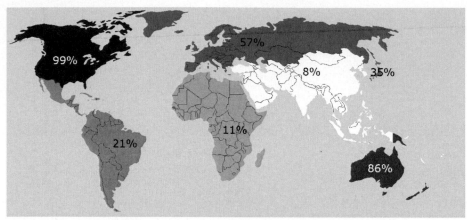

Figure 26.2 Cancer registry coverage: geographical coverage (percentage of total population) of cancer registries by region[4]

due to external causes) and the most common cause of death by disease, with the exception of Africa and some Asian countries.

Cancer in children is often not preventable. Prenatal factors are considered to affect the incidence of tumours in children under the age of 5 years. It is generally accepted that cancer results from genetic changes. The carcinogenic process in children is much shorter than in adults. Childhood cancer incidence rates are highest during infancy, so it is reasonable to assume that many paediatric cancers result from aberrations in early developmental stages and in utero.

An increased risk of childhood cancers has been reported to be associated with certain genetic conditions or syndromes such as chromosomal abnormalities, DNA-repair disorders, congenital anomalies, hereditary immune deficiency states and other hereditary syndromes. Racial differences have been observed in childhood tumours, even within industrialized countries. A peak incidence in acute lymphoblastic leukaemia (ALL) usually occurs between the ages of 2 and 3 years in white American children and from 1 to 4 years in European children, but not among African–Americans. Ewing's sarcoma is another well-established example of a cancer with racial differences, with the lowest incidence rate in black children (African or American).[7]

Overall, childhood cancer is about 20% more common among boys than among girls. The male predominance is greater for lymphomas, liver tumours and nasopharyngeal carcinoma, and less marked for leukaemia, brain tumours, neuroblastoma and soft tissue sarcomas. Boys and girls have a similar incidence of retinoblastoma and Wilms' tumour. The incidence in girls is only greater for extragonadal germ cell tumours, malignant melanoma, and adrenal cortex and thyroid carcinomas.

There are also marked variations between populations in the incidence of specific types of childhood cancers. Nearly one-third of all childhood neoplasms are leukaemias. International variation occurs in the rate of ALL, and the higher incidence of ALL in early childhood has usually been associated with higher levels of socio-economic status, suggesting that environmental factors play a role. Although a considerable number of environmental or exogenous factors have been suggested as risk factors for childhood cancers, only a few have been proven, and they are mostly infectious agents, including Epstein–Barr virus, hepatitis B virus, human immunodeficiency virus and human herpesviruses. These infections are probably responsible for the international variation in the incidence of some childhood cancers, such as lymphoma, nasopharyngeal carcinoma, hepatic cancer and Kaposi's sarcoma. In addition, some parasitic infections have been implicated, particularly malaria in tropical Africa, acting as a cofactor for Burkitt's lymphoma, and schistosomiasis in Egypt, causing bladder cancer. [7]

The EUROCARE collaboration has revealed considerable variation in survival between European countries,[8] but, unlike those for adults, the survival rates of children with cancer in Western Europe are similar to those in the USA.[9] In the developing countries, where 80% of the world's children with cancer live, they are often diagnosed too late or not diagnosed at all and, without access to life-saving treatment, more than one in two of these children diagnosed with cancer will die.

The increases in survival rates occurred during a period of great technical advances in childhood cancer treatment, but there were also major changes in referral patterns. At one time, most children with cancer were treated at local hospitals, there were few specialists in paediatric oncology, and opportunities for participation in collaborative studies of treatment were limited. Treatment has gradually become more centralized, and more children have been entered in national and international clinical trials and studies.[10] For several types of cancer, survival has been found to be higher among children who were treated at specialist centres or who were entered in national or international clinical trials.

As a consequence of the improved survival rates described above, the number of adult survivors of childhood cancer has increased substantially (Figure 26.3). In 1961, there were only about 15 survivors in Britain aged 30 or above, and none above 40, while in 2000, there were over 26 000 survivors, of whom almost 7000 (about 25%) were aged over 30 years. In 1971, there were 5500 survivors, with over 1000 above age 20 and 100 aged 30 or above. In 1981, there were nearly 3000 survivors aged 20 and above, but fewer than 100 of them were aged over 40 years, while in 2000, almost 2500 (almost 20% of those aged 20 and above) were aged over 40 years. Eventually, more than 1 in 1000 adults of all ages will be survivors of childhood cancer. [11]

Cancer information on the Internet

The Internet has become an increasingly common source of medical information for patients with cancer. For example, over 50% of adults in the USA have searched online for health information and 80% of all US Internet users have searched online for at least one major health topic.[12]

Use of the Internet to access cancer information is related to age (being more common in those aged under 60 years), higher income, higher education and being white.[13] However, there has been little research on Internet cancer information use among minority racial/ethnic groups in the USA and Western Europe, or in populations of developing countries, or on the appropriateness of the websites available to

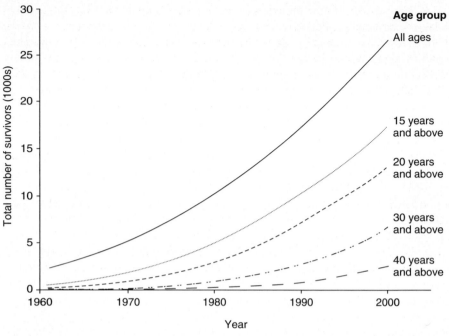

Figure 26.3 Number of (past or current) childhood cancer patients (by age group) alive at the end of each year in the UK, 1961–2000[11]

such populations.[12,13] Many cancer organizations have created patient-centred websites to provide comprehensive information about specific cancers, but most of the information available is in English, limiting its use for non-speakers.

A study of cancer patients' self-reported attitudes to the Internet came to the following conclusions:[14]

- Patients are comfortable giving as well as receiving cancer information and support online; they are also comfortable in evaluating it.
- They are interested in the experiences of other patients and derive benefit by interacting with them directly, through venues such as discussion boards and email lists or, indirectly, through activities such as reading biographies.
- They perceive better outcomes after using online health information and support.
- Cancer patients have a certain level of trust in online information, primarily for information obtained from established reputable sources such as studies in journals and advice given by medical doctors; they also trust websites endorsed by health authorities.
- They are confident in their ability to evaluate information, including comprehension of research reports.
- They display a healthy scepticism when presented with the option of divulging personal health information. However, some patients are willing to provide email addresses and, if they receive personalized information, they are comfortable in disclosing their identity.

Another study evaluating cancer patients' and caregivers' interests about the Internet indicated that most patient and caregiver respondents were interested in Internet-based cancer-related services such as information related to treatment (80%), conversations with physicians via the Internet (70%) and online support groups (65%). In addition, respondents reported that they would be likely to use such services (70%) and were interested in home health care services delivered via PCs (60%). No differences were found between ethnic groups, geographical settings or patient status (patient versus caregivers) on these variables. Minorities, older individuals and less-educated individuals were less likely to have knowledge of and to have used the Internet.[15]

In the last few years, there have been efforts to improve online cancer information quality. Good examples include the International Cancer Information Service (established in 2001), the American Society of Clinical Oncology (ASCO) website People Living with Cancer (launched in 2002) and the Oncopediatria.org portal[16] (launched in 2004).

Online information about childhood cancer and web-based initiatives on the subject are less common, even in industrialized countries. This may be a reflection of the lower incidence of the disease on this age group or may be a misconception about the similarity of the disease between adults and children.

International initiatives

While most international initiatives that focus on paediatric oncology are from cooperative groups in Western Europe or North America, there are some good examples that focus on developing countries. These include the following.

SLAOP

The Latin American Society of Paediatric Oncology (SLAOP) provides information for general paediatricians and paediatric oncologists by publishing articles, news and presentations in paediatric and evidence-based oncology on its website.[17] SLAOP is also developing a Latin-American Paediatric Oncology Registry, and has launched the Latin-American Paediatric Promyelocytic Leukaemia Registry, a web-based registry available through its website.

St Jude Children's Research Hospital

The St Jude's Hospital in Tennessee has an International Outreach programme with the object to improve the survival rates of children with catastrophic illnesses worldwide, through the transfer of knowledge, technology and organizational skills. This is achieved through twinning programmes and through two websites: Cure4Kids[18] and POND4Kids.[19]

The Cure4Kids website was launched in October 2002 and provides medical education for physicians, nurses, scientists and health care workers in countries with limited resources who treat children with catastrophic diseases. The main functions are:

- online education about catastrophic childhood illnesses
- collaborative work spaces for document sharing and online meetings; several countries, including Brazil, Lebanon, Morocco, Guatemala, El Salvador, Honduras and Mexico, participate in these international meetings
- access to consultation and mentoring by staff of St Jude's Hospital
- technology and training for better management of patient information.

The core of Cure4Kids is an online digital library of reference material, a discussion area for exchange of advice and information between doctors, and access to online seminars and lectures. The website is also used to host live meetings via web conferencing (video and voice-over-IP).[18] In September 2007, there were 11 490 registered users in 157 countries.

The Paediatric Oncology Networked Database (POND4Kids) is an online, multilingual database for paediatric haematology/oncology patients. The aim is to improve the care of paediatric oncology patients in countries with limited resources by the exchange of information and experience among oncologists who practise in a similar medical environment. The major objectives of POND4Kids are to:

- store patient data for easy retrieval and analysis in a way that ensures quality control
- provide uniform data collection to facilitate comparison of information among centres
- provide a single tool for data storage and retrieval to facilitate training of data managers
- develop a multilingual online system that is available to users at no cost.

POND4Kids is hosted on a web server and is divided into several virtual sites. Clinicians at different POND4Kids sites can share information about individual patients, groups of patients with the same disease or all patients. Shared records have personal identifiers removed, but retain a unique POND identification number. Information sharing facilitates analysis by colleagues of specific diseases treated at multiple centres in low-income countries. Information can also be shared with international experts to assist with analysis and quality improvement.

Ten centres in nine countries (seven in Central America, two in Morocco and one in Jordan) currently use the POND4Kids website. In the first two years of operation (2004–2006), over 9000 patient records were entered into POND4Kids.[20] Many paediatric oncology services in developing countries have adopted these websites for registering and discussing their patients, instead of developing a website of their own.

SIOP

The International Society of Paediatric Oncology (SIOP) provides information for professionals by publishing best practice guidelines on its website[21] and by making available the SIOP educational books and conference lectures on the Cure4Kids website.

International agencies

The IARC publishes the *International Classification of Childhood Cancer*,[22] currently in its third revision, and adopted worldwide in childhood cancer registries. The IARC also publishes the *Cancer Incidence in Five Continents* report that is updated every 5 years,[2-4] and publishes cancer registration manuals and papers on the social inequalities of cancer. Almost all publications are available at the agency's website.[23]

The IACR has designed a suite of computer programs to meet the needs of population-based cancer registries in developing countries. The software is in its fourth version, named CanReg4, and can be used in a Windows-based network environment. It is available in English, Spanish, French, Italian, Turkish, Chinese, Thai, Arabic and Farsi. The software is free and is available at the IACR website.[24]

Twinning programmes

Twinning programmes are partnerships between institutions in industrialized countries and those in developing countries with the goal of improving survival rates among children with cancer. These programmes have reduced the rates of abandonment of treatment, relapse and death due to toxic effects of treatment. The investments that they have attracted have led to improvements in access to treatment and hospital infrastructure. The best results have been obtained when local oncologists were recruited as programme directors and asked to promote the idea of a strong paediatric oncology unit among their peers and to coordinate the training of providers.[25]

Most twinning programmes have a telemedicine component, usually videoconferencing, web-based case report forms or continuing medical education (CME). Examples are the programme between the King Hussein Cancer Centre (KHCC) in Amman, Jordan and the Hospital for Sick Children in Toronto, Canada in paediatric neuro-oncology[26] and the MISPHO Consortium initiatives in Central America.[27]

Online childhood cancer registries in developing countries

Although online cancer registries have became more common in the last few years, only a few childhood cancer registries have been implemented by developing nations, and even fewer with a web-based interface. Examples include the following.

Brazil

The Oncopediatria portal was launched in 2004 and is a web-based system that offers services and information on paediatric cancer.[16] It maintains a secure online patient registry, a web-based bone marrow transplant registry tool and online cooperative treatment protocols for the Brazilian Society of Paediatric Oncology. It is part of a national telemedicine network of universities, research institutes and medical institutions that has been established in Brazil to support distance medical practice in oncology, called ONCONET.[28-30]

The main objectives are:

- to improve the information flow in research programmes and cooperative treatment protocols
- to disseminate and harmonize treatments through the use of protocols that produce the highest cure rates
- to establish the basis for a national demographic record of paediatric cancer
- to make available statistics, demographic data and analyses of the results of treatments using the protocols.

The system is hosted on clusters of computers. It is based on open-source software, designed to provide high performance, fault tolerance and high availability.

Some of the Brazilian Society's cooperative protocols have been implemented. The first online treatment protocol targets the treatment of high-risk neuroblastoma.[29] A protocol for multiple subtypes of non-Hodgkin's lymphoma and another for paediatric bone marrow transplantation[30] are also available. In these protocols, much of the data is textual, but parts of the record are medical images. The system allows images to be stored in several common image formats such as JPEG and DICOM (digital imaging and communications in medicine).

In June 2007, there were 310 registered paediatric oncologists from 53 out of 58 treatment centres in 23 states; there were 7000 registered patients.

Argentina

The Argentinean Paediatric Oncology Hospital Registry (ROHA) was established in 2000 using the WHO/IARC standards for cancer registration. It registers children with solid and haematological malignancies. Registered data can be consulted online at the ROHA website.[31]

Eastern Europe

The Automated Childhood Cancer Information System (ACCIS) is a project developed by the IARC and supported by the European Commission, with the objectives of collecting, presenting, interpreting and disseminating data on childhood cancer in Europe. The ACCIS database contains some 160 000 records on childhood and adolescent cancer cases registered over the last 30 years in 78 European population-based cancer registries, covering 2.6 billion person-years. The Eastern European countries with information stored in this database are Belarus, Estonia, Hungary, Slovakia, Slovenia and Turkey.[32]

Belarus

The childhood population-based cancer registry of the Republic of Belarus was created in August 1999 and registered cases retrospectively to the year 1989. It was created as one of the international health care initiatives after the Chernobyl disaster. Consolidated data can be consulted online at the registry's website.

Serbia

The Childhood Cancer Registry of Central Serbia was created by the Institute of Public Health of Serbia 'Dr Milan Jovanović Batut'. The registry has consolidated data from 1997 to 2005, available online at the Institute's website.[34]

India

The non-governmental organization South Asian Marrow Foundation –'Matchpia' – has a web-based initiative named Project India,[35] which launched the United South Asian Donor Registry (USADR), an online bone marrow donor registry. This is probably India's largest registry. The foundation also performs matching between donors and patients, including those with paediatric cancer.

Singapore

The Singapore Childhood Cancer Registry (SCCR) was established in September 1997 under the auspices of the Paediatric Oncology Group (Singapore), and registers all children, aged 18 years and below, who have been diagnosed with haematological or solid malignancies. Physicians voluntarily register the patients through a secure web-based form on the registry's website.[36]

Paediatric oncology web-based information

Most childhood cancer information websites from developing countries belong to parents' associations and support groups. The information content on these websites is usually focused on the activities and objectives of the organization, and there is limited information on the most common types of childhood cancer and only general information about therapy options. For more complete information, there are usually links to North American, local governmental or international websites. There are a few exceptions to this rule, which are mentioned below.

Government websites usually offer general cancer information targeting adults with cancer. In Brazil and South Africa, local childhood cancer medical associations and some treatment centres have websites with more detailed cancer information for parents and professionals.

Latin America

The Brazilian National Cancer Institute (INCA) has a subsection of its website[37] dedicated to childhood cancer information for parents and professionals, including statistics, treatment guidelines, early detection and an overview of the cancer types. There are also many cancer-related publications available for download.

Over 20 childhood cancer support groups in Brazil offer websites with disease information for the general public. For example, the Brazilian Lymphoma and Leukaemia Association (ABRALE) has a website[38] that offers detailed information on leukaemia and lymphoma for parents and health professionals. It has a subsection dedicated to cancer in children. Distance learning tools, legal support information, forums and downloadable information booklets are also available.

The Oncopediatria website[16] from Brazil has an open information section for parents and health professionals that includes cancer information, articles, summaries of treatment studies and a biweekly newsletter.

The Organization of Parents of Children with Cancer and Related Diseases (OPNICER) from Colombia offers on its website[39] legal information for parents and a roadmap of the challenges faced by children and parents from cancer diagnosis to cure.

The Natalí Dafne Flexer Association from Argentina offers detailed information for parents, patients, volunteers and professionals, as well as articles, downloadable booklets and other childhood cancer resources on its website.[40]

Eastern Europe

The Romanian Association of the Parents with Cancer and Leukaemia Ill Children (P.A.V.E.L.) has an information section on its website[41] with diagnostic information, nutritional orientation and support information for parents and professionals, as well as best practice guidelines for doctors.

Asia

The Children's Cancer Foundation of Singapore offers detailed information and resources for parents and teachers, and downloadable booklets in three languages on its website.[42]

Africa

The South African Children's Cancer Group (SACCSG) has a web portal[43] with information for general practitioners on early diagnosis of cancer. It also provides information and support for parents, in partnership with the Childhood Cancer Foundation of South Africa.

Conclusion

The field of oncology is vast, and knowledge is increasing rapidly. The main gap between industrialized and developing countries in this field is not the availability of the newest medications; rather, it is differences in the information about the types of cancer afflicting the population and on the best ways to treat them. The increases that have occurred in the cure rate of children with cancer are mainly due to the use of better combinations of existing drugs, rather than the use of new ones.

The Internet offers great potential for bridging the knowledge gap. The instant availability of up-to-date information for medical practitioners can increase the speed of diagnosis. The availability of accurate cancer profiles in each country, resulting from work done by the national registries, can guide professionals to the most likely diagnosis, and help governments and private initiatives to direct their resources to treat cancer more effectively.

Acknowledgements

I thank Adilson Yuuji Hira, Marcelo Knörich Zuffo and the staff of the Telemedicine and Bioinformatics Unit from the Laboratory of Integrated Systems of the University of São Paulo for their advice and support.

References

1. Clemmesen J. Statistical studies in the aetiology of malignant neoplasms. *Acta Pathol Microbiol Scand Suppl* 1974; **247**: 1–266.
2. Doll R, Payne P, Waterhouse J, eds. *Cancer Incidence in Five Continents: A Technical Report.* New York: Springer, 1966.
3. Parkin DM, Whelan SL, Ferlay J, Raymond L, eds. *Cancer Incidence in Five Continents,* Volume VII. Lyon: IARC, 1997.
4. Parkin DM, Whelan SL, Ferlay J et al, eds. *Cancer Incidence in Five Continents,* Volume VIII. Lyon: IARC, 2002.
5. International Agency for Research on Cancer. *Biennial Report 1994–95.* Lyon: IARC, 1995.
6. Berrino F, Sant M, Verdecchia A et al, eds. *Survival of Cancer Patients in Europe: The EUROCARE Study.* Lyon: IARC, 1995.
7. Stiller CA. Epidemiology and genetics of childhood cancer. *Oncogene* 2004; **23**: 6429–44.
8. Gatta G, Corazziari I, Magnani C et al. Childhood cancer survival in Europe. *Ann Oncol* 2003; **14**(Suppl 5), v119–27.
9. Gatta G, Capocaccia R, Coleman MP et al. Childhood cancer survival in Europe and the United States. *Cancer* 2002; **95**: 1767–72.
10. Mott MG, Mann JR, Stiller CA. The United Kingdom Children's Cancer Study Group – the first 20 years of growth and development. *Eur J Cancer* 1997; **33**: 1448–52.
11. Children's Cancer and Leukaemia Group. Available at: www.ukccsg.org.uk.
12. Fogel J. Internet use for cancer information among racial/ethnic populations and low literacy groups. *Cancer Control* 2003; **10**(Suppl 5): 45–51.
13. Nguyen KD, Hara B, Chlebowski RT. Utility of two cancer organization websites for a multiethnic, public hospital oncology population: comparative cross-sectional survey. *J Med Internet Res* 2005; **7**: e28.
14. LaCoursiere SP, Knobf MT, McCorkle R. Cancer patients' self-reported attitudes about the Internet. *J Med Internet Res* 2005; **7**: e22.
15. Monnier J, Laken M, Carter CL. Patient and caregiver interest in internet-based cancer services. *Cancer Pract* 2002; **10**: 305–10.
16. Oncopediatria. Available at: www.oncopediatria.org.br.
17. SLAOP. Available at: www.slaop.org.
18. Cure4Kids. Available at: www.cure4kids.org/ums/home.
19. POND4Kids. Available at: www.pond4kids.org.
20. Quintana Y, Howard S, Norland M et al. Pond4Kids – a multi-site online pediatric oncology research database for collaborative protocol research. *AMIA Annu Symp Proc* 2005: 1090.
21. International Society of Paediatric Oncology. Available at: www.siop.nl.
22. Steliarova-Foucher E, Stiller C, Lacour B, Kaatsch P. International Classification of Childhood Cancer, third edition. *Cancer* 2005; **103**: 1457–67.
23. International Agency for Research on Cancer. Available at: www.iarc.fr.
24. International Association of Cancer Registries. Available at: www.iacr.com.fr.
25. Ribeiro RC, Pui CH. Saving the children – improving childhood cancer treatment in developing countries. *N Engl J Med* 2005; **352**: 2158–60.
26. Qaddoumi I, Mansour A, Musharbash A et al. Impact of telemedicine on pediatric neuro-oncology in a developing country: the Jordanian–Canadian experience. *Pediatr Blood Cancer* 2007; **48**: 39–43.

27. Howard SC, Marinoni M, Castillo L et al. Improving outcomes for children with cancer in low-income countries in Latin America: a report on the recent meetings of the Monza International School of Pediatric Hematology/Oncology (MISPHO) – Part I. *Pediatr Blood Cancer* 2007; **48**: 364–9.
28. Hira AY, Lopes TT, de Mello AN et al. Establishment of the Brazilian telehealth network for paediatric oncology. *J Telemed Telecare* 2005; **11**(Suppl 2): 51–2.
29. Hira AY, Lopes TT, de Mello AN et al. Web-based patient records and treatment guidelines in paediatric oncology. *J Telemed Telecare* 2005; **11**(Suppl 2): 53–5.
30. de Mello AN, Trautenmüller P, Hira AY et al. Development of a Web-based bone marrow transplant registry system. *J Telemed Telecare* 2006; **12**(Suppl 3): 64–6.
31. Registro Oncopediátrico Hospitalario Argentino (ROHA). Available at: www.roha.org.ar.
32. Steliarova-Foucher E, Kaatsch P, Lacour B et al. Quality, comparability and methods of analysis of data on childhood cancer in Europe (1978–1997): report from the Automated Childhood Cancer Information System project. *Eur J Cancer* 2006; **42**: 1915–51.
33. Child Health International Foundation. *A Childhood Cancer Registry for Belarus.* Available at: www.pghfree.net/~chif/registry.html.
34. Institute of Public Health of Serbia 'Dr Milan Jovanović Batut'. Available at: www.batut.org.yu/english.html.
35. Matchpia. Available at: www.matchpia.org.
36. Singapore Childhood Cancer Registry. Available at: sccr.pogs.org.sg.
37. Instituto Nacional de Câncer (INCA). Available at: www.inca.gov.br.
38. Associação Brasileira de Linfoma e Leucemia (ABRALE). Available at: abrale.org.br.
39. Organización de Padres de Niños con Cáncer y Enfermedades Relacionadas (OPNICER). Available at: www.opnicer.org.
40. Fundación Natalí Dafne Flexer. Available at: www.fundacionflexer.org.
41. Romanian Association of the Parents with Cancer and Leukaemia III Children (P.A.V.E.L.). Available at: www.asociatiapavel.home.ro.
42. Children's Cancer Foundation. Available at: www.ccf.org.sg.
43. South African Children's Cancer Study Group (SACCSG). Available at: www.saccsg.co.za.

27 E-health in international networks: New opportunities for collaboration

Shariq Khoja and Azra Naseem

Introduction

In recent years, there has been a substantial reduction in the availability of health professionals in developing countries, which has been accompanied by a rise in the demand for high-quality health care. This combination has forced health care institutions to collaborate and share their resources to provide comprehensive, high-quality and accessible health care at a reasonable cost.

The Aga Khan Development Network (AKDN) is an international network that comprises several institutions, working for the development of poor nations in Asia and Africa, in social development (health, education and housing), disaster relief, economic development and preservation of cultures. Most of the development in the health sector is carried out through the Aga Khan Health Services (AKHS) and the Aga Khan University (AKU).

The AKHS operates a private, not-for-profit health care system. It includes more than 200 health care facilities, including 9 hospitals. The AKHS provides primary health care and curative medical care in Afghanistan, India, Kenya, Pakistan and Tanzania. It also provides technical assistance to governments in health service delivery in Kenya, Syria and Tajikistan. The community health programmes of the AKHS are designed to reach vulnerable groups in society, especially childbearing women and young children, through low-cost, proven medical technologies. Experience has confirmed the efficacy of these services in improving health status and their cost-effectiveness.[1]

The AKU is an international university with 11 teaching sites in 8 countries: Afghanistan, Kenya, Pakistan, Tanzania, Uganda, Syria, Egypt and the UK. The AKU is also associated with university hospitals in Pakistan and Kenya. The largest of these is the Aga Khan University Hospital, Karachi (AKUH, K), which has 542 beds and provides services to 38 000 inpatients and 500 000 outpatients annually. The Aga Khan University Hospital, Nairobi (AKUH, N) also provides tertiary- and secondary-level health care services in East Africa.

The extent and scope of the AKDN's health activities require considerable networking between the different agencies. For decades, this networking was maintained by traditional means of communication and extensive travel by health professionals between various institutions. In the last five years, some institutions within the AKDN have begun to adopt information and communication technology (ICT) to enhance their educational, research, information exchange and health provision activities. All these activities can be grouped under the umbrella of 'e-health'. Although, e-health in the AKDN is still in its infancy, activities directed towards learning, care provision and information exchange have already begun.

Benefits of e-health

Institutions within the AKDN have shown interest in adopting e-health to enhance their education, research, information exchange and health provision activities. The following benefits are anticipated:

- *Improved clinical care.* An e-health network will encourage rapid adoption of e-health applications that will facilitate improved clinical care. For example, common access to clinical practice guidelines will aid standardization of care, and use of specific e-health applications such as teleconsulting will raise the confidence and skills of clinicians in rural and remote locations.
- *Greater knowledge sharing.* An e-health network, with an emphasis on knowledge rather than simply information, will ensure greater knowledge sharing.
- *Greater scope for research.* Interaction through an e-health network will enhance partnerships and sharing of resources, which will in turn contribute to a greater scope for research.
- *Greater capacity building.* Capacity building, in particular, will be strengthened through an e-health network. Institutions with a common focus (within or outside the AKDN) could join and contribute their respective skills and experiences.
- *Administrative resilience.* A successful e-health network will strengthen administrative resilience.

Although, e-health in the AKDN is still at its beginning, activities directed towards learning, care provision and information exchange have already begun. These activities are described briefly below.

Learning

The AKU and the AKHS have worked in collaboration to develop asynchronous learning for medical and nursing students, and to develop continuing medical education (CME) for health care providers. Efforts are also being made to introduce the use of live e-learning software at the AKU. Two distinct instructional settings can be identified where ICT is used for learning:

- In technology-enhanced classroom teaching, teachers use PowerPoint slides to illustrate concepts in their face-to-face lectures and later distribute them to the class by email. Students submit word-processed assignments for assessment.

- In distance education, nurses and other health care providers, particularly in East Africa, complete formal educational programmes at remote locations. In such programmes, email messages are used, together with online discussions via video-conferencing or through web-conferencing.

There is also blended or distributed learning as a combination of these two approaches, with an increasing emphasis on the use of online learning technologies. E-learning in blended courses can take many different forms. Examples include:

- repository of learning objects
- web-based virtual learning environment
- a database of Internet links
- synchronous e-learning through Elluminate
- remote access for health professionals.

Repository of learning objects

In 2003, a searchable Library of Images was developed at the AKU. The aim was to create a repository of learning objects, which could be searched, reused and shared over the network to avoid duplication of effort in developing learning resources. Initially, the pictures and other images were digitized and catalogued with appropriate metadata information. Later, registered users, including students, faculty members, clinicians, residents and allied health staff, were also able to contribute images with associated metadata information. A committee was set up to review each contribution in order to ensure its relevance and accuracy and to avoid redundancy and duplication. Moreover, ethical issues such as concealing the identity of patients were also considered. Currently, 1500 digitized items (clinical photographs, radiological images, operative findings, microscopy slides, ECG and EEG charts, animations, and video-clips) are available[2] for AKU faculty members, staff, students and other health care providers through the Internet.[3] The images from the Library of Images are used in class lectures, presentations and assignments, and are also linked with course materials available via AKUMed. The material is shared with other institutions within the network with access to the AKU intranet.

Web-based virtual learning environment

The need for a system that would allow access to course information, lecture notes and a discussion forum for students of the MBBS programme was felt by the faculty at the AKU Medical College, and led to the development of an asynchronous virtual learning environment (VLE) called AKUMed. VLE refers to the components in which learners and tutors participate in online interactions of various kinds, including online learning.[4] With growing numbers of faculty members using AKUMed, its popularity has increased, and similar systems are being designed for the School of Nursing and the Department of Community Health Sciences, in order to offer courses with strong online components.

Database of Internet links

A portal with links to websites on various health-related topics has been developed. The portal is accessible through the AKU intranet and is regularly updated. It is used by the students and faculty members of the AKU.

Synchronous e-learning

Elluminate Live has been introduced as a live e-learning tool in all campuses of the AKU. It was chosen because it can be used from areas with low-bandwidth Internet connections. The software allows recording, and permits sharing of audio, video, text and image data. Elluminate also allows the use of white board and document sharing, to facilitate online discussions. Finally, it supports transfer of medical data and live teleconsultations, which may be an important feature for the AKU. Several pilot projects have been initiated in different campuses of the AKU in Asia, Africa and Europe. A summary of the pilot projects at each campus is given in Table 27.1.

Remote access for health professionals

Remote access for health staff was conceived as a structured educational programme for health care providers, which focused on problem-based learning via a web-based distance learning system. The purpose of this programme was to facilitate evidence-based practice of medicine and nursing at the Aga-Khan Hospital in Dar-es-Salaam and its five affiliated primary care centres in Tanzania. A phased approach was planned, followed by the introduction at other AKHS institutions. The web interface allows multiple threaded discussions based on specific interest areas, including sub-specialties such as paediatrics, cardiology and nursing. This makes it possible for health professionals in North America to share journal articles, PowerPoint presentations, quality assurance tools and weblinks to various resources with staff in Tanzania. The long-term goal is to make this method of learning accessible to health care professionals associated with the AKHS in East Africa or with other private and public sector hospitals, to improve health care delivery in those countries.

Care provision

Two examples of telehealth in AKDN agencies are:

(1) email-based teleconsultations in Tanzania
(2) a teleradiology link in Afghanistan.

Email-based teleconsultations

In 2004, a pilot telemedicine programme began that allowed communication between doctors working at the Aga Khan Hospital in Dar-es-Salaam and clinicians in North America. The goal was to create partnerships that would improve the delivery and quality of health care in the region. The pre-defined turnaround time for queries was 24–72 hours.

Table 27.1 Summary of the pilot projects at each AKU campus

	AKU-IED, Karachi	AKU-CHS, Karachi	AKU-ISMC, London	AKU-SON, Karachi and AKU-EA, Nairobi
Objective	Understand changing needs and plan accordingly	Look into all possible options where Elluminate will be useful	Gain confidence with Elluminate	Pilot Elluminate use for continuing education courses offered from AKU-SON Karachi to East Africa, Afghanistan and Egypt
Areas	Distance education courses Meetings with Professional Development Centres Other uses by faculty members in teaching-related activities	Work in progress (WIP) Online CME course with East Africa Web seminar on health problems in Pakistan Postgraduate education programmes	Meetings with different departments, e.g. Finance, IT and Provost's Office, once a month or more Lectures, cultural hour and lunch-hour seminars (Wednesday afternoons once a month) Faculty Assembly (first Saturday), although time and day difference could be a problem Lectures organized by Research Department, Special Lecture Series and AKU-IED AKU 25th Anniversary Planning Committee Meeting	Continuing education programme for practising nurses Online courses for nursing students Meetings and resource sharing between nursing faculty staff from different locations
Expected outcomes	Identify problems relevant to the implementation of Elluminate Live in order to plan for wider implementation of Elluminate Live at AKU-IED	Skill enhancement of the faculty, staff and students User satisfaction (through the help of feedback forms)	Attendance at meeting, seminar or workshop that would otherwise have been missed Work closely with other AKDN institutions to share intellectual or material resources and strengthen the relationship with other AKDN entities Follow-up with students and distance education	Number of online teaching sessions using live teaching tools Evaluation of online tools by moderators and participants for online learning Identifying problems with online learning in different locations

In practice, the programme was under-utilized by the professionals in Dar-es-Salaam. Over a 3-year period, approximately 80 teleconsultations occurred, whereas the estimated number of consultations at the time of the launch was 2500. The main reasons for this underutilization were insufficient bandwidth for an effective Internet-based education programme, discomfort among Dar clinicians in Dar-es-Salaam due to inadequate exposure to the use of computers, and practice behaviours and the environment preventing the use of technology to its fullest capacity. The evaluation team found that the leadership at the Aga Khan Hospital in Dar-es-Salaam was very positive with respect to the use of technology for the training of health care providers. This led to the new programme of remote access for health care professionals that has been described above.

Teleradiology link

The AKUH in Karachi has a partnership with the French Medical Institute for Children (FMIC), which is an 85-bed paediatric hospital in Kabul. The primary aim of the telemedicine project was to provide access to high-quality diagnostic services. As a first step, the project used broadband technology and wireless video consultation with digital image transfer to provide teleradiology services. CT scans and X-ray images can be diagnosed and interpreted and treatment can be suggested from Karachi. A combination of fibre-optic and radio links is used to transfer images from the FMIC to the AKUH in Karachi (Figure 27.1). Four or five images are transferred to the AKUH every day, and reports are sent back to the FMIC in less than 24 hours.

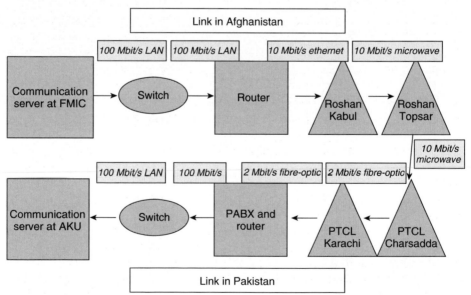

Figure 27.1 Teleradiology link between the French Medical Institute for Children, Kabul and the Aga Khan University Hospital, Karachi

Information exchange

Since its inception, the AKU has made patient information available to all care providers, while being careful to maintain the confidentiality of patient records. Several programmes have been introduced to capture medical information electronically and make this available in all patient care areas. Laboratory records, radiology reports, nursing and physician records and order entries, and several types of administrative information have been computerized for rapid access by all care providers. There are still several missing elements, such as physician notes, outpatient records, decision support systems and sharing of patient records between campuses. The university has therefore developed a detailed plan to achieve this. The ultimate goal of electronic health records is to integrate computerized medical records and ordering systems with routine care, and avoid any duplication of work in the form of generating paper records. This will lead eventually to a paperless organization where all information will be available in electronic form, guided by policies to ensure privacy and confidentiality of patient data, yet ensuring rapid access to information for the care providers.

Opportunities and challenges

The above examples of e-health work show that the AKDN has increased the availability of learning resources, health care and information for its own institutions, with a view to making health services more affordable and accessible in the developing world generally. E-health also offers opportunities for the network institutions to build on each other's strengths and expertise by sharing knowledge, expertise, best practices and information. For example, the doctors and nurses in East Africa possess specialist knowledge and skills in certain tropical diseases, which could be shared with doctors and nurses in other institutions of the network. Such collaboration is likely to encourage the development of a strong knowledge base founded on indigenous, culturally sensitive, e-health applications.

No innovation is free of challenges, especially if it involves bringing a change in the everyday practices, attitudes and beliefs of people. Stemming from the use of new technologies for e-health, there are challenges associated with the development, delivery and sustainability of such programmes. For instance, the above examples represent the efforts of small groups of doctors and nurses from the AKU and the AKHS who are enthusiastic about the use of ICT for learning and are also familiar with modern technology. However, there is a wide spectrum of technological access and expertise among other potential users. Likewise, expertise in teaching and learning, providing patient care and sharing information through technology also vary considerably between the network institutions. Moreover, since there has been no previous experience of such programmes among the participating institutions, there are no formal polices and procedures to guide the implementation. Furthermore, in most cases, no systematic evaluation has yet been conducted to assess the outcomes. While funding for the current projects has been provided through the AKDN, the availability of funds for future research, development and evaluation of e-health applications could represent a problem. Clearly, there is a need for network-wide resource sharing, accountability and coordination for the development and implementation of e-health programmes, policies and strategies for AKDN institutions.

Next steps

To enhance the use of e-health in the AKDN, it is important to develop a network-wide strategy for e-health. Such a strategy would allow collective learning and sharing of knowledge and experience among people providing health care within the AKDN. To develop a network approach to e-health, the following principles have been proposed:

- E-health initiatives should increase access to health care information and services for communities, and enhance the quality of care among network institutions and partners through knowledge transfer and educational programmes.
- E-health initiatives should address the needs of health care institutions, identified and prioritized using sound techniques. The prioritized needs should also guide external institutions and health care professionals interested in working in the field of e-health to focus on interventions addressing the most important health needs of the community.
- All e-health initiatives for the network and partners should ensure that knowledge and experience gained from these projects are measured, and that the results are disseminated to the broader community.
- All e-health initiatives should be standardized and planned to enhance networking among AKDN institutions and partners.
- E-health initiatives for the network and partners should identify suitable platforms and systems that have universal applications. Proprietary software should be avoided whenever possible.
- E-health initiatives should promote collaboration with other partner institutions, especially public institutions, without compromising the quality of care or the safety and confidentiality of patients receiving services from AKDN institutions.
- All e-health projects should focus on the sustainability of the initiatives by demonstrating a return on investment and integration with the existing programmes.

To confirm the above principles, a process of needs and readiness assessment has been started in all the countries where the AKDN operates. This will:

- identify the current and future needs of health care institutions that can be addressed by using e-health
- define the available alternatives and provide justification for the use of e-health
- determine the infrastructure, awareness, willingness, capacity, sociocultural environment and institutional polices required for e-health
- define the process of e-health planning leading to enhanced readiness of health care institutions in the relevant countries
- develop a model for e-health needs and readiness assessment for AKDN institutions and partners in other countries (and for other similar institutions).

The needs and readiness assessment exercise is currently being carried out in Tanzania and Afghanistan. These two countries were selected based on their needs and existing collaborations between network institutions. The readiness assessment is focusing initially on teleconsultations and tele-education. However, the needs assessment will capture institutional needs in information and knowledge management as well.

The following activities are being conducted during the needs and readiness assessment exercise in the two countries:

1. *Developing a stakeholder team in each country*. Separate teams of key stakeholders are being formed in each country to plan the needs and readiness assessment in these countries. The stakeholder team decides on the process of needs and readiness assessment by identifying the relevant instruments, supervising data collection and compiling results for guiding e-health implementation in each country.
2. *Training the stakeholder team in each country*. Once the teams have been formed, the members will be exposed to e-health terminologies and concepts. These are required to carry out the planning of needs and readiness assessment. The training programmes in each country will last for two days each.
3. *Conducting the needs assessment in AKDN institutions*. Identifying the needs of AKDN institutions that could be addressed though e-health will be conducted using (i) discussions with the stakeholder team members to document their views and suggestions and (ii) focus group discussions with different groups of health care providers and managers of health care institutions. The participants for focus group discussions will be identified by the stakeholder team, and the sessions will be conducted by team members from AKU.
4. *Identifying appropriate e-health solutions for the suggested needs*. On the basis of the identified needs, appropriate e-health solutions will be selected by the stakeholder team. The process will be carried out in consultation with the team from the AKU and a consultant. Efforts will be made to identify simple, low-cost, low-bandwidth and culturally sensitive e-health solutions for AKDN institutions.
5. *Prioritizing e-health solutions*. In the next step, the stakeholder team will prioritize the e-health solutions. This step will help in assessing and building the readiness of health care institutions for the e-health applications that have been identified, and avoid wasting time on applications that may not be required in the short term.
6. *Conducting readiness assessment of network institutions*. Finally, the stakeholder team will choose among the existing tools for e-health readiness assessment that have already been validated and tested in developing countries. The teams will also finalize the plan for analysing the information collected.

Conclusion

The AKDN represents an interesting example of agencies and institutions working in several different countries towards a common development goal. Health is a component of the overall development of the communities, which makes it necessary for the health care institutions to build strong relationships with institutions involved in other facets of development. Better coordination within, among and between these agencies, and with the communities, is necessary for provision of health care in these countries. E-health offers great potential to enable a network of this size to achieve its goals of better access and high quality of care, while operating within the available resource constraints.

The AKDN has developed a plan to move from pilot trials to routine operations, by developing a network approach guided by an overall strategy. The strategy is based on the principles of needs and readiness assessment, community and community-centeredness, knowledge transfer, networking, open platforms, standardization and evaluation. A broad-based needs and readiness assessment has already been started in two countries.

Further reading

Aga Khan Development Network. Available at: www.akdn.org.

Harambee: Reinforcing African Voices through Collaborative Processes. Available at: www.uneca.org/aisi/picta/HarambeeOverview-v1.pdf.

Ministry of Economic Development, New Zealand. *Strengthening Networks and Partnerships.* Available at: www.gif.med.govt.nz/aboutgif/networks.asp.

United Nations Development Programme (UNDP). *Networks for Development: Lessons Learned from Supporting National and Regional Networks on Legal, Ethical and Human Rights Dimensions of HIV/AIDS.* Available at: www.undp.org/hiv/publications/networks.htm.

United Nations Economic and Social Commission for Asia and the Pacific. *Handbook on Strengthening the Women's Information Network for Asia and the Pacific through Computer Networking.* Available at: www.unescap.org/esid/GAD/Publication/computer.pdf.

Wiley D. *Connecting Learning Objects to Instructional Design Theory: A Definition, a Metaphor, and a Taxonomy.* Available at: www.reusability.org/read/chapters/wiley.doc.

References

1. Fort V, Obonyo B, Madhavan S. *Strengthening the Institutional Capacity of Aga Khan Health Service, East Africa's Community Health Department to Support Organizations Working in Community Health Service.* Available at: pdf.dec.org/pdf_docs/Pdacf019.pdf.
2. Aga Khan University. Available at: www.aku.edu.
3. Library of Images, Aga Khan University. Available at: loi.aku.edu/loi.
4. Joint Information Systems Committee (JISC). *Circular 7/00: MLE in Further Education: Progress Report.* Available at: www.jisc.ac.uk/news/stories/2000/07/circular700.aspx.

SECTION 5

THE FUTURE

28 The future use of telehealth in the developing world

Richard Wootton

Introduction

Much has been written about the potential for telemedicine in the developing world. However, after reviewing the literature, it is clear that the evidence base supporting its practical utility is rather slender, and that most of the material published to date has been in the form of comments, letters, discussions, product reports, news items or case reports.[1] None the less, in preparing this book, the implicit thesis was that telemedicine can have a positive effect on health care delivery in developing countries, and that ultimately it can reduce the global burden of disease. The latter could perhaps be regarded as the Holy Grail for workers in the field. How does the experience reported in the book reflect this ideal?

The examples in this book show unequivocally that useful services can be delivered in the developing world using telehealth. None the less, viewed from the perspective of telehealth activity in the world as a whole, it is clear that there has been relatively little use of telehealth in developing countries so far. One obvious reason is the information and communication technology (ICT) environment, where there are evident challenges to the more widespread use of telehealth and to the use of e-health generally. These are, in fact, general problems concerning the use of ICT anywhere, including:

- the cost of IT hardware and software
- the limited availability of fast broadband and mobile networks
- the slow development of software in languages other than English.

These and other factors add up to the so-called 'digital divide' between the developing world and the industrialized world (see Chapter 2).

ICT barriers

A useful framework for considering access to ICT is provided by the Real Access criteria.[2] These criteria have been used to analyse the factors concerning access to ICT and its use, including the 'soft' aspects that are often overlooked. The criteria are designed to help understand the reasons why ICT development projects fail to achieve their goals, and to identify the reasons why such projects succeed. There are 12 criteria, which are inter-related:

(1) physical access to technology
(2) appropriateness of technology
(3) affordability of technology and technology use
(4) human capacity and training
(5) locally relevant content, applications and services
(6) integration into daily routines
(7) socio-cultural factors
(8) trust in technology
(9) local economic environment
(10) macroeconomic environment
(11) legal and regulatory framework
(12) political will and public support.

An understanding of these factors can be used to improve the way that ICT-based development policies and initiatives are planned, monitored and evaluated.

Other barriers

Telehealth, of course, is a complex matter. A satisfactory ICT environment is a necessary, but not sufficient, condition for the successful practice of telehealth. There are other barriers to the use of telehealth, and they apply in the industrialized world as well. The barriers include:

- organizational factors, e.g. changing the way in which hospitals and doctors work
- human factors, e.g. lack of staff with the appropriate skills
- medicolegal matters, including ethical concerns.

As the examples in this book show, it is possible to overcome all these obstacles and bring about successful, and in some cases sustainable, telehealth operations.

Telemedicine examples

In summarizing telehealth work, it is usual to categorize the applications under three headings: clinical, educational and administrative. These categories are not mutually exclusive.

Administrative

This book contains only a few examples of telehealth work in the administrative category. This is surprising, since facilitating administrative work – conducting meetings at a distance, providing web-based data collection forms and supplying online reports, for example – are all perfectly proper forms of telehealth, and ones that are likely to provide major benefits in terms of avoided staff travel and improved information flows. Perhaps this is the unglamorous, and therefore under-reported, face of e-health.

Education

Although relatively little mention is made of administrative telehealth work, this book contains more examples of education. One of the most successful educational projects, and one that appears to be sustainable, is led from Geneva by the organization Réseau Afrique Francophone de Télémédecine (RAFT), which provides services in French-speaking African countries. Education is delivered in real time using interactive web-casting.[3] A successful example of the opposite modality, asynchronous education, is the Pacific open-learning network of the World Health Organization (WHO).[4] The open-learning network provides online (web-based) courses, course materials and other resources to health professionals in the Pacific region. In addition, 15 learning centres have been established in 11 Pacific Island countries to increase access to online materials and resources.

Although they are not explicitly identified in this book, there are two other significant educational resources that deserve mention. First, there is the HINARI project (Health Internetwork Access to Research Initiative), which was established in 2002 by the WHO, when it secured agreement from many of the world's scientific publishers to make their journals available in developing countries at no cost to the reader.[5] Over 3750 journal titles are now available to health institutions in 113 countries. Second, the US National Library of Medicine made the Medline database freely available to the world via the Internet in the mid-1990s. Using the PubMed search engine, more than 17 million citations and abstracts of biomedical research articles can be searched via the web. The ready availability of the Medline database via PubMed, and free access to several thousand journals via HINARI, are splendid examples of how the industrialized world can assist less fortunate countries. The indirect health gains of these initiatives remain to be quantified, but can confidently be assumed to be substantial.

The educational projects described in this book are undoubtedly successful. None the less, they should be viewed in a global health care context. Many countries face critical shortages of health service providers, such as doctors, nurses and midwives (Figure 28.1).[6] This is important because, unsurprisingly, the number of health workers and their skills are positively correlated with population health outcomes. The WHO has set out a framework for improving the global health workforce, by focusing on strategies related to the stage when people enter the workforce, the period of their lives when they are part of the workforce, and the point at which they make their exit from it. The strategy focuses on:

- *entry*: preparing the workforce through strategic investments in education and effective and ethical recruitment practices
- *workforce*: enhancing worker performance through better management of workers in both the public and private sectors
- *exit*: managing migration and attrition to reduce wasteful loss of human resources.

Telemedicine has an obvious role to play in improving access to education, and perhaps in allowing better supervision of a dispersed workforce. One might expect

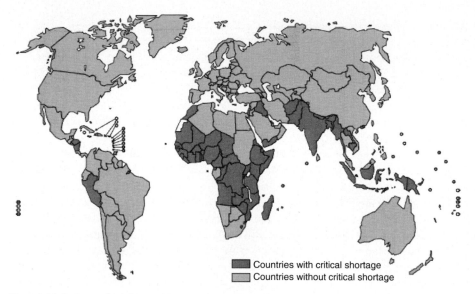

Figure 28.1 Countries with a critical shortage of health service providers. There is an estimated shortage of almost 4.3 million doctors, midwives, nurses and support workers worldwide. (Reproduced from *World Health Report 2006*;[6] data taken from *Global Atlas of the Health Workforce*[15])

that greater access to education could be achieved at lower cost by pooling of resources and by expanding the use of telemedicine and distance education. Clearly, education represents a fruitful potential area for telehealth in the developing world.

Clinical

In clinical telehealth, there has been little use of videoconferencing in developing countries, for the obvious reasons of the cost of the requisite technology and the restricted availability of suitable telecommunications. The Medical Missions for Children has a videoconferencing network to a number of hospitals in developing countries, although a good deal of the telehealth activity that takes place is educational in nature, for example mentoring of local doctors, rather than direct patient care (see Chapter 10).

In practice, a substantial proportion of clinical telehealth work in developing countries is done by email or by web messaging (Table 28.1). Successful examples of the use of email include the Cambodia work managed from Boston (see Chapter 13) and the global e-referral network operated by the Swinfen Charitable Trust (see Chapter 19). The latter has recently moved from a system based on plain email to one based on a secure web server. Long-running examples of the use of the web for delivering clinical consultations include the US Army's system in the Pacific[7] (see Chapter 15) and the highly regarded iPath system for case discussions among groups of pathologists.[8]

Table 28.1 General-purpose second-opinion telemedicine networks providing services in the developing world

Operator	Referring sites	Expert sites	Date of first operation	Mechanism	Description
Partners Health care, Boston, Massachusetts, USA	Rovieng Health Centre, Cambodia; Rattanikiri Hospital, Cambodia	Sihanouk Hospital, Phnom Penh; Harvard Medical School, Boston	2001	Email	Email consultations are used to support health workers at a rural clinic in northern Cambodia. The email advice comes from specialists at a tertiary hospital in Phnom Penh and from the Massachusetts General Hospital in Boston. In 2003, a second site at a small hospital in northern Cambodia began referring cases
Tripler Army Medical Center, Honolulu, Hawaii, USA	US-associated Pacific islands	Tripler Army Medical Center, Hawaii	1997	Web	A web-based teleconsulting system is used by the main US Army hospital in Hawaii to support referrers in hospitals (mainly military hospitals) around the Pacific
iPath Association, University of Basel, Basel, Switzerland	Several (mainly telepathology), e.g. Cambodia, Solomon Islands, Bangladesh. Also more recent teleconsultation work, e.g. Ukrainian Swiss Perinatal Health Project	Mainly Swiss, European	2001	Web	The iPath software was originally developed for telepathology case conferences (for which it is an excellent tool, and several tens of thousands of case conferences have now been conducted – technically by a number of different organizations who all use the same software). More recently, the software has begun to be used for general teleconsulting (i.e. non-pathology work)
Swinfen Charitable Trust, Canterbury, UK	Global (34 countries)	Global (13 countries)	1999	Email and Web	A simple email teleconsultation system was established at a single hospital in Bangladesh by a UK-based charity. Specialist opinions were obtained from a small panel of volunteer consultants. The operation has now grown to service over 100 hospitals around the world, with a panel of nearly 400 consultants. An automatic message handling system is employed, supplemented by a more recent web-messaging system
Geneva University Hospitals, Geneva, Switzerland	Africa (nine countries)	Geneva	2001	Web via satellite	The RAFT project provides services from Geneva to nine French-speaking African countries. The core activity is distance education via webcasting of interactive courses. Some teleconsultation work also takes place, mainly involving specialists in Geneva

Intermediate between the two poles of real-time videoconferencing and store-and-forward messaging lies the VHF radio network installed in the Peruvian jungle to facilitate communications with remote health centres.[9]

Cost-effectiveness

Although the above examples should all be considered to be successful demonstrations of telehealth in the developing world, it has to be admitted that strict evidence for cost-effectiveness remains elusive. Analysis of cost-effectiveness is a health economics tool that enables comparisons to be made between alternative interventions in terms of their costs and consequences. For example, is it preferable to spend resources on a PACS system at the national referral hospital, or to implement a programme of directly observed treatment of tuberculosis? To answer this question requires not only that the costs be known, but also that the consequences – the health gain – can be calculated. The latter may be done in terms of life-years gained, for example; if so, the situation is relatively straightforward. If the health gain includes other advantages – perhaps improved quality of life or reduced incidence of medical complications – then assigning a monetary value to the benefits is likely to be more difficult.

Telehealth research workers know only too well that it is hard enough to obtain evidence for cost-effectiveness in telehealth work in industrialized countries; it is even harder to do so in developing countries. Yet the matter of cost-effectiveness remains a serious question hanging over the potential future use of telehealth. More than a decade ago, the question was posed whether it is ethical to devote significant resources to telehealth in the developing world if the costs and benefits are largely undocumented when there are health measures, such as vaccination, sanitation and clean drinking water, with characteristics that are well understood.[10]

The WHO has provided examples of interventions that, if implemented properly, can substantially reduce the burden of disease, especially among the poor, and do so at a reasonable cost (Table 28.2).[11] What is striking about this list is how little telehealth has yet been applied in these areas. Telehealth may have a place in directly observed treatment of tuberculosis (DOTS),[12] but little is yet known about its feasibility on a wide scale, never mind its cost-effectiveness. It is true that telehealth has been used successfully to provide HIV/AIDS services (see Chapter 9), but again it remains to be seen how easy it will be to scale up the pilot programmes.

In this connection, it is worth noting the Peruvian telemedicine network that is based on email transmission by VHF radio link. A recent study has documented fewer urgent patient transfers from health posts and health centres,[9] and there is emerging evidence of cost-effectiveness.[13]

A strategy for telemedicine

Given the above, and the need to obtain quantitative evidence of cost-effectiveness, what is the right strategy for telehealth in the developing world? The key aspects appear to be:

Table 28.2 Interventions with a large potential impact on health outcomes[11]

Examples of interventions	Main contents of interventions
Treatment of tuberculosis	Directly observed treatment schedule (DOTS): administration of standardized short-course chemotherapy to all confirmed sputum smear-positive cases of tuberculosis under supervision in the initial (2–3 months) phase
Maternal health and safe motherhood interventions	Family planning, prenatal and delivery care, clean and safe delivery by trained birth attendant, postpartum care, and essential obstetric care for high-risk pregnancies and complications
Family planning	Information and education; availability and correct use of contraceptives
School health interventions	Health education and nutrition interventions, including anti-helmintic treatment, micronutrient supplementation and school meals
Integrated management of childhood illness	Case management of acute respiratory infections, diarrhoea, malaria, measles and malnutrition; immunization, feeding/breastfeeding counselling, micronutrient and iron supplementation, anti-helmintic treatment
HIV/AIDS prevention	Targeted information for sex workers, mass education awareness, counselling, screening, mass treatment for sexually transmitted infections, safe blood supply
Treatment of sexually transmitted infections	Case management using syndrome diagnosis and standard treatment algorithm
Immunization (EPI Plus)	BCG at birth; OPV at birth, 6, 10, 14 weeks; DPT at 6, 10, 14 weeks; HepB at birth, 6 and 9 months (optional); measles at 9 months; TT for women of childbearing age
Malaria	Case management (early assessment and prompt treatment) and selected preventive measures (e.g. impregnated bed nets)
Tobacco control	Tobacco tax, information, nicotine replacement, legal action
Non-communicable diseases and injuries	Selected early screening and secondary prevention

1. Concentrate on areas identified by the WHO as being likely to affect the disease burden.
2. Work with local staff.
3. Try and establish within-country telehealth networks.
4. Evaluate the costs and consequences, to provide evidence of cost-effectiveness.

In 2006, Lord Crisp examined how the UK experience and expertise in health could best be used to help improve health in developing countries.[14] He made a number of detailed recommendations, but pointed out that it was necessary for developing countries to take the lead and to 'own' the solutions, which could be supported by international, national and local partnerships based on mutual respect.[14] This surely epitomizes any potential use of telehealth.

Conclusion

What then is the future for telehealth in the developing world? Clearly, telemedicine does not represent 'the answer' to all public health challenges in developing countries. However, it can provide value, particularly when it is employed to strengthen and support a local team, rather than simply being used to import expertise from outside to supplement or supplant local efforts. One important role for telemedicine is in the training of local health professionals. The place of telemedicine in direct patient care delivery remains to be established, although there are promising indications of its success in certain circumstances. Consultations via email and the web should form an essential part of health partnerships.

The long-term goal of telehealth work must remain the demonstration of its efficacy in comparison with well-understood measures such as the provision of safe drinking water and immunization (Figures 28.2 and 28.3). One unanswered question is the future design of telehealth networks. Whether resources should be concentrated into a single network or into several, it is clear that the long-term aim should be to establish within-country telemedicine networks (supported from out of country where appropriate) that:

- demonstrably alter health outcomes
- can be shown to be cost-effective and sustainable
- will act as a model for other countries to copy.

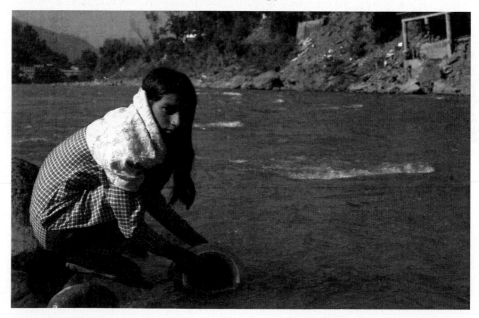

Figure 28.2 People forced to use one water source for all daily chores – like this girl in Pakistan – face increasing risks of gastrointestinal infections and other waterborne diseases. Together, these diseases kill around 2.2 million people globally each year, mostly children in developing countries. (Photograph courtesy of WHO/Christopher Black)

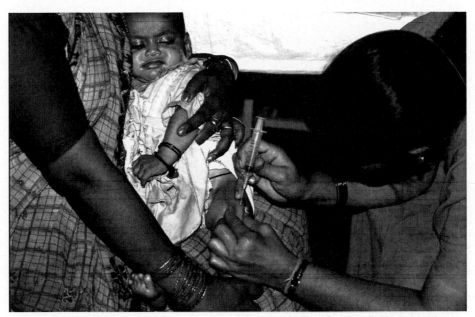

Figure 28.3 Child immunization at the Malipur Maternity Home in Delhi, India. Immunization is considered to be one of the most cost-effective health interventions. There is a well-defined target group; contact with the health system is only needed at the time of delivery; and vaccination does not require any major changes of lifestyle. (Photograph courtest of WHO/P Virot)

This will enable the success of the telemedicine second-opinion work that has been performed to date to be exploited on a global scale.[1] Telemedicine is a small but significant component of ICT in health care delivery. In the future, it is to be hoped that telemedicine will develop into a proven tool for facilitating learning and for capacity building, in addition to its role in direct clinical care.

References

1. Wootton R. Telemedicine support for the developing world. *J Telemed Telecare* 2008; **14**: 109–14.
2. Bridges.org. *Real Access/Real Impact Criteria*. Available at: www.bridges.org/Real_Access.
3. Geissbuhler A, Bagayoko CO, Ly O. The RAFT network: 5 years of distance continuing medical education and tele-consultations over the Internet in French-speaking Africa. *Int J Med Inform* 2007; **76**: 351–6.
4. POLHN. *Pacific Open Learning Health Net*. Available at: www.polhn.com.
5. World Health Organization. *HINARI Access to Research Initiative*. Available at: www.who.int/hinari/en.
6. World Health Organization. *The World Health Report 2006 – Working Together for Health*. Available at: www.who.int/whr/2006/en.
7. Callahan CW, Malone F, Estroff D, Person DA. Effectiveness of an Internet-based store-and-forward telemedicine system for pediatric subspecialty consultation. *Arch Pediatr Adolesc Med* 2005; **159**: 389–93.
8. Brauchli K, Oberli H, Hurwitz N et al. Diagnostic telepathology: long-term experience of a single institution. *Virchows Arch* 2004; **444**: 403–9.
9. Martínez A, Villarroel V, Seoane J, del Pozo F. A study of a rural telemedicine system in the Amazon region of Peru. *J Telemed Telecare* 2004; **10**: 219–25.

10. Wootton R. The possible use of telemedicine in developing countries. *J Telemed Telecare* 1997; **3**: 23–6.
11. World Health Organization. *The World Health Report 2000 – Health Systems: Improving Performance.* Available at: www.who.int/whr/2000/en.
12. DeMaio J, Schwartz L, Cooley P, Tice A. The application of telemedicine technology to a directly observed therapy program for tuberculosis: a pilot project. *Clin Infect Dis* 2001; **33**: 2082–4.
13. Martínez A, Villarroel V, Puig-Junoy J et al. An economic analysis of the EHAS telemedicine system in Alto Amazonas. *J Telemed Telecare* 2007; **13**: 7–14.
14. Crisp N. *Global Health Partnerships: The UK Contribution to Health in Developing Countries* ('The Crisp Report'). Available at: www.dh.gov.uk/en/Publicationsandstatistics/Publications/PublicationsPolicyAnd-Guidance/DH_065374.
15. World Health Organization. *Global Atlas of the Health Workforce.* Available at: www.who.int/globalatlas/default.asp.

Index